MULTIMODALITY TREATMENT OF LUNG CANCER

LUNG BIOLOGY IN HEALTH AND DISEASE

Executive Editor

Claude Lenfant
Director, National Heart, Lung and Blood Institute
National Institutes of Health
Bethesda, Maryland

ADDITIONAL VOLUMES IN PREPARATION

The opinions expressed in these volumes do not necessarily represent the views of the National Institutes of Health.

MULTIMODALITY TREATMENT OF LUNG CANCER

Edited by

Arthur T. Skarin

Dana-Farber Cancer Institute
Brigham and Women's Medical School
and Harvard Medical School
Boston, Massachusetts

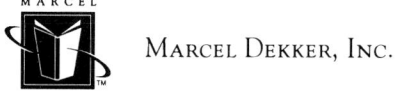

MARCEL DEKKER, INC. NEW YORK · BASEL

ISBN: 0-8247-0236-0

This book is printed on acid-free paper.

Headquarters
Marcel Dekker, Inc.
270 Madison Avenue, New York, NY 10016
tel: 212-696-9000; fax: 212-685-4540

Eastern Hemisphere Distribution
Marcel Dekker AG
Hutgasse 4, Postfach 812, CH-4001 Basel, Switzerland
tel: 41-61-261-8482; fax: 41-61-261-8896

World Wide Web
http://www.dekker.com

The publisher offers discounts on this book when ordered in bulk quantities. For more information, write to Special Sales/Professional Marketing at the headquarters address above.

Current printing (last digit):
10 9 8 7 6 5 4 3 2 1

PRINTED IN THE UNITED STATES OF AMERICA

INTRODUCTION

> When meditating over a disease, I never think of finding a remedy for it, but instead, a means of preventing it.
>
> —Louis Pasteur

This is indeed an extraordinary statement! On the one hand, one can only applaud such zeal for preventing diseases, and certainly among all of those who pursued this goal, Louis Pasteur was one of the greatest. On the other hand, saying that one would not "think of finding a remedy" is almost an admission of defeat.

Lung cancer is an enormous public health problem in the United States, and it will soon be an even greater one in the rest of the world. Preventing it is everyone's dream, especially because it sounds so easy—"get rid of tobacco smoking and other inhalable carcinogens and the problem will be solved." The reality is that it is not so easy; undoubtedly the main causes of lung cancer will be with us for a long time, and even if they disappeared today, their impact would remain for years to come.

There is no question that epidemiologists, clinicians, and researchers have recognized that the war against lung cancer must be fought on both the prevention front and the treatment front. Although no cure is in sight, many breakthrough advances based on molecular biology and molecular genetic approaches have greatly contributed to the progress that we are witnessing.

In the more than 20 years of its existence, the Lung Biology in Health and Disease series of monographs has included several volumes about lung cancer, each looking at different aspects and reporting on the latest advances. This volume, however, is unique because it brings together all the therapeutic modalities that have been developed: surgery, radiation therapy, chemotherapy, etc. As pointed out by the editor, Dr. Arthur Skarin, in the preface, "Progress in improving the cure rate of lung cancer is slow but definite." If Pasteur had known then what is known today, he would have been "thinking of finding a remedy." Today, the clinician hopes for the prevention of lung cancer, but also knows too well that, in the meantime, one must use the best we have to help the patient. This book will bring clinicians up to date on the options that are available.

Dr. Skarin has assembled a roster of contributors who are well-recognized experts in the field. They all bring years of experience and of success in applying the available treatments. Physicians caring for lung cancer patients and the patients themselves should benefit from the experience reported in this volume. As the editor of this series of monographs, I am proud to present this volume and grateful to Dr. Skarin and his contributors for the opportunity to do so.

Claude Lenfant, M.D.
Bethesda, Maryland

PREFACE

Over the past decade, considerable progress has been made in understanding the molecular biology of lung cancer and in the development of multimodality treatment programs. Several promising new chemotherapy agents, including those with novel mechanisms of action, have become available, and data from activity in advanced disease are rapidly accumulating. It is often difficult for the busy physician to keep up with progress in this field. This new volume of the Lung Biology in Health and Disease series should lead to a better understanding of the molecular events in the pathogenesis of lung cancer as well as the results of treatment of all stages of disease. The current staging evaluation guidelines are thoroughly reviewed and the most recent International TNM staging system is summarized in detail.

Deaths from lung cancer exceed deaths from breast, colon, and prostate cancers combined. Although elimination of cigarette smoking is the best way to reduce this epidemic, chemoprevention is an important strategy in the fight against lung cancer. Completed, ongoing, and future trials are reviewed by Khuri et al. (Chapter 2). For example, synthetic retinoids can activate biological responses that result in apoptosis of human lung cancer cell lines. A large, randomized U.S. Intergroup study has recently been completed, testing whether *cis*-retinoic acid can prevent new lung cancers (compared to a placebo group) in patients with resected stage I disease. Results will not be available for several years.

The revised International Lung Cancer Staging System, published in 1997 by Mountain (1), differs from the earlier 1986 version (2) by identification of several subgroups that have prognostic importance. For example, stage I is separated into stage IA (T1N0) and IB (T2N0), stage II into IIA (T1N1) and IIB (T2N1 and T3N0). Clinical radiologic staging assessment is reviewed in detail by Shaffer (Chapter 3), and surgical-pathological staging is discussed by Flores et al. (Chapter 4), including the important role of VATS (video-assisted thoracoscopic surgery) and closed thoracotomy. The role of VATS in staging as well as in therapy is further addressed by Mentzer (Chapter 5).

Multimodality treatment is available for all stages of lung cancer. Although many patients are given an individualized course of treatment for various reasons, the use of clinical trials is encouraged in order to answer important questions. For example, chemotherapy may be utilized in every stage of lung cancer, but its role has been established only in advanced unresectable stage III and IV disease. Randomized Phase III trials in stage IV disease have shown improvement in patient survival compared to best supportive care only. In unresectable stage IIIA and IIIB disease, chemotherapy improves the results of radiotherapy, compared to radiotherapy alone. Overall patient survival beyond 5 years in one large series was double that of radiotherapy (3).

In resectable stage IIIA disease numerous single-institution Phase II efficacy studies have shown improvement in survival (30–35% at 5 years) compared to 5–15% survival noted in earlier studies utilizing radiotherapy and surgery only. At the Dana-Farber Cancer Institute, one of the first studies of induction chemotherapy, utilizing CAP (cyclophosphamide, adriamycin, and cisplatin) with pre- and postoperative radiotherapy and further CAP chemotherapy, showed a rather high response rate of 72% prior to surgery (4). Long-term overall survival beyond 3–5 years plateaus at 34% (Fig. 1). Additional studies using other induction chemotherapy regimens have confirmed high rates of initial remission and resection, significant downstaging at the time of surgery (5), and similar prolonged survival rates for all patients (6) (Strauss and Baldini, Chapter 10). The best survival occurs in patients who are downstaged to stage 0 or I disease (79%) or stage II disease (42%) as reported in one recent study (7). In this last study, concurrent chemoradiotherapy was utilized along with twice-daily radiation, a schedule that is under current evaluation in several randomized trials.

Two randomized trials were conducted in stage IIIA disease with similar study designs, comparing induction or no induction chemotherapy followed by surgery (and radiotherapy). About 30 patients were entered in each group, with similar results (8,9). Both studies were closed by early stopping rules because of the inferior results when preoperative chemotherapy was not used. Although patients receiving induction chemotherapy had similar favorable projected survivals of over 30–40% in the original reports, longer follow-up has shown a decrease in survival. Variable factors in stage subcategories, gender, and other prognostic factors may explain the initial good results. However, induction chemotherapy appears to affect the biology of stage III disease, with a shift in median survival. Larger international randomized trials are ongoing and the final multimodality strategy remains to be determined. Of interest, a Phase III Cancer and Leukemia Group B (CALGB) trial initiated in 1991, with chemotherapy as the study variable, had to be closed early due to difficulty in adding patients after publication of the two positive studies mentioned above. Preliminary analysis of the CALGB study, with about 30 patients in each arm, shows no major differences in outcome when induction chemotherapy

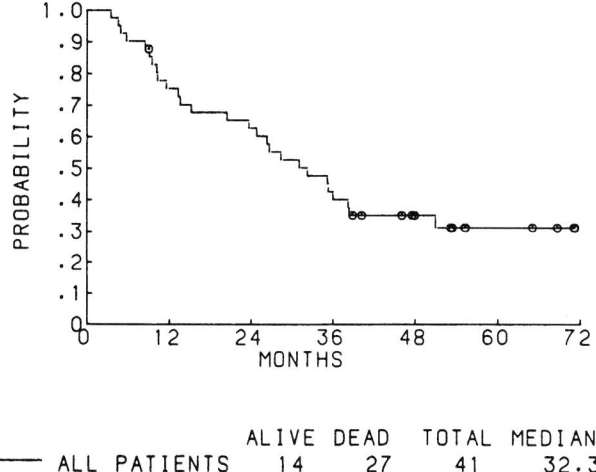

Fig. 1 Survival for all 41 patients with stage IIIA NSCLC treated at DFCI and affiliated hospitals. Long-term survival plateaus at 34% beyond 3–5 years. Median survival is 32.3 months. (From Ref. 4; reprinted with permission of Alan R. Liss.)

is compared to no chemotherapy, along with surgery and radiotherapy (12). Other groups are evaluating induction chemotherapy with and without surgery, and with and without radiation followed by surgery as well as chemoradiotherapy (sequential versus concomitant). Also being tested are variables in radiotherapy technique (stereotactic), scheduling (hyperfractionation), and dosing. Finally, induction chemotherapy is being utilized in feasibility studies in not only stage III disease but high-risk stage I and II disease (13).

The treatment of advanced stage IIIB and IV non-small-cell lung cancer (NSCLC) has had a more optimistic outcome since cisplatin-containing regimens became available. Meta-analysis of almost 10 randomized trials has revealed statistically significant improved survival rates for use of cisplatin-based regimens compared to supportive care only (14) (Dang et al., Chapter 12). Owing to the availability of several new combination-chemotherapy regimens, large Phase III trials are being conducted to compare these newer regimens to traditional combinations (15; and Chapter 12). For example, the Eastern Cooperative Oncology Group is comparing cisplatin/taxol versus cisplatin/gemcitabine versus cisplatin/taxotere versus carboplatin/taxol, while a large trial sponsored by Rhône-Poulenc Rorer is evaluating cisplatin/navelbine versus cisplatin/taxotere versus carboplatin/taxotere. Quality of life is also improved when chemotherapy is utilized and economic feasibility has been demonstrated (15). Various new active single agents are now available, with response rates of 20–30% in previously untreated patients. These drugs, many with novel mechanisms of action, include the taxanes (Paclitaxel and Docetaxol), gemcitabine, navelbine, and CPT-11 (Chapter 12). Exciting agents that may become available in the future include matrix metalloproteinase inhibitors, antiangiogenesis compounds, small molecules interrupting vital steps in the cell cycle of tumor cells, antisense oligonucleotides, monoclonal antibodies, and highly specific vaccines.

An excellent review of preclinical animal models that can be employed in the development of new therapeutic regimens for lung cancer is provided by Teicher and Frei (Chapter 14). This comprehensive treatise gives the rationale for and results of combining "multimodality" programs (e.g., radiation and antiangiogenesis drugs, as well as chemotherapeutic agents with different mechanisms of action) in killing tumor cells in animal systems before use as Phase I/II programs in humans.

The evaluation and management of small cell lung cancer (SCLC) are explored in Chapters 1–4. Although surgery has a limited role, some patients benefit from resection, particularly those with early-stage disease (Donahue and Mathisen, Chapter 15). The important role of radiotherapy, as demonstrated by recent randomized trials that show improvement in local control of both thoracic and occult CNS disease, is covered in detail in Chapter 16 (Kumar). Improvement in survival with use of radiation therapy has now been demonstrated. Recent data from use of new chemotherapeutic agents are discussed in Chapter 17 (Boral and Lynch), and overall treatment strategies for limited and extensive disease categories are presented. Finally, the encouraging impressive improvement in survival (50% or greater at 5 years) for selected patients treated with high-dose chemotherapy with marrow or peripheral blood stem cell support is discussed in Chapter 18 (Elias).

Progress in improving the cure rate of lung cancer is slow but definite. In some cases, Hamlet's observation that "disease desperate grown is relieved by desperate appliances or not at all" may apply to many patients, but the major impact on improving survival of established disease will undoubtedly result from not only a multimodality (team) approach but use of various agents and molecules that attack the cancer cell (seed) and tissues (soil) at multiple target sites. Elimination of tobacco smoking and industrial carcinogen exposure along with chemoprevention and improved early detection will ultimately be the most effective ways of eradicating the lung cancer epidemic.

I would like to dedicate this volume to Carol M. Lowe, in memory of her vivacious and courageous life as well as her concern for the health of others, who, with her husband Philip C. Lowe, established the Lowe Center for Thoracic Oncology at the Dana-Farber Cancer Institute and Brigham and Women's Hospital. Their generosity will ensure the continued support of clinical and laboratory research efforts in the war against lung cancer.

Arthur T. Skarin

REFERENCES

1. Mountain CF. Revisions in the international system, for staging lung cancer. Chest 1997; 111:1710–1717.
2. Mountain CF. A new international staging system for lung cancer. Chest 1986; (Suppl 4):2255–2335.
3. Dillman RO, Herndon J, Seagren SL, Eaton WL, Green MR. Improved survival in stage III non-small cell lung cancer: seven-year follow-up of cancer and Leukemia Group B (CALGB) 8433 trial. J Natl Cancer Inst 1996; 88:1210–1215.
4. Skarin AT, Jochelson M, Sheldon T, Malcolm A, Oliynyk P, Overholt R, Hunt M. Neoadjuvant chemotherapy in marginally resectable stage III M_0 non-small cell lung cancer: long term follow-up in 41 patients. J Surg Onc 1989; 40:266–274.
5. Martini N, Kris MG, Flehinger BJ, et al. Preoperative chemotherapy for stage IIIA (N2) lung cancer: the Sloan-Kettering experience with 136 patients. Ann Thorac Surg 1993; 55:1365–1374.
6. Albain KS. Induction chemotherapy with/without radiation followed by surgery in stage III non-small-cell lung cancer. Oncology 1997; 11 (suppl.): 51–57.
7. Choi NC, Carey RW, Daly W, Mathisen D, Wain J, Wright C, Lynch T, Grossbard M, Grillo H. Potential impact on survival of improved tumor downstaging and resection rate by preoperative twice-daily radiation and concurrent chemotherapy in stage IIIA non-small-cell lung cancer. J Clin Oncol 1997; 5:712–722.
8. Rosell R, Gomez-Codina J, Camps C, et al. A randomized trial comparing preoperative chemotherapy plus surgery with surgery alone in patients with non-small cell lung cancer. N Engl J Med 1994; 330:153–158.
9. Roth J, Fossella F, Komaki R, et al. A randomized trial comparing perioperative chemotherapy and surgery with surgery alone in resectable stage III non-small cell lung cancer. J Natl Cancer Inst 1994; 86:673–680.
10. Elias AD, Herndon J, Kumar P, Sugarbaker D, Green MR. A phase III comparison of "best local regional therapy" with or without chemotherapy (CT) for stage IIIA T1-3N2 non-small cell lung cancer (NSCLC): preliminary results. ASCO Proc 1997; 16:1611.
11. Pisters KMW, Ginsberg RJ. Phase II trial of induction paclitaxel and carboplatin (PC) in early stage (T2 NO, T1-2 N1, and selected T3 N0-1) non-small cell lung cancer (NSCLC). ASCO Proc 1998; 17:1738.
12. Herbst RS, Dang NH, Skarin AT. Chemotherapy for advanced non-small cell lung cancer. Hematol Oncol Clin North Am 1997; 11:473–517.
13. Evans WK, Will BP, Berthelot JM, Earle CC. Cost of combined modality interventions for stage III non-small-cell lung cancer. J Clin Oncol 1997; 15:3038–3048.
14. Eberhardt W, Wilke H, Stamatis G, et al. Preoperative chemotherapy followed by concurrent chemoradiation therapy based on hyperfractionated accelerated radiotherapy and definitive surgery in locally advanced non-small-cell lung cancer: Mature results of a Phase II trial. J Clin Oncol 1998; 16:622–634.
15. Bonner JA, McGinnis WL, Stella PJ, et al. The possible advantage of hyperfractionated thoracic radiotherapy in the treatment of locally advanced non-small cell lung carcinoma. Cancer 1998; 82:1037–1048.

CONTRIBUTORS

Eben Alexander III, M.D.   Professor, Department of Neurosurgery, Brigham and Women's Hospital, and The Children's Hospital, Boston, Massachusetts

Elizabeth H. Baldini, M.D., M.P.H.   Department of Radiation Oncology, Brigham and Women's Hospital, Dana-Farber Cancer Institute, Boston, Massachusetts

Peter McL. Black, M.D., Ph.D.   Neurosurgeon-in-Chief, Department of Neurosurgery, Brigham and Women's Hospital, and The Children's Hospital, Boston, Massachusetts

Anthony L. Boral, M.D., Ph.D.   Instructor in Medicine, The MGH Cancer Center, Massachusetts General Hospital, Boston, Massachusetts

Raphael Bueno, M.D.   Associate Thoracic Surgeon, Department of Surgery, Brigham and Women's Hospital, Boston, Massachusetts

Nam H. Dang, M.D.   Dana-Farber Cancer Institute, Boston, Massachusetts

Malcolm M. DeCamp, Jr., M.D.   Assistant Professor of Surgery, Harvard Medical School, Divison of Thoracic Surgery, Brigham and Women's Hospital, Boston, Massachusetts

Dean M. Donahue, M.D.   Assistant in Surgery, The MGH Cancer Center, Massachusetts General Hospital, and Instructor in Surgery, Division of Thoracic Surgery Harvard Medical School, Boston, Massachusetts

Victoria J. Dorr, M.D.   Assistant Professor of Medicine, Department of Hematology/Oncology, University of Missouri, Ellis Fischel Cancer Center, Columbia, Missouri

Anthony D. Elias, M.D.   Assistant Professor of Medicine, Department of Medicine, Dana-Farber Cancer Institute, Harvard Medical School, Boston, Massachusetts

Raja M. Flores, M.D.   Chief Resident, Division of Thoracic Surgery, Brigham and Women's Hospital, Harvard Medical School, Boston, Massachusetts

Emil Frei III, M.D.   Dana-Farber Cancer Institute and the Joint Center for Radiation Therapy, Boston, Massachusetts

Rodolfo Hakim, M.D.   Assistant Professor, Department of Neurosurgery, Fundación Santa Fe de Bogotá, Bogotá, Columbia

Roy S. Herbst, M.D.*   Department of Medical Oncology, Dana-Farber Cancer Institute, Boston, Massachusetts

Waun Ki Hong, M.D.   Professor of Medicine, Department of Thoracic/Head and Neck Medical Oncology, University of Texas, M.D. Anderson Cancer Center, Houston, Texas

Michael T. Jaklitsch, M.D.   Instructor in Surgery, Division of Thoracic Surgery, Brigham and Women's Hospital, Harvard Medical School, Boston, Massachusetts

Faldo R. Khuri, M.D.   Assistant Internist and Assistant Professor of Medicine, Department of Thoracic/Head and Neck Medical Oncology, University of Texas, M.D. Anderson Cancer Center, Houston, Texas

Parvesh Kumar, M.D.   Chairman and Associate Professor, Department of Radiation Oncology, Robert Wood Johnson Medical School/UMDNJ, Cancer Institute of New Jersey, New Brunswick, New Jersey

Jay S. Loeffler, M.D.   Professor, Department of Radiation Oncology, Harvard Medical School, and Massachusetts General Hospital, Boston, Massachusetts

---

*Present affiliation: University of Texas, M.D. Anderson Cancer Center, Houston, Texas.

Thomas J. Lynch, Jr., M.D. Assistant Professor of Medicine, The MGH Cancer Center, Massachusetts General Hospital, Boston, Massachusetts

Douglas J. Mathisen, M.D. Visiting Surgeon, General Thoracic Surgery Department, Massachusetts General Hospital, and Professor of Surgery, Harvard Medical School, Boston, Massachusetts

Steven J. Mentzer, M.D. Associate Professor of Surgery, Harvard Medical School, Division of Thoracic Surgery, Brigham and Women's Hospital, Boston, Massachusetts

José J. Norberto, M.D. Fellow in Cardiothoracic Surgery, Department of Cardiothoracic Surgery, Ohio State University Medical Center, Columbus, Ohio

Michael C. Perry, M.D., M.S., F.A.C.P. Nellie B. Smith Chair of Oncology, Professor and Director, Division Head of Hematology/Oncology, University of Missouri, Ellis Fischel Cancer Center, Columbia, Missouri

Ravi Salgia, M.D., Ph.D. Assistant Professor of Medicine and Associate Physician, Department of Adult Oncology, Dana-Farber Cancer Institute, Brigham and Women's Hospital, Harvard Medical School, Harvard Medical School, Boston, Massachusetts

Kitt Shaffer, M.D., Ph.D. Clinical Director of Radiology, Department of Radiology, Dana-Farber Cancer Institute, Harvard Medical School, Boston, Massachusetts

Arthur T. Skarin, M.D., F.A.C.P., F.C.C.P. Medical Director, Thoracic Oncology Program, and Associate Professor of Medicine, Department of Adult Oncology, Dana-Farber Cancer Institute, Brigham and Women's Hospital, Harvard Medical School, Boston, Massachusetts

David J. Sugarbaker, M.D. Chief, Division of Thoracic Surgery, Brigham and Women's Hospital, and Chief of Surgical Services, Dana-Farber Cancer Institute, Harvard Medical School, Boston, Massachusetts

Gary M. Strauss, M.D. Chief of Hematology-Oncology, Dana-Farber Cancer Institute, Harvard Medical School, Boston, and Department of Hematology/Oncology, Memorial Hospital, Worcester, Massachusetts

Scott J. Swanson, M.D. Assistant Professor of Surgery, Harvard Medical School, and Associate Chief, Division of Thoracic Surgery, Brigham and Women's Hospital, Boston, Massachusetts

Lamya R. Tannous-Khuri, Ph.D. Visiting Scientist, Department of Thoracic/Head and Neck Medical Oncology, University of Texas, M.D. Anderson Cancer Center, Houston, Texas

Beverly A. Teicher, Ph.D.* Lilly Research Laboratories, Indianapolis, Indiana

Harold C. Urschel, Jr., M.D. Departments of Thoracic and Cardiovascular Surgery, University of Texas Southwestern Medical School and Baylor University Medical Center, Dallas, Texas

---

Formerly at: Dana-Farber Cancer Institute and the Joint Center for Radiation Therapy, Boston, Massachusetts.

CONTENTS

Part One

INTRODUCTION

1

Molecular and Cellular Biological Abnormalities in Lung Cancer and the Potential for Novel Therapeutics

RAVI SALGIA and ARTHUR T. SKARIN

Dana-Farber Cancer Institute
Brigham and Women's Hospital
Harvard Medical School
Boston, Massachusetts

I. Introduction

Lung cancer is a common and an extremely lethal cancer in the United States and the world. Multiple abnormalities of lung cancer cells have been described, and the molecular and cellular biology of normal and cancerous cells is just beginning to be appreciated. Over the course of the past decade, considerable understanding has been obtained on the molecular mechanisms of transformation in lung cancer. Molecular abnormalities include chromosomal aberrations, expression of onco-genes, and loss of tumor suppressor genes. On a cellular level, lung cancer cells can have growth factor and cell surface epitope abnormalities. A common finding in lung cancer is metastatic spread of the original carcinoma. The mechanisms of metastasis involve the interaction of the lung cancer cell with the extracellular matrix, changes in cell adhesion, proteinase production, intravasation and extrava-sation from the circulatory system, colonization in the distant site, and angio-genesis.

Described in this chapter are chromosomal abnormalities that can occur with emphasis on recent findings of the role of telomerase, alteration of oncogenes and tumor suppressor genes, and abnormal molecular biomarkers in lung cancer.

3

Also, some of the metastatic mechanisms involving matrix metalloproteinases and angiogenesis are discussed. Based on the understanding of the abnormalities at the cellular and molecular levels, newer therapies are being pursued. Novel therapies based on translational research described herein include gene therapy, immunological therapy, antiangiogenesis agents, and matrix metalloproteinase inhibitors.

II. Molecular Biological Abnormalities in Lung Cancer

A. Model of Lung Cancer Development

For any tumor to become cancerous, various mutations/alterations occur in the cell which render it neoplastic. To understand the mechanisms for transformation, we will briefly describe several pathways which can be activated or suppressed in the pathogenesis of lung cancer (Figs. 1, 2). As illustrated in the figures, the cell is surrounded by other cells and extracellular matrix. The extracellular matrix and various molecules in the circulation can communicate with the cell through receptors such as growth factor receptors, adhesion molecules (such as cadherins), and integrins. Once a transducing signal is achieved in the cell, different pathways may be activated which can lead to dramatic changes that could affect the cytoskeleton, morphology, or migration of the cell. Eventually, the signal is transmitted to the nucleus, and certain genes can be activated or suppressed, which results in malignant transformation.

When a cell becomes neoplastic, many changes occur inside and outside the cellular environment. The cell not only changes its internal homeostatic mechanisms, but also changes the extracellular environment. Eventually, the cancerous population multiplies and, thereafter, may metastasize and colonize in different sites. For a carcinoma to metastasize, many events occur such as: invasion with changes in tumor cell adhesion, proteinase production, and locomotion; intravasation and extravasation from the circulatory system; colonization in the distant site; and angiogenesis in the new site of implant. Many of these alterations and mechanistic concepts in lung cancer will be described.

B. Chromosomal Abnormalities, Telomerase Activation, and Implications

Using both actual tumor specimens and cell lines, various chromosomal and oncogene abnormalities have been identified. There have been a number of reports on the various chromosomal abnormalities (including loss of complete chromosomes or portions thereof) that can occur in lung cancer. For example, in non-small-cell lung cancer (NSCLC), chromosomal aberrations have been described on 3p, 8p, 9p, 11p, 15p, and 17p with deletions of chromosomes 7, 11, 13, or 19. Also, in

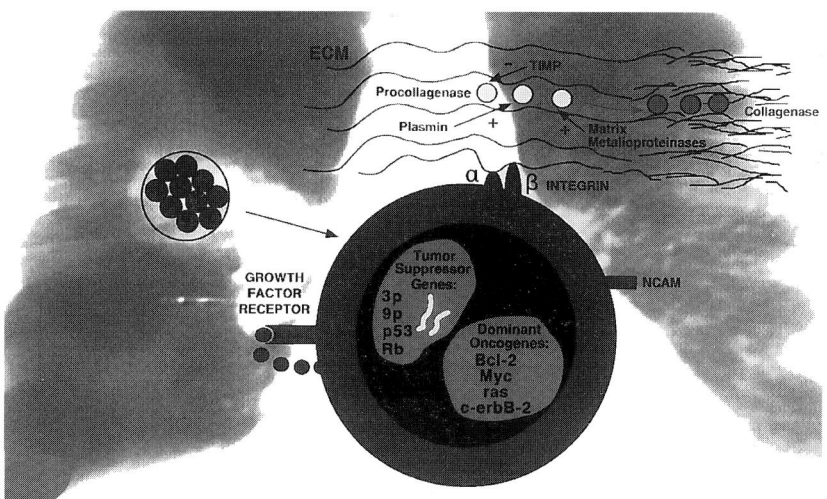

Figure 1 Molecular and biochemical abnormalities in a lung cancer cell and its interaction with the extracellular matrix. Represented is a group of lung cancer cells and magnification of a solitary tumor cell. The cell surface depicts growth factor receptor, α,β subunits of integrin, and the neural cell adhesion molecule (NCAM). Integrins interact with the extracellular matrix (ECM). Shown are how plasmin, matrix metalloproteinases, and tissue inhibitors of metalloproteases (TIMP) regulate the conversion of procollagenase to collagenase with the degradation of the ECM. The nuclear area depicts tumor suppressor genes such as those located on chromosomes 3p and 9p, *p53,* and *Rb.* See text for details.

small-cell lung cancer (SCLC), chromosomal abnormalities have been described on 1p, 3p, 5q, 6q, 8q, 13q, or 17p (1).

One of the most consistent chromosomal abnormalities in lung cancer has been the loss of the short arm of chromosome 3 (3p[14–25] (2). The loss of alleles at 3p is observed in >90% of SCLC tumors and approximately 50% of NSCLC tumors (3). As many as three tumor-suppressor genes may contribute to SCLC pathogenesis. Most recently, the *FHIT* gene (for fragile histidine triad) has been localized to 3p 14.2, and about 80% of SCLC tumors show abnormalities of this gene (4). The protein product of the *FHIT* gene is involved in the metabolism of diadenosine tetraphosphate into ATP and AMP. Loss of *FHIT* gene results in the accumulation of diadenosine tetraphosphate and could lead to the stimulation of DNA synthesis and proliferation. The *FHIT* gene may represent one of several potential tumor suppressor genes located on chromosome 3p involved in the pathogenesis of SCLC.

Other genetic losses have, although not consistently, been identified in lung cancer. In NSCLC, these include genetic loss at chromosome 8p(21.3–22) and

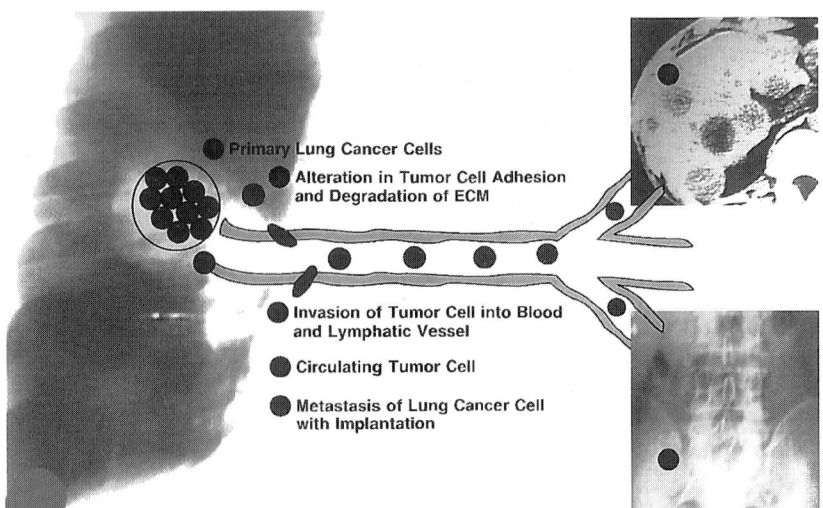

Figure 2 Mechanisms of lung cancer metastasis. Represented is how a tumor cell can metastasize from the original lung cancer. Stepwise, there is alteration in tumor cell adhesion with degradation of the extracellular matrix (ECM). Thereafter, there is invasion by tumor cell into the circulation vessel. Finally, there are implantation and new angiogenesis in distant sites such as liver and bone. See text for details of the mechanisms involved.

may affect in 50% of tumor samples (5). Genetic loss at 9p(21–22) could potentially involve the p16 (MTS1/p16^{INK4A}) and p15 (MTS2/p15^{INK4B}) tumor suppressor genes, which are involved in cell cycle regulation at the G1 checkpoint by inhibiting cyclin-dependent kinase CDK4 and maybe affected in 67% of tumor samples (6,7). Genetic loss at 11p (p13 and p15) may involve the Wilms' tumor suppressor gene at region p13 and can be affected in 20% to 46% of tumor samples (8). SCLC exhibits infrequent loss of 9p, but more losses than NSCLC of 3p, 5q, 13q, and 17p (3).

Telomeres, which are genetic elements at the ends of linear eukaryotic chromosomes consisting of tandem repeats of simple DNA sequences, are important in stabilizing chromosomes from degradation, illegitimate recombination, or cellular senescence (9). Longer telomeres are present in germ cells and most cancer cells via the telomerase enzyme, and this probably maintains the ability of the cells to divide indefinitely (10). Telomerase activity has been directly correlated with malignant and metastatic phenotype of a wide array of solid tumors. In one study, 80% of tumor tissue from lung cancer had telomerase activity (11). Since telomerase activation is essential for long-term growth of many malignancies, inhibition of this enzyme would be an attractive target for therapy.

Compared to the chronology of colon cancer development, it is quite difficult to arrive at the chronology of events for a normal cell to develop from a pre-neoplastic lesion to a frank neoplasia in lung cancer. It is possible that multiple synchronous molecular abnormalities occur in response to toxins such as cigarette smoke, which transform the normal lung cell into a cancerous cell.

C. Oncogenes and Tumor Suppressor Genes

Various oncogene expressions have been investigated in NSCLC and SCLC. There are two forms of oncogenes: dominant oncogenes, and tumor suppressor genes. Dominant oncogenes, such as *RAS, MYC, HER-2/NEU*, and *BCL-2*, exert their effect by overtaking the normal cellular growth function; tumor suppressor oncogenes exert their effect in controlling cellular growth. Once suppressor oncogenes such as *p53, Rb*, p16^{INK4A}, p15^{INK4B} and genes on chromosome 3p are deleted, normal control mechanisms are not available. None of the genes have been implicated in the etiology of lung cancer 100% of the time (12).

1. Oncogenes
a. RAS Genes.

The *RAS*-dominant oncogenes play an important role in signal transduction and cellular proliferation. The RAS proteins have a molecular weight of 21 kDa and consist of K-RAS, H-RAS, and N-RAS. RAS proteins are active when bound to guanosine triphosphate (GTP) and are inactivated by GTPase-activating protein (GAP) by hydrolyzing GTP to guanosine diphosphate (GDP). These proteins acquire transforming potential secondary to a point mutation at codon 12, 13, or 61 in the encoding gene. Mutations at or near the GTP-binding domain of RAS protein prevents the inactivation of GTP, thereby resulting in continuous RAS activity. K-*RAS* mutations are common in NSCLC, with a frequency of up to 30%; however, they have not been reported in SCLC. Increased expression correlates with decreased survival, especially in resectable cases (13,14).

b. MYC *Genes.*

The *MYC*-dominant oncogenes, c-*MYC*, N-*MYC*, and L-*MYC*, encode for nuclear DNA binding proteins which are involved in transcriptional regulation. The general mechanism of activation is gene amplification with resulting overexpression. The frequency of abnormal expression is low in NSCLC (10%) and variable in SCLC (10% to 40%). In a study of Japanese patients with NSCLC by Kawashima et al. (15), the restriction fragment/length polymorphism (RFLP) of the L-*MYC* gene was identified as a marker for metastatic potential. However, there may be geographical differences since no RFLP changes of the L-*MYC* gene were detected in NSCLC tumor samples from Australian, Norwegian or North American patients (8,16). Studies in SCLC have shown that amplification of c-*MYC* genes adversely affect survival (17–19).

c. HER2/NEU *Gene.*

c-*erbB-1* proto-oncogene encodes the epidermal growth factor receptor and has been a classic model for signal transduction events in normal and transformed cells. A related proto-oncogene, c-*erbB-2* (also known as *HER2/NEU*), encodes for a protein product of molecular weight 185 kDa (p185^{neu}), and also is a growth factor receptor. Frequency of abnormal expression of p185^{neu} in NSCLC is approximately 25%, and no abnormalities have been reported in SCLC. Overexpression of p185^{neu} has been shown to be associated with an adverse prognosis in adenocarcinoma of the lung (20).

d. BCL-2 *Gene.*

BCL-2 proto-oncogene product inhibits programmed cell death, termed apoptosis. *BCL-2* overexpressing cells have expansion of cell populations secondary to lack of apoptosis. In a group of patients with squamous cell carcinoma, 5-year survival was better for patients with *BCL-2*-positive tumors (78% vs. 48%; $P < .05$) (21). The better prognosis for *BCL-2*-positive tumors is unknown.

2. Tumor Suppressor Genes

a. p53 *Gene.*

The *p53* gene, located at chromosome 17p13.1, encodes a nuclear protein which acts as a transcription factor and blocks the progression of cells through the cell cycle late in the G1 phase. The most common genetic changes associated with cancer involve mutations of the *p53* gene. *p53* gene mutations cause a loss of tumor suppressor function, promoting cellular proliferation. Some *p53* mutant proteins also have transforming properties by binding and inactivating available wild-type (normal) *p53*. The Li-Fraumeni cancer syndrome that is typified by multiple tumors at an early age of onset is characterized by inherited forms of *p53* mutations. *p53* mutations can involve deletions, point mutations, and overexpression. In lung cancer, the prevalent type of point mutation is a GC to TA transversion and is related to adducts of benzo(a)pyrene from cigarette smoking. Frequency of mutations may be up to 50% in NSCLC and 80% in SCLC (22). Initially, it was believed that lung cancer has an adverse correlation with *p53* protein overexpression (23). However, recent data suggest that high expression of the *p53* oncoprotein may be a favorable prognostic factor in a subset of patients with NSCLC (24).

b. RB *Gene.*

The *RB* gene, located on chromosome 13q14.11, encodes for a nuclear protein which was determined to be abnormal in patients with retinoblastoma. Knudson predicted the tumor suppressor nature of this gene by studying inheritance patterns of familial retinoblastoma (25). The protein encoded for *RB* is 105 kDa and is important in regulating the cell cycle during G0/G1 phase. There is usually a deletion of the *RB* gene in >90% of SCLC, and approximately 15% of NSCLC. The expression of the tumor suppressor gene *RB* may be an adverse prognosticator in lung cancer (26,27).

c. *p16^{INK4A}* and *p15^{INK4B}* genes.

Certain lung cancer cells have a characteristic deletion of chromosome 9p21, thus implicating one or more tumor suppressor genes in this region as being important. From genetic analysis, *p16^{INK4A}* (hereafter designated *p16*) and *p15^{INK4B}* (designated *p15*) have been identified to map within 30 kb of each other in this region. p16 was originally identified as a binding protein to CDK4 in a yeast two-hybrid screen, and contains four ankyrin repeats (28). *p15* was thereafter cloned from a low stringency screen using *p16* with a human keratinocyte cDNA library, and has a very high homology with *p16* (29). In some cells stimulated by TGF-β, p15 induction is 30-fold greater than p16 (7). Both *p16* and *p15* encode for proteins that inhibit CDK4 involved in cell cycle control, thereby preventing progression from G1 to S phase.

Mutations or deletions of *p15,* but not of *p16,* were found in 8 of 25 primary lung tumors by Okamoto et al. (30). Five of 22 metastatic tumors had homozygous deletions of *p15,* and 6 of 22 tumors had mutations of *p16* (30). Shapiro et al. (31,32) have described no detectable p16 protein expression in 17 of 27 primary NSCLC tumors, and abundant protein in 4 of 5 SCLC tumors. In NSCLC cell lines, an inverse correlation exists between p16 expression and RB expression (33), thereby implicating a key role of these proteins in growth suppression.

III. Cellular Biological Abnormalities in Lung Cancer
A. Growth Factor Abnormalities

Besides abnormalities of oncogenes, neoplastic cells respond to growth factors in an abnormal fashion. In SCLC, many of the tumor cells produce neuroendocrine peptides, such as gastrin-releasing peptide (GRP), and respond to them in an autocrine or paracrine fashion. Other growth factors abnormal in SCLC are believed to be insulinlike growth factor I and transferrin. One hypothesis of how growth factors are important is that certain components of cigarette smoke may injure pulmonary neuroendocrine cells, leading to CD10/neutral endopeptidase secretion with resultant hyperplasia and eventual carcinogenesis (34,35). In NSCLC, factors such as epidermal growth factor, insulinlike growth factor, platelet-derived growth factor, and transforming growth factor α and β can be involved in abnormal neoplastic cell response.

Gastrin-releasing peptide was initially cloned from a human lung carcinoid tissue and SCLC cell lines. Located on chromosome 18q21, GRP is encoded to be a 145–amino acid peptide. It is a proliferative growth factor and transduces intracellular signals. GRP binds to the GRP receptor, which is a member of the G-protein family. In SCLC, GRP functions as an autocrine growth factor to stimulate cell growth (36–38).

Epidermal growth factor (EGF), a 53–amino acid peptide, is a ligand for the EGF receptor, a product of the erbB-1 proto-oncogene. The EGF receptor is expressed at high levels in patients with NSCLC (>50%) and at low levels in patients with SCLC (20,39,40).

Insulinlike growth factor I (IGF-I) is an insulinlike protein elevated in >95% SCLC and >80% NSCLC; it may modulate mitogenic signaling (41,42). As with IGF-I, transferrin may function as an autocrine growth factor in SCLC (43).

Steel factor, the ligand for the proto-oncoprotein tyrosine kinase receptor c-Kit, supports growth and survival of immature hematopoietic cells of multiple lineages. In SCLC, c-Kit and Steel factor are simultaneously expressed, thus forming an autocrine loop (44).

Transforming growth factor $\beta 1$ is part of the TGFβ family and initially recognized as a factor that causes fibroblasts to behave as transformed cells. TGFβ can stimulate growth and inhibit cellular proliferation in carcinogenesis (45). A number of growth factors thus appear to play a role in lung cancer pathogenesis and progression.

B. Cell Surface Epitopes

Lung cancer cells have been shown to express different cell surface epitopes. Recently, there has been a trend to cluster the antigens found on the lung cancer cell surface, similar to the cluster designation for leukocytes (46–48). Thus far, 15 clusters have been designated for antibodies that react against normal lung cells or lung cancer cells. Not all the antigens for the individual clusters have been fully characterized, however, this is one of the building blocks for categorizing the various cell surface antigens in lung cancer. As an example, by raising various antibodies to different epitopes of SCLC, neural cell adhesion molecule (NCAM) has been identified to be expressed on SCLC cells and has been designated under cluster 1 (49). NCAM belongs to a family of sialoproteins involved in cell-cell adhesions. In general, adhesion molecules are important in cell-cell and cell–extracellular matrix communications, and in an abnormal state may play a role in tumor invasion and metastasis. In some studies, 100% of SCLC tumors react with the NCAM antibodies, whereas only 9% of NSCLC tumors react with this antibody (50).

Along with cell surface adhesion molecule expression, lung cancer cells can express ABH blood group antigens, and this expression appears to confer prognostic significance. The ABH blood group antigens are expressed on the surface of most epithelial cells, in addition to red blood cells. The expression of blood group antigen A seems to confer better survival in NSCLC (51). The H/Le^y/Le^b antigen is a carbohydrate antigen related to blood group antigen H. Expression of H/Le^y/Le^b is high in certain cases of lung cancer. Expression of this antigen is thought to be related to deletion of the A and B blood group antigens, which are its precursor antigens on the surface of the cancer cells. Studies have shown that cancers in which this deletion occurs have a greater potential for invasion and thus a worse prognosis (52).

C. Tumor Markers

Tumor markers of lung cancer include hormones, fetoproteins, cell surface membrane antigens, and enzymes (34). The biomarkers are useful for staging and also for following the clinical course of the disease. Decrease in tumor marker levels generally parallels response to treatment. Elevation of the tumor marker may predate other evidence of relapse by several months.

CEA (carcinoembryonic antigen) and CA-125 are particularly useful in lung cancer (53–57). Studies at our institution showed elevation of both markers in about half the cases of NSCLC and SCLC (58). Neuron-specific enolase (NSE) and chromogranin-A (chrA) markers of neuroendocrine differentiation are more useful in SCLC (59,60). Other tumor markers of value in selected cases include hormones (e.g., ACTH, MSH, ADH), lipid-sialic acid (LSA), tissue polypeptide antigen (TPA), and neural cell surface adhesion molecule (NCAM) (34,61,62). Some of these tumor markers also prove to be important prognosticators in lung cancer, particularly when initially elevated (63).

IV. Metastasis
A. Paget's Seed and Soil Hypothesis

In his classic study, Paget (64) noticed that breast cancer cells metastasized widely, with a predilection to the bones. This metastasis pattern to the skeletal system was different for a variety of tumors. From his observations Paget concluded that metastasis occurred when certain tumor cells ("seed") had special affinity for the growth environment provided by certain specific organs ("soil"). Fidler (65) has defined three principles of the "seed and soil" hypothesis for any tumor to metastasize. Tumor cells are heterogeneous and have different angiogenic, invasive, and metastatic properties. The process of metastasis is selective for cells that succeed in invasion and survival in the circulation, and eventually multiply within the organ parenchyma. Eventually, the tumor cell can overtake the normal homeostatic mechanisms. For metastatic disease, therapy should in part be geared toward these concepts with interruption of propagation and spreading mechanisms noted above.

B. Extracellular Matrix and Proteinases

For a neoplastic cell to metastasize, it must interact with its extracellular matrix (ECM) and break the barrier to the circulation. The critical event of tumor invasion is the interaction of the neoplastic cell with the basement membrane. Basement membranes are composed of type IV collagen, laminin, and heparan sulfate proteoglycan as its major components. The ECM is composed of the basement membrane along with other large molecules such as fibronectin and vitronectin. Type IV collagen forms the basement membrane scaffolding on which laminin, heparan sulfate, proteoglycan, and other minor components of the basement membrane are assembled (66). Recent data show that degradation of type IV collagen is important for tumor cell invasion and subsequent metastasis.

Extracellular matrix degradation is a highly dynamic event and is dependent on the rate of production of the ECM components, production of proteinases, and production of proteinase inhibitors. Two families of proteinases, plasminogen activator (PA) and matrix metalloproteinase (MMP), are important in degradation of the ECM and will be discussed. The proenzyme plasminogen in the ECM can be cleaved by either tissue-PA (t-PA) or urokinase-type PA (u-PA) to produce the active plasmin. Fibronectin, laminin, fibrin, and type IV collagen can be degraded by plasmin proteolysis. u-PA is also released from cells in an inactive pro form which must be proteolytically cleaved to activate plasminogen. There is high expression of u-PA and/or t-PA in malignant tumors. At least four known inhibitors of PA exist: plasminogen activator inhibitor-1 (PAI-1); PAI-2; protease nexins; and α2-antiplasmin. It is the fine balance between PA and PA inhibitors that keeps the normal homeostasis, and once this is disrupted in malignancies, metastasis may occur (67).

Matrix metalloproteinases are another family of proteinases which are used mainly to degrade and remodel all components of the ECM. This family consists of 11 enzymes which are released as inactive pro forms which are activated in the extracellular environment. Three main subgroups are classified on their substrates: interstitial collagenases, stromelysins, and gelatinases (type IV collagenases). All MMPs contain (from N to C terminus of the molecule) a signal sequence, a profragment activation locus, a zinc atom binding domain, a catalytic domain typical of enzymes, a proline-rich hinge region, and a hemopexin-or vitronectinlike domain. Several members of the MMP family have been implicated in tumor invasion, including MMP-1 (type 1 collagenase), MMP-3 (stromelysin), and MMP-2 and -9 (type IV gelatinase/collagenase), in the active site and turnover extracellular matrix proteins. Substrates for MMP include fibrillar collagens of bone, skin, and interstitia, and the nonfibrillar collagens laminin and fibronectin of the basal laminina (68,69).

MMPs are regulated by general and specific inhibitors in the cells. There are general protease inhibitors such as α2-macroglobulin in the serum, or specific inhibitors such as TIMPs (tissue inhibitors of metalloproteases) (67). The TIMP-1 gene is located on the X chromosome, is a 28-kDa glycoprotein, and forms irreversible noncovalent complexes. The TIMP:MMP ratio is usual, with a 1:1 molar stoichiometry, and the ratio is very critical. TIMP-1 is considered to function as a metastasis suppressor gene (70). TIMP-2 is a nonglycosylated 21-kDa protein and blocks the hydrolytic activities of all activated MMPs (71). Finally, TIMP-3 is not secreted from cells and remains soluble and localized to the ECM (72). As for other proteinases and their inhibitors, a fine balance must exist within the cell for normal cellular machinery. In tumorigenesis, this is completely disrupted and can lead to angiogenesis around the tumor nidus.

C. Angiogenesis and Tumor Invasion

Inducing angiogenesis may be an important mechanism for a tumor cell to proliferate and eventually metastasize. For tumor proliferation, initially there is a long-lasting prevascular phase with local invasion of the primary tumor. Thereafter, there is a short-lasting vascular phase with blood and lymphatic vessel invasion. Angiogenic factors cause ingrowth of new capillaries, and these have leakiness due to fragmented basement membranes. This then allows for tumor cells to enter into the circulation. Angiogenesis can be measured with factor VIII immunostaining of microvessels (73).

Tumor cells themselves as well as inflammatory cells at the tumor site can mediate angiogenesis. Factors include fibroblast growth factor, vascular endothelial cell growth factor, interleukins 8 and 12, angiogenin, angiotropin, platelet-derived endothelial growth factor, transforming growth factor α,β, and tumor necrosis factor α (74). One or more of these factors may act in concert responding to tumorigenesis. Angiogenesis inhibition would be an ideal tool in clinical chemotherapeutics.

Accumulating data indicate that angiogenesis is a significant prognostic factor in stage I lung cancer. For example, Harpole et al. (75) examined tumors from 275 patients with stage I NSCLC and compared survival via multivariate analysis using angiogenesis, proto-oncogene c-*erbB*-2, tumor suppressor gene p53, and the proliferation marker KI-67. Of these factors, excessive angiogenesis was the most significant prognostic factor in stage I lung cancer.

Tumor cells can also penetrate preexisting vessels, thereby leading to metastasis. Roberts et al. (76) showed that arterial or venous vascular invasion by tumor was present in 67 of 87 patients (77%) who underwent lobectomy or pneumectomy for adenocarcinoma or squamous cell carcinoma. There was no correlation of degree of invasion with survival. However, Macchiarini et al. (77) analyzed 45 patients with peripheral, node-negative NSCLC, treated with wedge resection alone; patients with tumor invasion (15%) had a poor survival and higher recurrence rate.

V. Novel Therapeutics in Lung Cancer

From the above knowledge of the basic biology of lung cancer and how a tumor can metastasize, various novel therapies are being utilized. The following is not intended to be a comprehensive review of the various therapies in lung cancer; however, examples of some novel therapeutics are presented to reflect how the knowledge of basic science is being translated into potentially beneficial chemotherapy.

A. Gene Therapy

Gene therapy utilizes genetic material as a therapeutic agent. In order to therapeutically deliver genes to tumor cells, viral or physical means are commonly utilized. Viral vectors include retrovirus, adenovirus, adenovirus-associated virus, and vaccinia virus. Each of these viral vectors has its own advantages and disadvantages. For example, retrovirus vectors integrate in the chromosome and allow sustained gene expression; however, this requires dividing cells, and retroviruses are difficult to grow to a high viral titer. Adenovirus vectors have the ability to transduce postmitotic cells and have a higher achievable titers; however, the gene expression is only transient, peaking in 3 to 5 days. Genes can also be introduced into tumor cells by nonviral techniques such as electroporation, liposomes, and calcium phosphate coprecipitation among others. There are basically two types of potential therapeutic genes that are used: directly tumoricidal, and immunity-inducing. Tumoricidal genes act by inducing growth arrest or killing of cells; examples include p53 and ras, which are being utilized in lung cancer. The other therapeutic gene mechanism is immunity-inducing, which is described below (78–80).

B. Immune Therapy

A longstanding goal of cancer research has been to induce the immune system to reject tumors. This goal is based on strong experimental evidence that many neoplasms express tumor antigens that could potentially be recognized by the immune system, leading to tumor cell destruction. An immune response occurs when T-cell receptors bind to a small antigenic peptide located in a groove of an MHC molecule on an antigen-presenting cell (APC). Endogenous antigens, regardless of their intracellular location, are processed into peptides and are usually presented to T cells in association with class I MHC molecules. Exogenous antigens are endocytosed by APCs such as macrophages, B cells, or dendritic cells, and are presented to T cells in the context of class II MHC molecules. MHC restriction is a consequence of the fact that certain peptides bind better than others to individual, polymorphic, MHC gene products. Self-antigens are presumably presented to T cells early in life, and self-reactive clones are deleted through poorly understood mechanisms. Later in life, self-reactive T cells cause autoimmune diseases, and mechanisms to eliminate such clones probably exist.

Antigen presentation by itself, however, is not sufficient for expansion of a T-cell clone and generation of an immune response. Recent data on the mechanisms of T lymphocyte activation indicate that both an antigen-specific signal delivered through the T-cell receptor (TCR) and a second antigen-nonspecific costimulatory signal are required (81). Costimulation may involve several molecules on APCs which are recognized by T-cell surface receptors. One of the most important is the B7-1 surface protein expressed by activated B cells, macrophages, and dendritic cells (82). B7-1 binds to CD28 and CTLA4 receptors on T cells, costimulates CD4+ T cells to proliferate, and is now known to be a member of a small family of molecules that can bind to CD28 and CTLA4, including B7-2 and at least one additional, uncloned member (83,84). The functional differences between CD28 and CTLA4 are unknown. Signals transduced by CD28 are required for production of IL-2, and can determine whether antigen activation of the TCR results in a productive immune response. CD28 signals may function in part to stabilize IL-2 mRNA and thus promote IL-2 production by an activated T cell. In some experimental systems, costimulation can be replaced by the addition of IL-2. Importantly, activation of the TCR by antigen in the absence of B7 costimulation results in clonal anergy or death (81).

For an immune response to be generated against a tumor, the tumor must have a suitable antigen, and either tumor cells must be able to effectively present antigen themselves or normal APCs must act as intermediates after acquiring antigen secreted or released from dead tumor cells. Since many tumors have antigens, failure to present antigen properly has been implicated as a cause of anergy to tumor antigens. There are now a number of model systems in which B7-1(–) tumors have been transfected with B7-1, resulting in the induction of a CTL response to both B7-1(–) and B7-1(+) tumors (85,86).

Cytokines can also provide costimulatory signals important in T-lymphocyte activation. Using B16 melanoma cells, Dranoff et al. (87) compared 10 cytokines (IL-1, 2, 4, 5, and 6); granulocyte macrophage colony stimulating factor (GM-CSF); γ interferon; tumor necrosis factor (TNF); intracellular adhesion molecule; and CD2 for enhancing immunogenicity. It was found that GM-CSF most effectively stimulated long-lasting and specific antitumor immunity requiring CD8+ T lymphocytes. In human melanoma, Rosenberg (88,89) took autologous tumor cells, established them in culture, and then immunized the donors after tranducing the IL-2 or TNF genes. After several weeks, draining lymph nodes were removed and CTL was expanded in culture and then reintroduced into the patient. This adoptive immunotherapy has been shown to be feasible in advanced melanoma and ovarian carcinoma (90–92). Similar studies are being planned for patients with lung cancer.

Recently Ratto et al. (93) evaluated adoptive immunotherapy using TIL expanded in vitro and rIL-2 in the postoperative treatment of resected NSCLC. There was no benefit observed in patients with stage II as compared with standard therapy. However, for patients with stage III NSCLC, local relapse was significantly reduced as compared with patients who received standard therapy ($P < .05$). The toxic effects of adoptive immunotherapy were secondary to the rIL-2 administration. Certainly, this is a preliminary study and more studies are needed to confirm these findings; however, adoptive therapy may be of potential benefit in lung cancer (94).

C. Antisense Therapy

With the advances in the knowledge of oncogenes in lung cancer, one novel method by which to downregulate the oncogene expression is antisense technology. A gene can be transduced into a cell in the antisense orientation, or antisense oligodeoxyribonucleotides (ASODNs), which are synthetic analogs, can be utilized. The strategy is designed to bind to the RNA transcripts of target genes in a sequence-specific manner. The resulting reaction interrupts translation of messenger RNA into protein, thereby specifically blocking gene expression. As an example, K-RAS gene in antisense orientation was used to transduce human lung cancer cell lines using a retroviral vector (95), and tumor growth suppression was seen. There were technical issues in that five to seven exposures were required to obtain transgene expression in 95% of the tumor cells. Also, this has not been done in human lung cancer.

As an example of a study inhibiting oncogene expression in lung cancer utilizing specific ASODNs complementary to mRNA of c-*MYC*, *BCL2*, and *p53*, Robinson et al. (96) determined cellular proliferation in three NSCLC cell lines. All three ASODNs were found to inhibit proliferation. Even though this study presents only preliminary data in cell lines, there is hope that it may be applicable to actual tumor samples.

D. Antibody Therapy

Since there are unique antigens that may be identified in lung cancer, it seems reasonable to design therapy that recognizes these antigens by specific antibodies and thereafter destroy the tumor cells. Recently, unique antibodies that recognize antigens in lung cancer have been conjugated to toxins such as diphtheria toxin and ricin. For example, using this concept and the observation that SCLC express the NCAM antigen, an antibody N901 (which recognizes the NCAM antigen on SCLC cells) has been conjugated with blocked ricin (N901-bR) and initially tested in Phase 1 study for extensive disease SCLC (97–99).

N901-bR is an immunotoxin composed of the chemically conjugated N901 monoclonal antibody and blocked whole ricin. N901 is a high-affinity murine monoclonal antibody that recognizes the NKH1 antigen, an NCAM isoform (100). NKH1 is expressed on SCLC cell lines and fresh human tumors (101). Thus, it is an ideal target for an immunotoxin for SCLC. Ricin is a highly potent, two-chain, plant toxin extracted from castor beans. The A chain of the toxin is responsible for ribosomal inactivation leading to inhibition of protein synthesis and cell death. The B chain of the toxin is responsible for binding to cell membranes and translocating the A chain across cell membranes. Under usual circumstances, ricin binds to and kills cells indiscriminately through binding the B chain to cell membranes. By chemically blocking the sites on the B chain that bind to cell membranes, ricin becomes dramatically less toxic to normal cells (102). Finally, by attaching the N901 monoclonal antibody to the B chain, the resultant compound binds to cells that are NKH1-positive, allowing the A chain to enter and kill the cell. The resultant compound, N901-bR, has the specificity of the N901 antibody and the cytotoxicity of blocked whole ricin (99,101).

A Phase I study of N901-bR in patients with relapsed or refractory SCLC was carried out at the Dana-Farber Cancer Institute (99,103). All of the 21 patients entered in the Phase 1 study were heavily pretreated with chemotherapy and radiation. All the patients had received cisplatin and vincristine prior to study entry. Detectable serum drug levels were seen at doses of N901-bR ranging from 5 µ/kg/day × 7 days to 40 µ/kg lean body weight/day × 7 days. N901-bR was well tolerated by the majority of patients in the study. In this Phase 1 design, the dose-limiting toxicity (DLT) was reached at 40 µ/kg lbw (lean body weight)/day × 7 days. The DLT was capillary leak syndrome. Two of the three patients treated at the DLT experienced capillary leak syndrome with weight gain of > 10 kg, peripheral edema, hypotension, and shortness of breath. One patient at the DLT also experienced thrombocytopenia, which may be related to the capillary leak syndrome. Notable toxicities included one patient with preexisting cardiac risk factors who suffered a silent myocardial infarction on day 7 of therapy, and one patient who died of respiratory failure secondary to progressive tumor on day 2 of therapy (103). One partial response was observed in the Phase 1 study. Even though there was only one partial response seen in SCLC, this unique immunoconjugate points to further therapies that can be designed in lung cancer based on specific antibodies and immunotoxins.

E. Antiangiogenesis Agents

Neovascularization for growth of tumors and metastases at distant sites is an ideal situation for therapeutic intervention. There have been some agents that inhibit angiogenesis; however, they have proven to be too toxic for clinical applications (104). One class of drug is designed on inhibition of angiogenic factors. For example, a naturally secreted antibiotic fumagillin of *Aspergillus fumigatus frescenius* was shown to cause endothelial cells in culture to round up and inhibit angiogenesis (105). Unfortunately, in vivo, fumagillin was too toxic to animals. Fortunately, though, synthetic analogs of fumagillin were tested, and TNP-470 (O-(chloroacetyl-carbamoyl) fumagillol) was found to be the most potent angiogenesis inhibitor and nontoxic to animals (105). In various assays, TNP-470 was a potent inhibitor of endothelial cell migration, endothelial cell proliferation, and capillary tube formation (106). Also, TNP-470 inhibits growth of certain primary and metastatic murine tumors along with human tumor xenografts. TNP-470 is currently in Phase 1 trials, and results are awaited. It is possible that as a single agent, angiogenesis inhibitors may not have a high activity; however, in combination with cytotoxic agents, they may prove to be quite efficacious (107).

F. Matrix Metalloproteinase Inhibitors

As discussed in the above sections, MMPIs have an important role in regulating MMPs and the extracellular matrix. The TIMPs are naturally occurring molecules which control the function of various proteinases. Even though they are native inhibitors, TIMPs have not been ideal antineoplastic agents, because of their high molecular weights and strong antigenic properties (69). As a natural progression to develop drugs to prevent cartilage and bone breakdown in rheumatoid arthritis, several synthetic MMPIs have been characterized. Of these, batimastat has been the most characterized, and this agent has been used in Phase 1 studies performed in cancer patients. Batimastat acts as a reversible inhibition substrate of MMPs. It has a weak cytostatic effect on cell lines, but no cytotoxic effects. Treatment with batimastat of mice harboring the B16 melanoma tumor, with metastases to the lungs, inhibited tumor growth and resulted in a significant reduction in lung colony number (68% inhibition; $P < .001$) (108). There was also inhibition of tumor progression with batimastat in xenograft models of human ovarian carcinoma and human colorectal carcinoma (109,110).

In clinical trials, the bioavailability of batimastat when given by oral formulation was quite disappointing. However, from animal data it was noted that intraperitoneal or intrapleural delivery of the drug may be effective in palliation. In patients with symptomatic pleural effusions, batimastat 15 to 135 mg/m^2 was given intrapleurally after aspiration of the effusion. This was tolerated quite well, and in patients receiving 60 to 135 mg/m^2 batimastat there was a significant reduction in the number of aspirations (111). Even though this is the only MMPI to have made it to such extensive clinical trials, this may be an important start in the applications of MMPIs. It is quite feasible to combine the various therapeutic modalities with MMPIs to obtain synergistic effects. For example, the weak broad-spectrum MMPI minocycline, the inhibitor of angiogenesis TNP-470, and cyclophosphamide in combination were more effective in reducing local invasion and distant metastases in murine Lewis lung carcinoma model (106).

VI. Conclusions

Lung cancer is a devastating illness, and there is great impetus to determine the molecular and cellular abnormalities in transformation of normal to malignant cells. A considerable amount has been learned about normal cellular homeostatic mechanisms and the aberrations leading to cancer. Lung cancer is a unique illness in that a majority of the tumors are related to toxins from cigarette smoking. One of our goals should be to continue defining abnormalities of the lung cancer cell and eventually translating this knowledge to novel therapies. However, elimination of tobacco products must be the first and foremost goal to stop the worldwide epidemic of lung cancer, particularly in third-world countries.

References

1. Devereux TR, Taylor JA, Barrett JC. Molecular mechanisms of lung cancer. Chest 1996; 109:14S–19S.
2. Hibi K, Takahashi T, Yamakawa K, et al. Three distinct regions involved in 3p deletion in human lung cancer. Oncogene 1992; 7:445–449.
3. Otterson G, Lin A, Kaye F. Genetic etiology of lung cancer. Oncology 1992; 6:97–112.
4. Sozzi G, Veronese M, Negrini M, et al. The *FHIT* gene at 3p14.2 is abnormal in lung cancer. Cell 1996; 85:17–26.
5. Ohata H, Emi M, Fujiwara Y, et al. Deletion mapping of the short arm of chromosome 8 in non-small cell lung carcinoma. Genes Chrom Cancer 1993; 7:85–88.
6. Merlo A, Gabrielson E, Askin F, et al. Frequent loss of chromosome 9 in human primary non-small cell lung cancer. Cancer Res 1994; 54:640–642.
7. Shapiro G, Rollins B. p16INK4A as a human tumor suppressor. Biochim Biophys Acta 1996; 1242:165–169.
8. Fong F, Zimmerman P, Smith P. Lung pathology: the molecular genetics of non-small cell lung cancer. Pathology 1995; 27:295–301.
9. Harley C, Kim N. Telomerase and cancer. In: DeVita VJ, Hellman S, Rosenberg S, eds. Important Advances in Oncology. Philadelphia: Lippincott-Raven, 1997:1–11.
10. Carbone D. The biology of lung cancer. Semin Oncol 1997; 24:388–401.
11. Hiyama K, Ishioka S, Shirotani Y, et al. Alterations in telomeric repeat length in lung

cancer are associated with loss of heterozygosity in p53 and rb. Oncogene 1995; 10:937–944.

12. Salgia R, Skarin A. Molecular abnormalities in lung cancer. J Clin Oncol 1998; 16:1207–1217

13. Slebos R, Kibbelaar R, Dalesio O, et al. K-ras oncogene activation as a prognostic marker in adenocarcinoma of the lung. N Engl J Med 1990; 323:561–565.

14. Harada M, Dosaka-Akita H, Miyamoto H, et al. Prognostic significance of the expression of ras oncogene product in non-small cell lung cancer. Cancer 1992; 69:72–77.

15. Kawashima K, Nomura S, Hirai H, et al. Correlation of the L-myc RFLP with metastasis, prognosis and multiple cancer in the lung cancer patients. Int J Cancer 1992; 50:557–561.

16. Mountain CF. New prognostic factors in lung cancer—biologic prophets of cancer cell aggression. Chest 1995; 108:246–254.

17. Brennan J, O'Connor T, Makuch R, et al. myc family DNA amplification in 107 tumors and tumor cell lines from patients with small cell lung cancer treated with different combination chemotherapy regimens. Cancer Res 1991; 51:1708–1712.

18. Noguchi M, Hirohasi S, Hara F. Heterogeneous amplification of myc family oncogenes in small cell lung carcinoma. Cancer 1990; 66:2053–2058.

19. Funa K, Steinholtz L, Nou E, et al. Increased expression of N-myc in human small cell lung cancer biopsies predicts lack of response to chemotherapy and poor prognosis. J Clin Pathol 1986; 88:216–220.

20. Kern J, Schwartz D, Nordberg J, et al. p185[neu] expression in human lung adenocarcinomas predicts shortened survival. Cancer Res 1990; 50:5184–5191.

21. Pezzella F, Turley H, Kuzu I, et al. *bcl*-2 protein in non-small-cell lung carcinoma. N Engl J Med 1993; 329:690–694.

22. Sidransky D, Hollstein M. Clinical implications of the p53 gene. Annu Rev Med 1996; 47:285–301.

23. Mitsudomi T, Oyama T, Kusano T, et al. Mutations of the p53 gene as a predictor of poor prognosis in patients with non-small-cell lung cancer. J Natl Cancer Inst 1993; 85:2018.

24. Lee J, Yoon A, Kalapurakal S, et al. Expression of *p53* oncoprotein in non-small-cell lung cancer: a favorable prognostic factor. J Clin Oncol 1995; 13:1893–1903.

25. Knudson A. Hereditary cancer: clues to mechanisms of carcinogenesis. Br J Cancer 1989; 59:661–666.

26. Yokota J, Akiyama T, Fung Y, et al. Altered expression of the retinoblastoma (*RB*) gene in small cell lung cancer of the lung. Oncogene 1988; 3:471–475.

27. Harbour J, Lai S, Whang-Peng J, et al. Abnormalities in structure and expression of the retinoblastoma gene in SCLC. Science 1988; 241:353–357.

28. Serrano M, Hannon GJ, Beach D. A new regulatory motif in cell-cycle control causing specific inhibition of cyclin D/CDK4. Nature 1993; 366:704–707.

29. Hannon GJ, Beach D. p15INK4B is a potential effector of TGF-beta-induced cell cycle arrest. Nature 1994; 371:257–261.

30. Okamoto A, Hussain SP, Hagiwara K, et al. Mutations in the p16INK4/MTS1/CDKN2, p15INK4B/MTS2, and p18 genes in primary and metastatic lung cancer. Cancer Res 1995; 55:1448–1451.

31. Shapiro GI, Edwards CD, Kobzik L, et al. Reciprocal Rb inactivation and p16INK4 expression in primary lung cancers and cell lines. Cancer Res 1995; 55:505–509.

32. Shapiro GI, Park JE, Edwards CD, et al. Multiple mechanisms of p16INK4A inactivation in non-small cell lung cancer cell lines. Cancer Res 1995; 55:6200–6209.

33. Otterson GA, Kratzke RA, Coxon A, et al. Absence of p16INK4 protein is restricted to the subset of lung cancer lines that retains wildtype RB. Oncogene 1994; 9:3375–3378.

34. Skarin A. Respiratory tract and head and neck cancer. In: Rubenstein E, Federman D, eds. Scientific America Medicine. New York: Scientific American, 1994:1–35.

35. Auerbach O, Stout A, Hammond E, et al. Changes in bronchial epithelium in relation to cigarette smoking and in relation to lung cancer. N Engl J Med 1961; 265:253–258.

36. Moody T, CB P, Gazdar A, et al. High levels of intracellular bombesin characterize human small cell lung carcinoma. Science 1981; 214:1246–1248.

37. Spindel E, Chin W, Price J, et al. Cloning and characterization of cDNAs encoding human gastrin-releasing peptide. Proc Natl Acad Sci USA 1984; 81:5699–5703.

38. Sausville E, Lebacq-Verheyden A, Spindel E, et al. Expression of the gastrin-releasing peptide genc in human small cell lung cancer. J Biol Chem 1986; 261:2451–2459.

39. Schneider P, Hung M, Chiocca S, et al. Differential expression of the c-erbB-2 gene in human small cell and non-small cell lung cancer. Cancer Res 1989; 49:4968–4971.

40. Weiner D, Nordberg J, Nowell P, et al. Expression of the neu gene encoded protein (p 185[neu]) in human non-small cell lung carcinomas of the lung. Cancer Res 1990; 50:421–425.

41. Reeve J, Payne J, Bleehen N. Production of immunoreactive insulin-like growth factor-1 (IGF-1) and IGF-1 binding proteins by human lung tumors. Br J Cancer 1990; 61:727–731.

42. Minuto F, Del Monte P, Barreca A, et al. Evidence for an increased somatomedin C/insulin-like growth factor-1 content in primary human lung tumors. Cancer Res 1986; 46:985–988.

43. Vostrcjs M, Moran P, Seligman P. Transferrin synthesis by small cell lung cancer cells acts as an autocrine regulator of cellular proliferation. J Clin Invest 1988; 82:331–339.

44. Hibi K, Takahashi T, Sekido Y, et al. Coexpression of the stem cell factor and the c-kit genes in small-cell lung cancer. Oncogene 1991; 6:2291–2296.

45. Sporn M, Roberts A, Wakefield L, et al. Some recent advances in the chemistry and biology of transforming growth factor-beta. J Cell Biol 1987; 105:1039–1045.

46. Souhami R, Beverley P, Bobrow L. Proceedings of the First International Workshop on Small Cell Lung Cancer. Lancet 1987; 2:325–326.

47. Souhami R, Beverley P, Bobrow L, et al. Antigens of lung cancer: results of the Second International Workshop on Lung Cancer Antigens. J Natl Cancer Inst 1991; 83:609–612.

48. Stahel R, Gilks W, Schenker T. Antigens of lung cancer: results of the Third International Workshop on Lung Tumor and Differentiation Antigens. J Natl Cancer 1994; Inst 86:669–672.

49. Moolenaar C, Muller E, Schol D. Expression of the neural cell adhesion molecule-

related sialoglycoprotien in small cell lung cancer and neuroblastoma cell lines H69 and CHP-212. Cancer Res 1990; 50:1102–1106.

50. Kibbelaar R, Moolenaar C, Michalides R, et al. Expression of the embryonal neural cell adhesion molecule N-CAM in lung carcinoma. Diagnostic usefulness of monoclonal antibody 735 for the distinction between small cell lung cancer and non-small cell lung cancer. J Pathol 1989; 159:23–28.

51. Lee J, Ro J, Sahin A, et al. Expression of blood group antigen A:a favourable prognostic factor in non-small cell lung cancer. N Engl J Med 1991; 324:1084–1090.

52. Mikaye M, Taki T, Hitomi S, et al. Correlation of expression of H/Le^y/Le^b antigens with survival in patients with carcinoma of the lung. N Engl J Med 1992; 327:14–18.

53. Laberge F, Fritsche H, Umsawasdi T, et al. Use of carcinoembryonic antigen in small cell lung cancer. Cancer 1987; 59:2047–2052.

54. Goslin R, Skarin A, Zamcheck N. Carcinoembryonic antigen. JAMA 1981; 246:2173–2176.

55. Sculier J, Feld R, Evans W, et al. Carcinoembryonic antigen: a useful prognostic marker in small-cell lung cancer. J Clin Oncol 1985; 3:1349–1354.

56. Kimura Y, Fujii T, Hamamoto K, et al. Serum CA-125 level is a good prognostic indicator in lung cancer. Br J Cancer 1990; 62:676–678.

57. Diez M, Cerdan F, Ortega M, et al. Evaluation of serum CA-125 as a tumor marker in non-small cell lung cancer. Cancer 1991; 67:150–154.

58. Salgia R, Skarin A, O'Day S, et al. CA 125: a useful tumor marker and an indicator of response to therapy in lung cancer. Proc ASCO 1994; 13:347a.

59. Said J, Vimadalal S, Nash G, et al. Immunoreactive neuron-specific enolase, bombesin, and chromagranin A as markers for neuroendocrine lung tumors. Hum Pathol 1985; 16:236–240.

60. Johnson P, Joel S, Love S, et al. Tumor markers for prediction of survival and monitoring of remission in small cell lung cancer. Br J Cancer 1993; 67:760–766.

61. Strauss G, Skarin A. Use of tumor markers in lung cancer. Hematol Oncol Clin North Am 1994; 8:507–532.

62. Strauss GM, Kwiatkowski DJ, Harpole DH, et al. Molecular and pathologic markers in stage I non-small-cell carcinoma of the lung. J Clin Oncol 1995; 13:1265–1279.

63. Salgia R, Skarin A. Lung cancer: from molecular biology to novel therapeutics. Hosp Phys 1996; 32:12–32.

64. Paget S. The distribution of secondary growths in cancer of the breast. Lancet 1889; 1:571–573.

65. Fidler I. Modulation of the organ microenviroment for treatment of cancer metastasis. J Natl Cancer Inst 1995; 87:1588–1592.

66. Yurchenco P, Cheng Y-S, Colognato H. Laminin forms an independent network in basement membranes. J Cell Biol 1992; 117:1119–1133.

67. Thorgeirsson U, Lindsay C, Cottam D, et al. Tumour invasion, proteolysis, and angiogenesis. J Neuro-Oncol 1994; 18:89–103.

68. Ray J, Stevenson W. The role of matrix metalloproteases and their inhibitors in tumour invasion, metastasis and angiogenesis. Eur Resp J 1994; 7:2062–2072.

69. Brown P, Giavazzi P. Matrix metalloproteinase inhibition: a review of anti-tumour activity. Ann Oncol 1995; 6:967–974.

70. Ponton A, Coulombe B, Skup D. Decreased expression of tissue inhibitor of metal-

loproteinases in metastatic tumor cells leading to increased levels of collagenase activity. Cancer Res 1991; 51:2138–2143.

71. Stetler-Stevenson W, Krutzsch H, Liotta L. Tissue inhibitor of metalloproteinase. J Biol Chem 1989; 264:17374–17378.

72. Staskus P, Masiarz F, Pallanck L, et al. The 21 kDa protein is a transformation-sensitive metalloproteinase inhibitor in chicken fibroblasts. J Biol Chem 1991; 266: 449–454.

73. Weinstat-Saslow D, Steeg P. Angiogenesis and colonization in the tumour metastatic process: basic and applied advances. FASEB J 1994; 8:401–407.

74. Folkman J, Klagsbrun M. Angiogenic factors. Science 1987; 235:442–447.

75. Harpole D, Richards W, Herndon J, et al. Angiogenesis and molecular biologic substaging in patients with stage I non-small cell lung cancer. Ann Thorac Surg 1996; 61:1470–1476.

76. Roberts T, Hasleton P, Musgrove C, et al. Vascular invasion in non-small lung carcinoma. J Clin Pathol 1992; 45:591–593.

77. Macchiarini P, Fontanini G, Hardin J, et al. Most peripheral, node-negative, non-small-cell lung cancers have low proliferative rates and no intratumoral and peritumoral blood and lymphatic vessel invasion. J Thorac Cardiovasc Surg 1992; 104:892–899.

78. Lee C-T, Chen HL, Carbone DP. Gene therapy for lung cancer. Ann Oncol 1995; 6:61–63.

79. Hussein A. The potential applications of gene transfer in the treatment of patients with cancer: a concise review. Cancer Invest 1996; 14:343–352.

80. Curiel DT, Pilewski JM, Albelda SM. Gene therapy approaches for inherited and acquired lung diseases. Am J Respir Cell Mol Biol 1996; 14:1–18.

81. Guinan E, Gribben J, Boussiotis V, et al. Pivotal role of the B7:CD28 pathway in transplantation tolerance and tumor immunity. Blood 1994; 84:3261–3282.

82. Freeman G, Freedman A, Segil L, et al. B7, a new member of the Ig superfamily with unique expression on activated and neoplastic B cells. J Immunol 1989; 143:2714–2722.

83. Freeman G, Jg G, Boussiotis V, et al. Cloning of B7-2: a CTLA4 counter-receptor that costimulates human T cell proliferation. Science 1993; 262:909–911.

84. Freeman G, Borriello F, Hodes R, et al. Murine B7-2, an alternative CTLA4 counter-receptor that costimulates T cell proliferation and interleukin 2 production. J Exp Med 1993; 178:2185–2192.

85. Townsend S, Allison J. Tumor rejection after direct constimulation of CD8+ T cells by B7-transfected melanoma cells. Science 1993; 259:368–370.

86. Nabel G, Chang A, Nabel E, et al. Immunotherapy for cancer by direct gene transfer into tumors. Hum Gene Ther 1994; 5:57–77.

87. Dranoff G, Jaffee E, Lazenby A, et al. Vaccination with irradiated tumor cells engineered to secrete murine granulocyte-macrophage colony-stimulating factor stimulates potent, specific, and long-lasting anti-tumor immunity. Proc Natl Acad Sci USA 1993; 90:3539–3543.

88. Rosenberg S. The immunotherapy and gene therapy of cancer. J Clin Oncol 1992; 10:180–199.

89. Rosenberg S, Anderson W, Blaese R, et al. Immunization of cancer patients using

autologous cancer cells modified by the insertion of the gene for interleukin-2. Hum Gene Ther 1992; 3:75–90.

90. Kradin R, Kurnick J, Lazarus D, et al. Tumor-infiltrating lymphocytes and interleukin-2 in treatment of advanced cancer. Lancet 1989; 1(8638):577–580.

91. Dillman R, Oldham R, Barth N, et al. Continuous interleukin-2 and tumor infiltrating lymphocytes as treatment of advanced melanoma. A national biotherapy study group trial. Cancer 1991; 68:1–8.

92. Aoki Y, Takakuwa K, Kodama S, et al. Use of adoptive transfer of tumor-infiltrating lymphocytes alone or in combination with cisplatin-containing chemotherapy in patients with epithelial ovarian cancer. Cancer Res 1991; 51:1934–1939.

93. Ratto G, Zino P, Mirabelli S, et al. A randomized trial of adoptive immunotherapy with tumor-infiltrating lymphocytes and interleukin-2 versus standard therapy in the postoperative treatment of resected nonsmall cell lung carcinoma. Cancer 1996; 78:244–251.

94. Karp D, Atkins M. Adoptive immunotherapy for nonsmall cell lung carcinoma. Cancer 1996; 78:195–198.

95. Zhang Y, Mukhopadhyay T, Donehower L, et al. Retroviral vector-mediated transduction of K-ras antisense RNA into human lung cancer cells inhibits expression of the malignant phenotype. Hum Gene Ther 1993; 4:451–460.

96. Robinson LA, Smith LJ, Fontaine MP, et al. c-myc antisense oligodeoxyribonucleotides inhibit proliferation of non-small cell lung cancer. Ann Thorac Surg 1995; 60:1583–1591.

97. Lynch T, Coral F, Shefner J, et al. Phase I trial of the novel immunotoxin N901-blocked ricin (N901-bR): demonstration of clinical activity in small cell lung cancer. Proc Annu Meet Am Soc Clin Oncol 1993; 12:A954.

98. Lynch T, Shefner J, Wen P, et al. Immunotoxin therapy with N901-blocked ricin (N901-BR) for small-cell lung cancer (SCLC): a Phase I study. Proc Annu Meet Am Soc Clin Oncol 1992; 11:A1063.

99. Lynch T. Immunotoxin therapy of small-cell lung cancer: N901-blocked ricin for relapsed small-cell lung cancer. Chest 1993; 103:436s-439s.

100. Griffin J, Hercend A, Beveridge R, et al. Characterization of an antigen expressed by human natural killer cells. J Immunol 1983; 130:2947–2951.

101. Epstein C, Lynch T, Shefner J, et al. Use of the immunotoxin N901-blocked ricin in patients with small-cell lung cancer. Int J Cancer 1994; 8(suppl):57–59.

102. Grossbard M, Lambert J, Goldmacher V, et al. Correation between in vivo toxicity and preclinical in vitro parameters for the immunotoxin anti-B4-blocked ricin. Cancer Res 1992; 52:4200–4207.

103. Lynch T, Lambert J, Coral F, et al. Immunotoxin therapy of small-cell lung cancer—a Phase I study of N901-blocked ricin. J Clin Oncol 1997; 15:723–734.

104. Malone T, Sharpe R. Development of angiogenesis inhibitors for clinical applications. Trends Pharmacol Sci 1990; 11:457–461.

105. Ingber D, Fujiti T, Kishimoto S, et al. Synthetic analogues of fumagillin that inhibit angiogenesis and suppress tumour growth. Nature 1990; 348:555–557.

106. Teicher B, Holden S, Ara G, et al. Potentiation of cytotoxic cancer therapies by tnp-470 alone and with other anti-angiogenic agents. Int J Cancer 1994; 57:920–925.

107. Kato T, Sato K, Kakinuma H, et al. Enhanced suppression of tumour growth by com-

bination of angiogenesis inhibitor O-(chloroacetly-carbamoy) fumagillol (TNP-470) and cytotoxic agents in mice. Cancer Res 1994; 54:5143–5147.

108. Chirivi R, Garofalo A, Crimmin M, et al. Inhibition of the metastatic spread and growth of B16-BL6 murine melanoma by a synthetic matrix metalloproteinase inhibitor. Int J Cancer 1994; 58:460–464.
109. Brown P. Matrix metalloproteinase inhibitors: a novel class of anticancer agents. Adv Enzyme Regul 1995; 35:293–301.
110. Watson S, Morris T, Robinson G, et al. Inhibition of organ invasion by the matrix metalloproteinase inhibitor batimastat (BB-94) in two human colon carcinoma metastasis models. Cancer Res 1995; 55:3629–3633.
111. Macaulay V, O'Byrne K, Saunders M, et al. Phase I study of matrix metallopro-teinase (MMP) inhibitor batimastat (BB94) in patients (pts) with malignant pleural effusions. Proc Annu Meet Am Soc Clin Oncol 1995; 14:A1580.

2

Chemoprevention of Lung Cancer

FADLO R. KHURI, LAMYA R. TANNOUS-KHURI, and WAUN KI HONG

University of Texas
M. D. Anderson Cancer Center
Houston, Texas

I.   Introduction

At the end of the 20th century, lung cancer is still the leading cause of cancer death in the United States (1). Although the 5-year survival rate for patients with lung cancer has improved since the early 1970s, this disease has retained a high mortality rate, making advance of lung cancer research a priority for clinicians, researchers, and the public. Ongoing clinical trials continue to be the forum in which new compounds and new combinations of chemotherapy and radiation treatments are evaluated. Lung cancer biology is the area in which much recent progress has been made, leading naturally to an increased focus on lung cancer prevention strategies.

II.   Lung Cancer and Smoking

The relationship between lung cancer and smoking has been established in an increasingly compelling fashion over the last five decades. This link has been carefully studied using extensive epidemiologic data initially, followed by a careful elaboration of the histologic changes in the bronchial epithelium that are associated with chronic smoke exposure and finally to the determination of the genetic damage that nicotine products can cause in the human genome. Initial observations date back to the 1940s, when an association between cigarette smoke and lung cancer was first observed. Subsequently, Ochsner and DeBakey cited this association in their landmark treatise on lung cancer in 1941 (2). In the 1950s, two large, well-designed epidemiologic studies established a strong link between smoking and lung cancer (3,4). However, the key understanding of the actual histologic changes that were observed in smokers with lung cancer would await the observations of Auerbach et al. (5,6), who sectioned the entire tracheobronchial trees of smokers and individuals who developed lung cancer. Here, Auerbach recorded three major types of epithelial changes: an increase in the number of cell rows, a primary loss of cilia, and the presence of atypical cells. Perhaps most striking was the finding of *carcinoma in situ,* a lesion composed entirely of atypical cells without cilia, whose average thickness was five or more cell rows, being observed in 15% of the tissue sections from patients who died of lung cancer. Of note, carcinoma in situ lesions were never found by Auerbach and his collaborators in the pathologic specimens of nonsmokers, and few were found in the bronchial trees of light smokers. Thus, they were observed in 4.3% of bronchial sections from patients who had smoked one to two packs of cigarettes per day and in 11.4% of the sections from those who smoked two or more packs of cigarettes per day. Others subsequently established that these findings were also reported in the bronchial tissue of passive smokers (7).

A. Epidemiologic Studies

Recent studies attribute approximately 87% of lung cancers to tobacco exposure. The relative risk for developing lung carcinoma in current smokers is 24-fold greater than that for people who never smoked (8). However, the relative lung carcinoma risk in all cohorts of former smokers, although lower than for current smokers, remains greater than for never smokers, even for those former smokers who quit in their 30s (8). This close correlation between smoking status and lung cancer resulted in the National Cancer Institute's Division of Cancer Prevention and Control's emphasis on instituting cancer prevention as the major strategy in the control of lung cancer, due to the poor 5-year survival rate of patients with lung cancer. Therefore, the major elements of the National Cancer Institute's program to reduce the number of deaths from lung cancer are the prevention of smoking and bringing about smoking cessation. The result of these massive campaigns to educate the public about the hazards of cigarette smoking has been a substantial reduction in the percentages of adults who actively smoke in the United States (9). A survey of data from 1965 through 1991 reveals that these and other campaigns have had a substantial impact. In fact, the most recent data available from 1991 reveal that 29.9% of adult men and 19% of adult women were estimated to be former smokers, representing a 77.2% decrease from 1965 in the percentage of Americans who actively smoke. This has been attributed not only to the fact that smoking cessation has almost doubled over the last three to four decades but also to a decrease in the number of people who actually commence smoking.

B. Lung Cancer and Former Smokers

In the most recent estimates, performed in 1991, 43.5 million adults in the United States were estimated to be former smokers, of whom 15.3 million are 45 to 64 years old, and 10.9 million are above age 65 (9). Therefore, among those in the current U.S. population who ever smoked, 48.5% are now considered former smokers. While it is clear that the risk of developing lung cancer decreases in individuals who stop smoking, the magnitude of the problem in former smokers was recently revealed when a survey of 980 lung cancer cases seen at either the University of Texas M.D. Anderson Cancer Center or the Harvard University–affiliated hospitals (10) revealed that more than 50% of these lung cancer cases occurred in former smokers. This clearly represents a significant public health problem for the United States, where there appears to be an increasing number of former smokers who will remain at substantial lifetime risk of developing cancer.

Recent data from the University of Texas M.D. Anderson Cancer Center appeared to indicate that smoking cessation or less lifetime smoking exposure predisposes individuals toward specific histologic subtypes of cancer, particularly adenocarcinomas in women. The same data revealed that smoking cessation appeared to postpone the age at which lung cancer occurred (11). Furthermore, this study revealed that individuals who had not smoked for more than 20 years were most likely to develop the adenocarcinoma histologic subtype of non-small-cell lung cancer, as opposed to squamous cell or small cell lung cancer in active current smokers (odds ratio [OR] ratio = 8.79) or squamous cell carcinoma (OR = 2.11). Interestingly, in examining these data, former smoking status was a positive predictor only for small cell carcinoma of the lung (OR = 5.50), a finding that is somewhat surprising in light of the fact that recent data suggest that there is an increasing correlation between adenocarcinoma and current smoking (12). The M.D. Anderson study also revealed that pack-years, a marker of overall tobacco use defined as the number of years of active smoking multiplied by the average number of packages of cigarettes consumed per day, appeared to be negatively associated with adenocarcinoma and positively associated with small cell carcinoma in all patients.

C. Field Cancerization: Current Genetic Evidence

The findings of Auerbach and the epidemiologic studies were strongly supported by recent molecular studies. These studies also fit nicely with Slaughter's previously defined theory of field cancerization (13). Hung et al. (14) demonstrated that highly specific deletions in the short arm of chromosome 3 occurred during hyperplasia, the earliest stage in the pathogenesis of lung cancer, and that they involved the respiratory tract. Furthermore, Kishimoto et al. (15) noted similar evidence for allele-specific losses of the short arm of chromosome 9 in the earliest stages of lung cancer pathogenesis. This work was consistent with earlier work by Sozzi et al. (16), who detected deletions of the short arm of chromosome 17 and of the p53 gene in premalignant lung lesions. Recent work by Sozzi et al. has followed up on Hung's previous work and has demonstrated that one of the genes that is most likely lost in lung carcinogenesis is the fragile histidine triad (FHIT) gene located on chromosome 3p (17,18). Along these lines, elegant work by Mao et al. (19) demonstrated that *ras* mutations could be detected in the sputum of smokers frequently prior to the actual diagnosis of lung cancer, thereby postulating a potential role for molecular screening where radiographic screening had previously failed to be effective.

This genetic evidence was further strengthened by the fact that the number of chromosomal or genetic alterations in lung cancers seem to involve both the activation of dominant cellular oncogenes and the inactivation or chromosomal deletion of tumor suppressor genes (20). Since the inactivation of tumor suppressor genes requires at least two genetic changes to inactivate both alleles, lung cancer cells must undergo several distinct genetic events to progress from the premalignant stage to lung cancer. Conservative estimates based on both the cytogenetic and molecular genetic changes place the total number of genetic events required for lung carcinogenesis between 10 and 20 events (21). The data supporting this rely on the facts that complex cytogenetic abnormalities are consistently found in tumor cells (22–25), and that similar genetic abnormalities are found in normal and nonmalignant lung tissue samples from patients with lung cancer (21). The sequence of these events is not precisely known at this time. However, recent data from Mao et al. (26) and from researchers at U.T. Southwestern Medical Center (27) have revealed that genetic changes, namely deletions of the short arms of chromosomes 3p, 9p, and also (but less frequently) 17p, are found not only in the lung tissue of patients who have cancer but also in the bronchial tissue of smokers and former smokers in whom there is no evidence of disease.

Further evidence supporting the field carcinogenesis theory comes from studies of genetic alterations in paraffin-embedded tissue sections using a chromosome in situ hybridization technique, (28–30) and in DNA content analyses after Feulgen staining (31). Using biotinylated chromosome 7-, 17-specific centromeric DNA probes, investigators at the University of Texas M.D. Anderson Cancer Center demonstrated that chromosomal polysomies were not only found in tumor cells but also in histologically defined premalignant lesions such as oral leukoplakia (30) and in nonmalignant epithelial lesions adjacent to tumors.

D.   A Direct Molecular Link Between Tobacco and Cancer

Perhaps the finding that most directly links lung carcinogenesis with tobacco has been the recent discovery by Denissenko et al. (32) that demonstrated that benzo(a)pyrene diol epoxide (BPDE) adducts are nonrandomly distributed along the exons of the *p53* gene in BPDE-treated HeLa cells and bronchial epithelial cells, and that these adducts map to the guanine positions in codons 157, 248, and 273 of the *p53* gene. The fact that there was strong and selective adduct formation that was found only at these sites and that these sites are the major mutational hot spots in lung cancer, offered direct proof that there is targeted adduct formation rather than phenotypic selection in the *p53* mutational spectrum of lung cancer. These results build on previous epidemiologic data in that they provide a direct molecular etiologic link between the major known chemical carcinogen found in tobacco and the development of human lung cancer. This unequivocal molecular evidence of tobacco's etiologic role in lung cancer, when taken with the evidence by Mao et al. (26) and Wistuba et al. (27) demonstrating persistent loss of heterozygosity (LOH) at chromosomes 3p, 9p, and 17p in bronchial biopsy samples obtained from current and former smokers, establishes tobacco as a cause of lung cancer and of the persistent genetic damage found in the airways of former smokers. Mao's data indicate that 67% of former smokers demonstrate evidence of persistent genetic abnormalities in bronchial epithelium. These data lead one to believe that there are stable genetic alterations that can persist in the airway long after smoking cessation. Most critically, the fact that LOH at 9p and 17p persists even in patients who quit smoking suggests that these may be markers of stable genetic damage caused by cigarette smoke, unlike LOH at 3p, which appears to be largely reversible following smoking cessation. Thus, the rationale for a chemopreventive intervention in former smokers is clear from the evidence of persistent genetic damage in the airway, as well as the etiologic role that tobacco plays in causing smoking related genetic changes.

III.   Toward a Model of Preneoplastic Disease

While multiple studies have reported that invasive squamous cell carcinomas of the lung arise in association with areas of *carcinoma in situ* (5,6,33,34), these studies note progressive changes from metaplasia to carcinoma that have been widely accepted to date as the hallmark of an orderly carcinogenic progress that ultimately leads to the development of squamous cell carcinoma. The initial findings in this regard were documented by Saccomanno et al. (35), who observed serial sputum samples of uranium miners: subsequent cytologic examination of exfoliated bronchial cells in the sputum of these miners led these researchers to conclude that human lung cancers developed through a series of readily identifiable stages. Saccomanno et al. further divided these stages into squamous cell metaplasia, squamous cell metaplasia with atypia (mild, moderate, or marked), *carcinoma in situ*, and invasive squamous cell carcinoma. Quantitative cytochemical studies in human and animal models have further supported these findings with the demonstration of increasing amounts of DNA in exfoliated cells from abnormal epithelia (36–38). Thus, mildly atypical cells are found to exhibit a diploid-tetraploid range of DNA content, thereby most likely representing normal proliferative activity, whereas moderately and severely dysplastic cells had DNA content that was far greater than that encountered in the diploid population.

Given current evidence, however, this sequential progression model appears to be far too simple to explain the complex carcinogenic process. As Saccomanno himself pointed out, not all bronchial metaplasia seems to follow the same pathway. Recent experimental studies and clinical observations of patients who stopped smoking after documentation of cytologic evidence of squamous metaplasia and various degrees of dysplasia all suggest that certain degrees of cytologic change detectable in human sputum are potentially reversible (35–38). While squamous metaplasia was initially identified as a potentially reversible premalignant lesion and was studied in multiple chemopreventive trials (36–38), the data of Mao et al. (26) and Wistuba et al. (27) demonstrated that persistent genetic abnormalities can be found even in the absence of squamous metaplasia. Therefore, the reliability of squamous metaplasia as a putative premalignancy model for lung cancer has become questionable. The development of a comprehensive model of premaligancy will likely require integration of recent molecular observations of persistent genetic abnormalities, such as those demonstrated by Mao et al. (26) with a reexamination of putative histologic subtypes of premalignancy, including bronchial metaplasia.

A. Chemoprevention Origins and Goals

With an increasing ability to detect genetic and histologic abnormalities in bronchial tissue, the goal is to develop an agent that can be effective as a chemopreventive compound. Chemoprevention was first defined by Michael A. Sporn, who coined the term to describe the use of natural or synthetic chemical agents to reverse, suppress, or prevent carcinogenic progression to invasive cancer (39).

Epidemiological studies have demonstrated that vitamin A deficiency is associated with an increased incidence of lung cancer in humans (40). Vitamin A deficiency also induces squamous metaplasia in the mucosa of the upper aerodigestive tract (41) that is similar to the premalignant changes in this mucosa found in heavy smokers (5). Dietary vitamin A supplementation reversed squamous metaplasia in the trachea of vitamin A–deficient animals *in vivo* (42), and various retinoids exhibited a similar activity *in vitro* (43).

Vitamin A derivatives, or retinoids, are a family of compounds that have complex biologic effects, including the modulation of differentiation, proliferation, and apoptosis within both normal and neoplastic tissues (44,45). The complexity of their function depends not only on the diversity of the retinoid ligands but also on the diversity of the nuclear retinoid receptors that mediate their activity. Retinoids bind and activate retinoid receptors to function as transcription factors. These receptors are expressed at varying levels in different cell types and thus this differential expression ultimately affects downstream gene expression.

There are two classes of nuclear retinoid receptors: the retinoic acid receptors (RARs), and the retinoid X receptors (RXRs). There are three subclasses: α, β, and γ, with each divided further into a large number of isoforms produced through differential promoter usage and alternative splicing of receptor transcripts (44,45). Specific isoforms of RARs and RXRs appear to have different functions, activating different downstream target genes. RXRs form homodimers and heterodimers with RARs or a host of other receptors such as those for vitamin D and thyroid hormones and with a variety of orphan receptors (44). Because RXR is a ligand-binding partner in combination with orphan receptors, RXR ligands appear to be more versatile than RAR ligands in the activation of retinoic and other pathways.

Natural and synthetic retinoids, including all-*trans,* 13-*cis,* and 9-*cis* retinoid acid, exist as stereoisomers, spontaneously interconverting in the intracellular space. For that reason, treatment with these retinoids nonselectively activates both RARs and RXRs. In contrast, newer synthetic retinoids are being developed that are capable of binding specifically to individual nuclear retinoids, thus allowing a degree of selectivity in the enhancement of the desired effects of certain retinoids and the reduction of the undesired effects. For example, a retinoid specific only for RAR-β may avoid inducing dermatologic side effects that have been caused by activation of RAR-γ. The goal is to enhance the potential therapeutic effects of specific retinoids while limiting the toxic effects caused by the widely used natural retinoids (46).

It is thought that retinoid receptors affect gene transcription either directly or indirectly. This phenomenon is illustrated by the receptor interaction with activator protein-1 (AP-1), an important regulator of cellular proliferation and inflammation (47–49). The mechanism of this interaction was recently elucidated by Kamei et al. (50), who demonstrated that retinoid-mediated inhibition of AP-1 activity appears to be the result of competition between nuclear retinoid receptors and AP-1 for binding to a transcriptional coactivator. This coactivator is found in limited quantities in the cell and is thus the rate-limiting step for both the retinoid receptors and AP-1 (50). Synthetic retinoids have been developed that selectively inhibit AP-1 without activating nuclear receptors (51). These AP-1-selective synthetic retinoids have been found to be potent antiproliferative agents in a number of tumor-derived cell lines (47–51) and are capable of reversing the squamous differentiation of bronchial epithelial cells (52). Their toxicity profile may be favorable, as retinoid toxicity has been linked to retinoid receptor activation.

Further work in the area of retinoid biology and pharmacology has focused on the study of retinoid resistance. Clinical *de novo* retinoid resistance occurs in 40% of oral premalignant lesions and appears to develop over time in many lesions that had previously responded to retinoid treatment (46). The mechanisms that underlie retinoid resistance are not yet well defined. However, the frequency with which clinical resistance is encountered has resulted in the evaluation of novel retinoids such as 4-*N*-(hydroxyphenyl) retinamide (4-HPR), which does not appear to bind any of the retinoid receptors but is a potent *in vitro* inducer of apoptosis (46,53). Retinoids also appear to have potent effects when combined with other cytotoxic or cytostatic agents. Shalinsky et al. (54) demonstrated that 9-cRA combined with cisplatin in human oral squamous carcinoma xenografts in nude mice shows enhanced antitumor efficacy bordering on synergism.

Thus, retinoids alone or in combination with other cytotoxic (54) or biologic (55,56) agents have the intriguing potential to reverse preneoplastic lesions. The preclinical demonstration of efficacy as well as the extensive epidemiologic data previously cited has led to the integration of retinoids into clinical chemoprevention trials in upper aerodigestive tract cancers as well as lung cancer.

1. Chemoprevention Trials

The ability of vitamin A derivatives to reverse premalignant lesions of the upper aerodigestive tract and to prevent SPTs in patients with an index squamous cell cancer of the head and neck forms much of the basis for the investigation of these same approaches in patients either at risk for or diagnosed previously with lung cancer.

2. Reversal of Premalignancy

One of the major problems in studies attempting to reverse premalignancy has been the difficulty in defining consistent premalignant changes in the bronchial epithelium. Investigators have used both cytologic changes in sputum and histologic changes in bronchial biopsy samples from metaplasia to dysplasia as markers of risk. Reversal of these premalignant changes to normal tissue has been regarded as a potential intermediate endpoint for the chemoprevention of cancer.

In general, studies focusing on sputum analysis from chronic smokers have shown wide spontaneous variation in the degree of atypia over time and no consistent effect from retinoids (36–38,57,79,80) (Table 1) In an effort to develop a more dependable, semiquantitative assay, Mathe et al. described the metaplasia index (MI) to quantitate the degree of squamous metaplasia in bronchial biopsies from six specific anatomic sites (58). The MI was defined as the number of samples with metaplasia divided by the total number of samples analyzed, multiplied by 100. MIs were documented pre- and posttreatment in a single-arm trial of smokers receiving etretinate 25 mg/day for 6 months (58). This trial demonstrated a decrease in the MI following etretinate therapy. These findings, however, are overshadowed by those of Lee et al. (38). In this trial, 93 smokers with metaplasia or dysplasia, quantitated at baseline using the MI, were randomized to 13-*cis* retinoic acid [13cRA] or placebo for 6 months. Posttreatment biopsy samples demonstrated a similar rate of decrease in the MI in both trial arms that was most strongly associated with smoking cessation, calling the findings of Mathe et al.

Table 1 Lung Cancer: Reversal of Premalignancy

Investigator (year)	Endpoint	No. patients	Compound	End result
Saccomanno (1982); Ref. 57	Sputum atypia	26	13-*cis*-retinoic acid (1–2.5 mg/kg//day)	Negative
Heimburger (1988); Ref. 36	Sputum atypia	73	Vitamin B$_{12}$ (500 µg/day), folic acid (10 mg/day)	Positive (atypical)
Arnold (1992); Ref. 79	Sputum atypia	150	Etretinate (25 mg/day)	Negative
Mathe (1982); Ref. 58	Squamous metaplasia	40	Etretinate (25 mg/day)	Positive
Lee (1994); Ref. 38	Squamous metaplasia	40	13-*cis*-retinoic acid (1 mg/kg/day)	Negative
McLarty (1995); Ref. 80	Squamous	1067	β-carotene (50 mg/day)	Negative

into question. Clearly, future trials of this sort will need to be placebo-controlled to correct for multiple variables such as smoking cessation, sampling differences, and spontaneous regression that can influence the final outcome.

B. Primary Prevention

Based on epidemiologic data, which indicated an inverse correlation between cancer risk and dietary β-carotene and serum retinol levels, β-carotene has been the major agent studied in primary prevention of lung cancer (59). Three large primary prevention trials using β-carotene with or without α-tocopherol or retinol have been completed, and two of the three trials have documented an increased incidence of lung cancer in the treatment arms with β-carotene (Table 2)

The Finnish ATBC trial randomized 29,133 male smokers aged 50 to 69 years to one of four regimens, using a 2×2 factorial design. The regimens were α-tocopherol (50 mg/day) alone, β-carotene (20 mg/day) alone, both agents, or placebo (60). The participants in the ATBC trial continued this intervention for 5 to 8 years. Over the course of the study, 876 new cases of lung cancer were diagnosed. Patients receiving β-carotene had an 18% increased incidence of lung cancer and an 8% increased mortality rate. α-Tocopherol administration failed to significantly alter either lung cancer incidence or overall mortality rate. Subsequent analysis of these data demonstrated a trend to increased risk for β-carotene treatment in heavy smokers (≥ 1 pack/day) and in those who had high ethanol intake (> 11 g/day) (61).

Accrual to one other primary prevention trial performed in the United States was stopped early due to similar findings. The CARET study randomized a total of 18,314 smokers, former smokers, and people with a history of asbestos expo-

Table 2 Completed Randomized β-Carotene Trials

Trial	Agents	Population	Duration of intervention	Endpoints	Outcome
ATBC (Ref. 60,61)	Vitamin E, β-carotene	Smokers (N = 29,133)	6 yr	Lung cancer	Harmful
CARET (Ref. 62)	β-carotene, vitamin A	Smokers (N = 18,344)	4 yr	Lung cancer	Harmful
Physician's Health Study (Ref. 63)	β-carotene	Healthy males (N = 20,071)	12 yr	Epithelial cancer	No benefit

ATCB, Alpha-Tocopherol, Beta-Carotene Cancer Prevention Study Group; CARET Beta-Carotene and Retinal Efficacy Trial.

sure to a combination of β-carotene (30 mg/day) and retinol (25,000 IU/day) in the form of retinyl palmitate or placebo in a double-blind trial (62). After a mean follow-up period of 4 years, accrual was suspended due to a relative risk of lung cancer and death from lung cancer in the treatment arm of 1.28 and 1.46, respectively. As in the ATBC trial, excess lung cancer incidence was associated with current smoking and the highest quartile of ethanol intake (62).

A third trial, of male physicians in the United States, of whom only 11% were current smokers, randomized 20,071 participants to β-carotene (50 mg qod) or placebo (63). Neither benefit nor harm was demonstrated from the intervention in terms of the incidence of malignant neoplasms, cardiovascular disease, or death from all causes.

The mechanism of enhancement of lung carcinogenesis by supplemental β-carotene (alone or in combination with retinol) in smokers has yet to be defined. The most plausible theory at this time implicates a potential pro-oxidant effect of β-carotene in the damaged lungs of individuals who continue to smoke heavily (64), but this has yet to be established. In light of the data from the CARET and ATBC trials, current smokers should not use β-carotene supplements. These results also emphasize that randomized clinical trials of patients at high risk should be the only setting for high-dose supplementation with compounds of unproven clinical efficacy.

C. Prevention of Second Primary Tumors

Three randomized trials designed to reduce the incidence of second primary tumors (SPT) in patients with an index cancer of the head and neck or lung have now been completed. Two of these three trials have demonstrated an impact on tobacco-related cancer with retinoid treatment (Table 3).

In a seminal study by Hong et al. (65), 103 patients with a prior diagnosis of squamous cell cancer of the head and neck were randomized to receive either

Table 3 Randomized Trials of Retinoids in Human Cancer Chemoprevention

Reference	Population	Intervention	No. patients	Endpoint	Result	*P* Value
Hong (1990, 1994); Ref. 65,66	US (prior HNSCC)	13 cRA (50–100 mg/ m²/day)	49	Second primary tumor	4% (32 mo); 14% (55 mo)	.005 (32 mo)
		Placebo	51		24% (32 mo); 31% (55 mo)	.042 (55 mo)
Pastorino (1993); Ref. 68	Italy (prior NSCLC)	RP (300,000 IU/day)	150	Second primary tumor	Longer time to SPT development	.045
		No treatment control	157			
Bolla (1994); Ref. 67	France (prior HNSCC)	Etretinate (50/25 mg/day)	156	Second primary tumor	18%	NS
		Placebo	160		18% (41 mo)	

HNSCC, head and neck squamous cell carcinoma; NSCLC, non-small-cell lung cancer; RP, retinyl palmitate; 13 cRA, 13-*cis*-retinoic acid.

high-dose 13cRA (50 to 100 mg/m²/day) or placebo for 1 year. Although originally conceived as an adjuvant trial, this study did not demonstrate any impact of treatment on locoregional recurrence or metastatic disease. However, with a median follow-up period of 32 months, second primary tumors developed in only two (4%) of the treated patients, as opposed to 12 (24%) of patients receiving placebo. Of particular note, 93% (13 of 14) of the second primary tumors observed were in the carcinogen-exposed field of the upper aerodigestive tract, lungs, and esophagus. Recent reanalysis of this trial at a median follow-up period of 4.5 years indicated the most striking results of the impact of 13cRA treatment on tumors in the "condemned" mucosa, with the development of 3 versus 13 SPTs in the retinoid and placebo arms, respectively (66). This effect of 13cRA persisted for approximately 3 years, after which time the annual incidence of SPT was approximately equivalent between the two arms. These promising results are offset somewhat by the significant toxic effects on mucocutaneous tissues associated with 13cRA that necessitated a marked dose reduction among one-third of the patients during 1 year of therapy.

A second trial, by Bolla et al. (67), randomized 316 patients with a prior squamous cell cancer of the oral cavity or oropharynx to etretinate (50 mg/day for 1 month, followed by 25 mg/day for 2 years) or placebo. After a median follow-up time of 41 months, treatment was not observed to affect incidence of either SPT or recurrent disease. The results of this trial were notable for the high rate of SPT (24% of patients), 79% of which were clearly tobacco-related.

In the only completed study of patients with an index diagnosis of lung cancer, Pastorino et al. (68) randomized 307 patients who had been surgically cured of stage I non-small-cell lung cancer to receive either retinyl palmitate (300,000 IU/day for 1 year) or placebo. The retinyl palmitate treatment was associated with an overall reduction in SPT—18 versus 29 in the retinyl palmitate and placebo arms, respectively. Considering only tobacco-related tumors, the data are more striking, with 13 SPT in the retinoid arm versus 25 in the placebo arm. In contrast to 13cRA, the retinyl palmitate was well tolerated, and compliance over 1 year of treatment exceeded 80%.

Building on the results of these two positive trials, current trials (see Table 4) include a National Cancer Institute (U.S.)-sponsored Phase III trial of low-dose 13cRA (30 mg/day for 3 years) versus placebo in patients who have undergone curative resection for Stage I non-small-cell lung cancer. Patients will receive follow-up care for 4 years after treatment ends to assess reduction in SPT incidence. Accrual of patients to this study was completed in April of 1997 with approximately 1450 patients registered (69). Data analysis awaits the completion of randomization. Similarly, the Euroscan study is evaluating the efficacy of retinyl palmitate (300,000 IU/day) and the antioxidant N-acetylcysteine (600 mg/day) in the prevention of SPT following the definitive therapy of early-stage squamous

Table 4 Selected Ongoing Chemoprevention Trials in Lung Cancer and Head and Neck Cancer

Trial	Patients	No. patients accrued/goal	Agents	Goals
Euroscan	Fully resected stage 1-111A NSCLC	2440/2600	Retinyl palmitate (300,00 IU/day) vs. placebo	Prevention of SPT
Intergroup study	Fully resected stage 1 NSCLC	1453/1453	13-*cis*-retinoic acid (30 mg.day) vs. placebo	Prevention of SPT
M.D. Anderson Cancer Center	Former smokers (quit for > 12 mo) with or without early-stage aerodigestive cancers	72/225	13-*cis*-retinoic acid (1 mg/kg/day) + α-tocopherol (1200 IU/day) vs. 9-*cis*-retinoic acid (50 mg/day) vs. placebo	Reversal of bronchia or dysplasia and g markers

cell carcinoma of the head and neck or fully resected stage I, II, or IIIA (T3N0 only) non-small-cell lung cancer. This study has a 2×2 factorial design; study participants received either retinyl palmitate alone or N-acetylcysteine alone, both drugs, or placebo for 2 years and then 4 years' follow-up care (70). As of January 1996, with data on 2440 participants (1449 head and neck cases; 991 lung cases), there have been 204 recurrences (~27%) in the patients with lung cancer. There were a total of 133 SPTs (5.5%) with 83 in the head and neck group (5.7%) and 50 in lung group (5.0%) (71).

IV. Future Directions

The magnitude of the cancer problem caused by tobacco use has inspired research into lung cancer causation and the active development of specific agents capable of reversing this striking carcinogenic process. That former smokers remain at increased risk for developing lung cancer (7–12) and that the genetic underpinnings of this process have been elucidated (26,27,32) have led to an increased focus on chemopreventive trials in former smokers. Particularly in light of the disturbing data that showed an increase in lung cancer incidence in active smokers who received β-carotene (60–62), chemopreventive interventions have no current place in standard practice outside the context of a clinical trial. Therefore, investigators at M.D. Anderson Cancer Center have launched a randomized, placebo-controlled, double-blind trial of 13-*cis*-retinoic acid plus α-tocopherol, a vitamin E derivative that may attenuate retinoid toxicity (72) versus a novel panagonist, 9-*cis*-retinoic acid, which binds both RAR-RXR heterodimers and RXR-RXR homodimers, versus placebo in former smokers with or without cancer. Because former smokers can have persistent genetic deletions even in the absence of visible histologic abnormalities, all former smokers who have smoked at least 20 pack-years are eligible for participation in this study. The study population should comprise 225 former smokers; 70 patients have been enrolled to date, and accrual is expected to be complete accrual in the year 2000 (73). Among the parameters being evaluated are the reversal of metaplasia, dysplasia, or both; the presence of persistent genetic lesions at the sites of specific tumor suppressor genes; and the loss of and possible upregulation of RAR-β. Xu et al.(74) have recently demonstrated progressive loss of RAR-β in non-small-cell lung cancers. The same group has also demonstrated that RAR-β may be upregulated by 13-cRA in a bronchial premalignancy trial, even in the absence of the reversal of metaplasia (75). This has led to an increasingly prominent role for this retinoid receptor as a putative intermediate endpoint marker in chemoprevention trials using classic retinoids that bind nuclear receptors.

Ironically, recent data from Oridate et al. (76) indicate that 4-HPR, a novel synthetic retinoid that does not appear to bind nuclear retinoid receptors, can induce apoptosis in cervical carcinoma cells by inducing reactive oxygen species.

This work has been applied to lung cancer cell lines, and it appears that 4-HPR may be more effective than all *trans* retinoic acid in inducing apoptosis in head and neck squamous cell lines (53). This has led to increased enthusiasm for the incorporation such novel and nontoxic retinoids into chemoprevention trials.

Furthermore, recent data from Lu et al. (51) identified several synthetic retinoids that can specifically turn on only precise portions of the complex retinoid response networks, thereby selectively activating specific biologic responses. These molecules appear to preferentially cause the induction of apoptosis in human lung cancer cells *in vivo* in an animal model, thereby providing a potential role for selective retinoids in lung cancer therapy as well as chemoprevention.

Finally, other small molecules and routes of delivery may be equivalent and possibly even superior to oral retinoids. Recent compelling data from Wiedmann et al. on the use of budesonide, an aerosolized glucocorticoid, in the reversal of lung adenomas in mice, suggest that aerosolized delivery of chemopreventive compounds may be a provocative and ultimately more successful approach to lung chemoprevention (77). A new era appears to be dawning where specific molecular targets for chemopreventive intervention are chosen and selective and highly specific chemopreventive compounds are utilized (78). It is the intermarriage of carefully conducted clinical chemoprevention trials, continued advances in the understanding of lung carcinogenesis, and the development of novel, increasingly effective compounds with improved drug delivery techniques that has brought about to recent striking advances in lung cancer chemoprevention.

Acknowledgments

Dr. Fadlo R. Khuri is the Recipient of an American Cancer Society Clinical Oncology Career Development Award, ACS CO CDA 96-41. Dr. Waun Ki Hong is an American Cancer Society Clinical Research Professor. This work was supported in part by the National Cancer Institute U19 CA68437. The authors gratefully acknowledge Julia Starr and the Department of Scientific Publications for editorial assistance, and Stephanie Johnson, LaShonda Holcombe, and Patricia Coldiron for the transcription of this chapter.

References

1. Ginsberg RJ, Kris MG, Armstrong JG. Cancer of the lung. *In*: DeVita VT, Hellman S, Rosenberg SA, eds. Cancer: Principles and Practice of Oncology. Ed 4. Philadelphia: J.B. Lippincott, 1994:673.
2. Ochsner A, DeBakey M. Carcinoma of the lung. Arch Surg 42:209, 1941.
3. Doll R, Hill AB. Smoking and carcinoma of the lung: preliminary report *BMJ* 2:739, 1950.

4.   Wynder EL, Graham EA. Tobacco smoking as a possible etiologic factor in broncho-
     genic carcinoma: a study of six hundred and eighty four proved cases. *JAMA* 143:329,
     1950.
5.   Auerbach O, Gere JB, Forman JB, et al. Changes in bronchial epithelium in relation
     to smoking and cancer of the lungs: a report of progress. *N Engl J Med* 256:97,
     1957.
6.   Auerbach O, Stout AP, Hammond EC, et al. Changes in bronchial epithelium in
     relation to cigarette smoking and in relation to lung cancer. *N Engl J Med* 256:253,
     1961.
7.   Trichopoulus D, Mollo F, Tomatis L, et al. Active and passive smoking and patholog-
     ical indicators of lung cancer risk in an autopsy series. *JAMA* 268:1697, 1992.
8.   Shopland DR, Eyre HJ, Pechacek TF. Smoking attributable cancer mortality in 1991.
     Is lung cancer now the leading cause of death among smokers in the United States? *J
     Natl Cancer Inst* 83(16):1142–8, 1991.
9.   Office of Smoking and Health, U.S. Centers for Disease Control. *Mobility and Mor-
     tality Weekly Report (MMWR)* 43:1994.
10. Kurie JM, Spitz MR, Hong WK. Lung cancer chemoprevention: targeting former
     rather than current smokers. *Cancer Prev Int* 2:55, 1995.
11. Tong L, Spitz MR, Fueger JJ, et al. Lung carcinoma in former smokers. *Cancer*
     78:1004, 1996.
12. Thun MJ, Lally CA, Flannery JT, et al. Cigarette smoking and changes in the
     histopathology of lung cancer. *J Natl Cancer Inst* 89:1580, 1997.
13. Slaughter DP, Southwick HW, Smejkal W. "Field cancerization" in oral stratified
     squamous epithelium: clinical implications of multicentric origin. *Cancer* 6:963,
     1953.
14. Hung J, Kishimoto Y, Sugio K, et al. Allele-specific chromosome 3p deletions occur
     at an early stage in the pathogenesis of lung cancer. *JAMA* 273:558, 1995.
15. Kishimoto Y, Sugio K, Hung JY, et al. Allele-specific loss in chromosome 9p loci in
     preneoplastic lesions accompanying non-small cell lung cancer. *J Natl Cancer Inst*
     87:1224, 1995.
16. Sozzi G, Miozzo M, Donghi R, et al. Deletions of 17p and p53 mutations in preneo-
     plastic lesions of the lung. *Cancer Res* 51:400–404, 1991.
17. Sozzi G, Rornielli S, Tagliabue E, et al. Absence of FHIT protein in primary lung
     tumors and cell lines with FHIT gene abnormalities. *Cancer Res* 57:5207–5212,
     1997.
18. Muller CY, O'Boyle JD, Fong KM, et al. Abnormalities of fragile histidine triad
     genomic and complementary DNA's in cervical cancer: association with human papi-
     lomavirus subtype. *J Natl Cancer Inst* 90:433–439, 1998.
19. Mao L, Hruban RH, Boyle JO, et al. Detection of oncogene mutations in sputum pre-
     cedes diagnosis of lung cancer. *Cancer Res* 54:1634, 1994.
20. Inman DS, Harris CC. Oncogenes and tumor suppressor genes in human lung car-
     cinogenesis. *Crit Rev Oncog* 2:161, 1991.
21. Ihde DC, Minna JD. Non-small cell lung cancer. Part I. Biology, diagnosis and stag-
     ing. *Curr Probl Cancer* 15:61, 1991.
22. Hittleman WN, Wang ZQ, Cheong N, et al. Premature chromosome condensation and
     cytogenics of human solid tumors. *Cancer Bull* 41:298–305, 1989.

23. Lee JS, Pathak S, Hopewood V, et al. Involvement of chromosome 7 in primary lung tumors and nonmalignant normal lung tissue. *Cancer Res* 47:6349–6352, 1987.

24. Miura I, Siegfried JM, Resau J, et al. Chromosome alterations in 21 non-small cell lung carcinomas. *Genes Chromosomes Cancer* 2:328–338, 1990.

25. Sozzi G, Miozzo M, Tagliabue E, et al. Cytogenetic abnormalities and overexpression of receptors for growth factors in normal bronchial epithelium and tumor samples of lung cancer patients. *Cancer Res* 51:400–404, 1991.

26. Mao L, Lee JS, Kurie JM, et al. Clonal genetic alterations in the lungs of current and former smokers. *J Natl Cancer Inst. J Natl Cancer Inst* 89:857–862, 1997.

27. Wistuba II, Lam S, Behrens C, et al. Molecular damage in the bronchial epithelium of current and former smokers. *J Natl Cancer Inst* 89:1366, 1997.

28. Kim SY, Lee JS, Ro JY, et al. Interphase cytogenetics in parafin sections of lung tumors by non-isotopic in-situ hybridization: mapping genotype/phenotype heterogenicity. *Am J Pathol* 142:307–317, 1993.

29. Lee JS, Kim SY, Hong WK, et al. Detection of chromosomal polysomy in oral leukoplakia, a premalignant lesion. *J Natl Cancer Inst* 85:1951–1954, 1993.

30. Voravud N, Shin DM, Ro JY, et al. Increased polysomies of chromosome 7 and 17 during head and neck multistage tumorigenesis. *Cancer Res* 53:2874–2883, 1993.

31. Gazdar AF, Hung J, Walker L, et al. Extensive areas of dysplasia and aneuploidy of the entire bronchial mucosal tract accompanies non-small cell lung cancers (NSCLC) and provides evidence for the field cancerization theory. *Proc Am Soc Clin Oncol* 12:334, 1993.

32. Denissenko MF, Pao A, Tung M, et al. Preferential formation of benzo [a]pyrene adducts at lung cancer mutational hotspots in p53. *Science* 274:430, 1996.

33. Auerbach O, Hammond EC, Garfinkel L. Changes in bronchial epithelium in relation to cigarette smoking, 1955–1960 vs 1970–1977. *N Engl J Med* 300:381, 1979.

34. Black H, Ackerman LV. Importance of epidermoid carcinoma in situ in histogenesis of carcinoma of carcinoma of the lung. *Ann Surg* 136:44, 1952.

35. Saccomanno G, Archer VE, Auerbach O, et al. Development of carcinoma of the lung as reflected in exfoliated cells. *Cancer* 33:256, 1974.

36. Heimburger DC, Alexander CB, Burch R, et al. Improvement in bronchial squamous metaplasia in smoking treated with folate and vitamin B_{12}. Report of a preliminary randomized, double-blind intervention trial. *JAMA* 259:1525, 1988.

37. Heimburger DC, Krumdieck CL, Alexander CB, et al. Localized folic acid deficiency and bronchial metaplasia in smokers: hypothesis and preliminary report. *Nutr Int* 2:54, 1987.

38. Lee JS, Lippman SM, Benner SE, et al. Randomized placebo controlled trial of isotretinoin in chemoprevention of bronchial squamous metaplasia. *J Clin Oncol* 12:937, 1994.

39. Sporn MB, Dulop NM, Newton DL, et al. Prevention of chemical carcinogenesis by vitamin A and its synthethic analogs (retinoids). *Fed Proc* 35:1332–1338, 1976.

40. Hong WK, Itri LM. Retinoids and human cancers, In: Sporn MB, Roberts AB, Goodman DS, eds. The Retinoids. New York: *Raven Press,* 1994:597.

41. Wolbach SB, Howe PR. Tissue changes following deprivation of fat-soluble A vitamin. *J Exp Med* 62:753, 1925.

42. Wolbach SB. Effects of vitamin A deficiency and hypervitaminosis in animals. In:

Sebrell WH, Harris RS, eds. The Vitamins. Vol. 1. New York: *Academic Press*, 1956: 106.

43. Sporn MB, Newton DL. Chemoprevention of cancers with retinoids. *Fed Proc* 38:2528, 1979.

44. Mangelsdorf DJ, Umesono K, Evans RM. The retinoid receptors. In: Sporn MB, Roberts AB, Goodman DS, eds. The Retinoids. New York: *Raven Press*, 1994: 319.

45. Chambon P. The retinoid signaling pathway: molecular and genetic analyses. *Semin Cell Biol* 5:115, 1994.

46. Mayne ST, Lippman SM. Retinoids and carotenoids. In: DeVita VT, Hellman S, Rosenberg SA, eds. Cancer: *Principles and Practice of Oncology.* 5th ed. Philadelphia: Lippincott, 1997.

47. Fanjul A, Dawson MI, Hobbs PD, et al. A new class of retinoids with selective inhibition of AP-1 inhibits proliferation. *Nature* 372:107–111, 1994.

48. Li JJ, Dong Z, Dawson MI, Colbum NI. Inhibition of tumor promoter-induced transformation by retinoids that transrepress AP-1 without transactivating retinoic acid response element. *Cancer Res* 56:483–489, 1996.

49. Angel P, Karin M. The role of Jun, Fos and the AP-1 complex in cell-proliferation and transformation. *Biochim Biophys Acta* 1072:129–157, 1991.

50. Kamei Y, Xu I, Heinzel T, et al. A CBP integrator complex mediates transcriptional activation and AP-1 inhibition by nuclear receptors. *Cell* 85:403–414, 1996.

51. Lu XP, Fanjul A, Picard N, et al. Novel retinoid-related molecules as apoptosis inducers and effective inhibitors of human lung cancer cells *in vivo. Nature Med* 3:686–690, 1997.

52. Lee HY, Dawson MI, Walsh GL, et al. Retinoic acid receptor—and retinoid x receptor-selective retinoids activate signaling pathways that coverage on AP-1 and inhibit squamous differentiaiton in human bronchial epithelial cells. *Cell Growth Diff* 7:997–1004, 1996.

53. Oridate N, Lotan D, Xu XC, et al. Differential induction of apoptosis by all-*trans*-retinoic acid and N-(4hydroxyphenyl) retinamide in human head and neck squamous cell carcinoma cell lines. *Clin Cancer Res* 2:855–863, 1996.

54. Shalinsky Dr, Bishoff ED, Gregory ML, et al. Enhanced antitumor efficacy of cisplatin in combination with ALRT 1057 (9-*cis* retinoic acid) in human oral squamous carcinoma xenografts in nude mice. *Clin Cancer Res* 2:511–520, 1996.

55. Lippman SM, Kavanagh JJ, Paredes-Espinoza M, et al. 13-*cis*-Retinoic acid plus interferon alpha-2a: highly active systemic therapy for squamous cell carcinoma of the cervis. *J Natl Cancer Inst* 84:241–245, 1992.

56. Lippman SM, Parkinson DR, Itri LM, et al. 13-*cis*-Retinoic acid and interferon alpha-2a: effective combination therapy for advanced squamous cell carcinoma of the skin. *J Natl Cancer Inst* 84:235–239, 1992.

57. Saccomanno G, Moran PG, Schmidt RD, et al. Effect of 13-*cis*-retinoic acid on premalignant and malignant cells of lung origin. *Acta Cytol* 26;78–85, 1982.

58. Mathe G, Gouveia J, Hercend TM, et al. Correlation between precancerous bronchial metaplasia and cigarette consumption, and preliminary results of retinoid treatment. *Cancer Detect Prev* 5:461–466, 1982.

59. Peto R, Doll R, Buckley JD, Sporn MB. Can dietary beta-carotene materially reduce human cancer rates? *Nature* 290:201–208, 1987.

60. Alpha-Tocopherol, Beta Carotene Cancer Prevention Study Group. The effect of vitamin E and beta carotene on the incidence of lung cancer and other cancers. *N Engl J Med* 330:1029–1035, 1994.

61. Albanes D, Heinonem OP, Taylor PR, et al. Alpha-tocopherol, beta carotene cancer prevention study: effects of baseline characteristics and study compliance. *J Natl Cancer Inst* 88:1560, 1996.

62. Omenn GS, Goodman GE, Thornquist MD, et al. Risk factors for lung cancer and for intervention effects in CARET, the Beta-Carotene and Retinol Efficacy Trial. *J Natl Cancer Inst* 88:1500–1509, 1996.

63. Hennekens CH, Buring JE, Manson JE, et al. Lack of long-term supplementation with beta-carotene on the incidence of malignant neoplasms and cardiovascular disease. *N Engl J Med* 334:1145, 1996.

64. Mayne ST, Handleman GJ, Beecher G. β-Carotene and lung cancer promotion in heavy smokers a plausible relationship. *J Natl Cancer Inst* 88:1513, 1996.

65. Hong WK, Lippman SM, Itri LM, et al. Prevention of second primary tumors with isotretinoin in squamous-cell carcinoma of the head and neck. *N Engl J Med* 323:795, 1990.

66. Benner SR, TF, Lippman SM, et al. Prevention of second primary tumors with isotretinoin in patients with squamous cell carcinoma of the head and neck: long-term follow-up. *J Natl Cancer Inst* 86:140–141, 1994.

67. Bolla M, Lefur R, Ton Van J, et al. Prevention of second primary tumors with etretinate in squamous cell carcinoma of the oral cavity and oropharynx. Results of a multicentric double-blind randomized study. *Eur J Cancer* 30:767–772, 1994.

68. Pastorino U, Infante M, Majoli M, et al. Adjuvant treatment of stage I lung cancer with high dose vitamin A. *J Clin Oncol* 11:1216–1222, 1993.

69. Winn RJ. CCOP Central Office, personal communication, November 1997.

70. Pastorino U, Van Zandwijk N, De Vries N, et al. Results of Euroscan trial. *Lung Cancer* 11:94–95, 1994.

71. Kirkpatrick A. EORTC Central Office, personal communication, August 1996.

72. Dimery IW, Hong WK, Lee JJ, et al. Phase I trial of alpha-tocopherol effects on 13-*cis*-retinoic acid toxicity. *Ann Oncol* 8:85–89, 1997.

73. Hong WK. Personal communication, February 1998.

74. Xu XC, Sozzi G, Lee JS, et al. Suppression of retinoic acid receptor β in non-small-cell lung cancer in vivo: implications for lung cancer development. *J Natl Cancer Inst* 89:624–629, 1997.

75. Xu XC, Lee JS, Lee JJ, et al. Decreased expression of retinoic acid receptor β in bronchial mucosa from heavy smokers and its up-regulation during chemoprevention trial with 13-*cis* retinoic acid. *Proc Am Assoc Cancer Res* 38:528, Abstract 3540, 1997.

76. Oridate N, Suzuki S, Higuchi M, et al. Involvement of reactive oxygen species in *N*-(4-hydroxyphenyl) retinamide-induced apoptosis in cervical carcinoma cells. *J Natl Cancer Inst* 89:1191–1198, 1997.

77. Wiedmann TS, Estensen RD, Zimmerman CL, et al. Chemoprevention of pulmonary carcinogenesis by aerosolized budesonide in female A/J mice. *Cancer Res* 57:5489–5492, 1997.

78. Hong WK, Sporn MB. Recent advances in chemoprevention of cancer. *Science* 278:1073–1077, 1997.

79. Arnold AM, Brownman GP, Levine MN, et al. The effect of synthetic retinoid etreti-
     nate on sputum cytology: results from a randomized trial. *Br J Cancer* 1992; 65:737–
     743.
80. McLaraty JW, Holiday DB, Girard WM, et al. Beta-carotene, vitamin A and lung can-
     cer chemoprevention: results of an intermediate endpoint study. *Am J. Clin Nutr*
     1995; 62:14315–14385.

3

Radiologic Staging of Lung Cancer

KITT SHAFFER

Dana-Farber Cancer Institute
Harvard Medical School
Boston, Massachusetts

I. Introduction

Imaging studies have historically played a crucial role in the detection and staging of lung cancer. This role is constantly changing as newer modalities become available. While at present, imaging cannot supplant surgical staging, it can act as a guide to the surgeon who will provide samples to the pathologist for definitive staging. Imaging studies can also play a role in detection of patients who are unlikely to benefit from surgical intervention. This may be on the basis of comorbid disease, extent of local disease, or detection of distant metastases. The surgeon, pathologist, and radiologist must work together to achieve the most appropriate care for each patient. In this article, the history of radiologic methods used in lung cancer staging will be reviewed, along with comparison of the various imaging studies, including plain films, CT, MR, and nuclear medicine techniques.

II. Historical Perspective

From the discovery of x-rays by Wilhelm Conrad Roentgen in 1895, one of the earliest clinical uses of the technique was in the chest. Because of the inherent contrast between air-filled lung and mediastinal/hilar structures, the chest is an ideal anatomic location for examination with x-rays. Within a few months of Roentgen's announcement of his discovery, reports were published of many astounding findings, primarily in the areas of tuberculosis, pneumonia, congestive heart failure, and pleural effusion (1). Early radiographs of the chest were limited by respiratory motion, since exposures of up to 45 min were required due to low output of the available x-ray tubes (1). With the development of more powerful and adequately shielded x-ray tubes, the chest radiograph became a practical and useful examination.

It is initially surprising that none of the earliest reports of utility of chest fluoroscopy and chest radiography mention the diagnosis of lung cancer. However, when one realizes that in the 1800s and earlier, lung cancer was a very rare disease, this deletion becomes clear. In a monograph on the disease published in 1912, it was noted that fewer than 400 cases had been reported in the entire world literature to that point, many of them in miners exposed to toxic dusts (2). However, the incidence of lung cancer began to rise in the 1930s, related to the increase in tobacco use. The death rate in men from this disease rose from fewer than 5 per 100,000 in 1930 to over 40 per 100,000 in the 1950s (3). These numbers have continued to rise. As at the beginning of this epidemic, the chest radiograph continues to play a crucial role in detection, staging, and follow-up. It remains the most common single type of radiologic examination overall in radiology departments, making up about half of all imaging studies performed (4).

Early radiologists were convinced that improvements in spatial resolution using standard radiographic techniques would solve all imaging problems. It soon became apparent that improved contrast resolution would be more helpful than improved spatial resolution, and that a cross-sectional method would offer distinct advantages. These realizations contributed to the development of computed tomography (CT) (5). The perception of the significance of CT scanning is reflected in the award of the Nobel Prize to Cormack for development of the equations used for image reconstruction and to Hounsfield for development of the first clinically practical machine for performing CT scanning (6,7).

A plain radiograph, while providing exquisite spatial resolution, has limited ability to resolve differences in tissue density. A typical CT slice can discriminate <0.5% difference in tissue density (8). In fact, since the range of detectable density differences is so wide, CT images are generally displayed at multiple contrast and brightness settings, to allow the viewer's eye to take advantage of this vast information set. A necessary prerequisite for development of CT was the availability of computers to handle quickly the vast number of calculations required. Conventional CT scanners acquire about 1 million pieces of information each second, and electron-beam scanners acquire 10 times as much (5).

The first use of mathematical modeling of data sets to produce axial tomographic slices was single photon emission tomography (SPECT). David Kuhl, at the University of Pennsylvania, produced the first emission tomographic image in 1959, and actually produced a transmission image in 1965, using a radioactive source under the patient, and a detector on the other side (9). In spite of this, there was little interest among radiologists in pursuing transmission tomography until the work of Hounsfield, a computer engineer employed by Electric and Musical Industry (EMI) Limited in England. In 1971, EMI installed a prototype head CT scanner in the Atkinson Morley's Hospital, where 70 head CTs were performed over 6 months. Each scan slice took 4 min to acquire, and data were analyzed over 2 days' time after completion of the study (5).

Despite intense excitement in the radiologic community regarding Hounsfield's first transmission tomographic images, EMI had difficulty initially arranging for manufacture of CT scanners. Radiologic equipment companies felt that there would be little use for the scans unless the spatial resolution of the images could be improved to a level comparable to radiographs. EMI manufactured the first scanners themselves, and wildly underestimated the demand for scanners throughout the world. Within 3 years of the publication of Hounsfield's initial article, more than 1000 CT scanners were in use in 50 countries (10).

Since that time, CT scanning has become the standard of care in imaging of many tumors, particularly lung cancer. In the past, up to 50% of thoracotomies for lung cancer were unsuccessful due to unexpectedly advanced disease. The number of "open and close" thoracotomies has dropped greatly in recent years, to about 10% (11). This improvement is due to a combination of advances in surgical technique and to improved imaging methods for screening patients for unresectable or metastatic disease.

III.   Chest Radiograph

The chest radiograph, while no longer the primary staging tool for lung cancer, remains a useful adjunct to other imaging studies since it provides an overview of the chest in a very compact form. To review a CT or MR of the chest may require considerable time, since such studies typically include from 25 to 100 separate images. The entire chest is available for viewing on two films with PA and lateral radiographs. These films may actually display certain anatomic structures in a clearer format than axial cross-sectional methods. This is particularly true of structures that run in a horizontal plane, such as the minor fissure or the vertebral bodies (Fig. 1).

Chest films remain a cost-effective way to follow patients undergoing treatment, or after completion of therapy. They are much less expensive than the other cross-sectional or nuclear medicine studies, and can be obtained in 1 to 2 min. They can be performed portably, and expose the patient to much less radiation than a chest CT. In the case of a patient with diffuse lung metastases, or bony

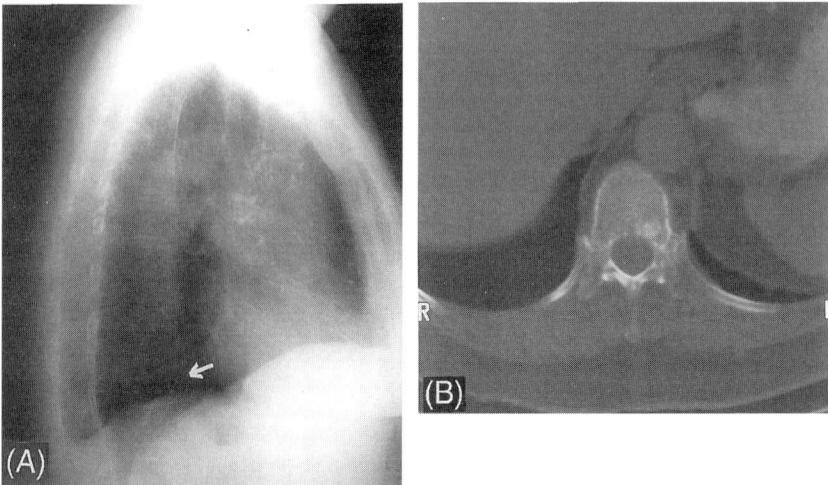

Figure 1   Advantages of chest film over CT for horizontally oriented structures. (A) Lateral chest film shows compression fracture in the thoracic region (arrow). (B) CT through the area does not demonstrate the abnormality as clearly. Additional thin sections reconstructed with bone algorithm might have shown the abnormality, but the chest film would be needed to direct attention to the region.

metastases visible in the chest, they may be the only staging study needed to exclude the patient from planned surgical treatment (Fig. 2).

As an adjunct to chest radiography, chest fluoroscopy can also play a role in staging lung cancer in certain specific circumstances. Fluoroscopy has the advantage of being a real-time examination. Thus it is useful in documenting rib lesions or fractures, or in distinguishing nodules from blood vessels. Because fluoroscopy is performed at a lower kV than routine chest radiography, it is more sensitive in detection of calcium (Fig. 3). Fluoroscopy can be used to observe moving structures, such as the diaphragm, and can therefore play a role in detection of tumor invasion of the phrenic nerve. Fluoroscopic guidance can also be used for lung or mediastinal biopsy.

IV.   Intrathoracic Staging with Chest CT

In order to better delineate the complex structures of the mediastinum and hila, CT scanning has generally replaced chest radiography. Most chest CT scanning can be performed without the use of intravenous contrast material because the location of vessels in the mediastinum is quite constant, and the vessels and nodes are usually outlined by mediastinal fat. However, hilar anatomy is more variable, and there is

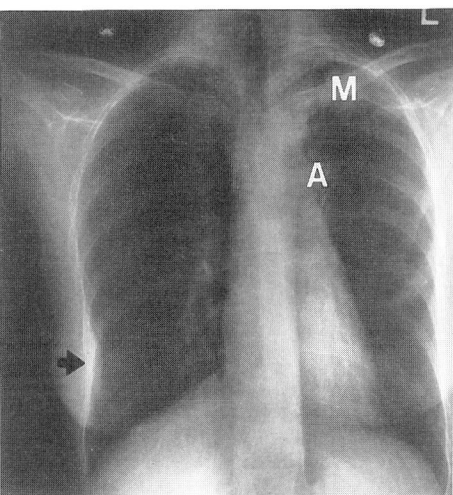

Figure 2 Occasionally, chest radiograph may be sufficient to stage the patient. This PA view shows a lung mass in the left upper lobe (M), aortico-pulmonic adenopathy (A), and a rib metastasis on the contralateral side (arrow), allowing determination that the patient is stage four.

not adequate fat in the hila to separate vessels from nodes. So, if detection and measurement of hilar nodes are deemed clinically important, intravenous contrast material should be administered (Fig. 4). Intravenous contrast material is also helpful in detection of compression or invasion of the great vessels by tumor (Fig. 5). For evaluation of lung parenchymal abnormalities, intravenous contrast material is generally not necessary, as natural contrast between air and parenchymal structures is sufficient (Fig. 6).

Standard CT scanners use a mechanically rotating gantry containing the x-ray generator, and a fixed ring of x-ray detectors. The patient is moved to a desired position within the gantry and the generator swings around 360° of rotation, while the detectors register the transmitted beam strength. The computer performs the necessary mathematical calculations, and an image is reconstructed. In spiral or helical scanning, the patient is slowly but continuously moved through the gantry, while the x-ray generator swings continuously around and around its 360° of rotation until it reaches a limit based on heat dissipation, usually 24 to 36 sec. This entire helical data set is then reconstructed into slices, spaced in whatever location the operator desires. The data set can be reconstructed again and again, using different starting points to obtain slices centered on particular structures of interest within the body.

In the chest, spiral or helical CT scanning has a distinct advantage in that a considerable portion of the chest can be examined in a single breath. With standard

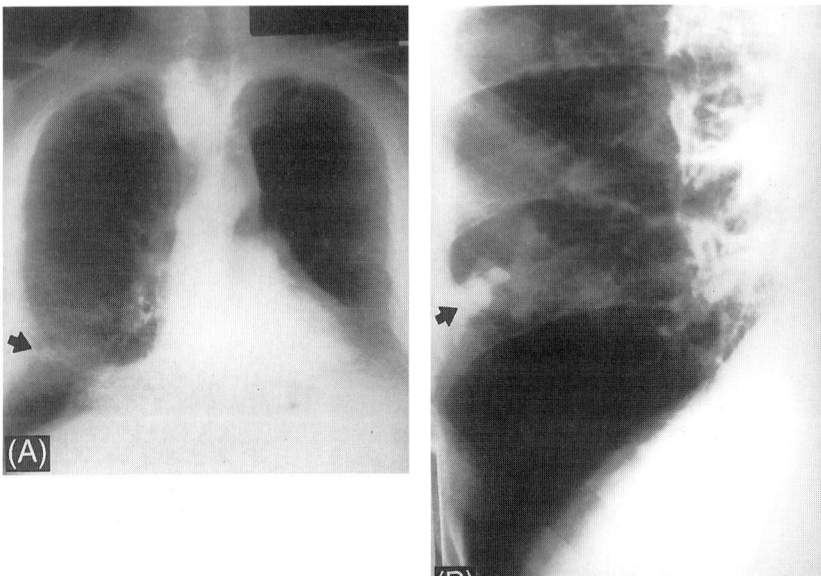

Figure 3 Utility of chest fluoroscopy for evaluation of lung nodules. (A) Chest radiograph shows a nodular density at the right base (arrrow). It is difficult on this film done with high kV to determine if the nodule is calcified. (B) Spot film at low kV from chest fluoroscopy clearly shows the lesion to be calcified (arrow), and therefore benign.

CT scanning, each slice or each group of two or three slices must be performed with the patient holding their breath, usually at maximum inspiration. This can lead to problems of misregistration of slices, if the patient takes in a different volume of air for each image. The main disadvantage of spiral or helical CT scanning is that there is some unavoidable degradation of image quality due to blurring from the constant motion of the patient through the gantry during the scan.

Another specialized CT technique is ultrafast, or electron beam, CT. In this method, the CT gantry contains both a fixed array of x-ray detectors and a ring of x-ray generators. During the scan, there is no mechanical motion of either part; the rotation of the x-ray beam is accomplished electronically. This allows collection of data for a slice in milliseconds rather than seconds, as in standard CT technique. With an ultrafast CT scanner, cine images of moving parts of the body, such as the heart, can be obtained (Fig. 7). The role of ultrafast CT is therefore most crucial in cardiac imaging; it offers no distinct advantage in lung cancer staging in most cases.

The basic limitation in use of CT in staging lung cancer is that it is a strictly anatomical technique. In other words, it detects the size and shape of objects in the chest, but cannot characterize them further, except in crude ways. Thus, CT can

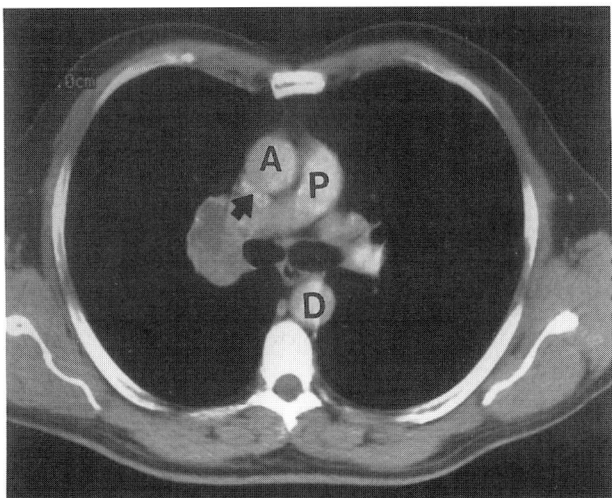

Figure 4 Use of intravenous contrast for evaluation of the hilum. This CT image after bolus contrast administration clearly shows a large right hilar mass that would have been difficult to separate from adjacent vascular structures without contrast. While the lesion would likely have been visible, accurate measurement for purposes of followup would have been impossible. Arrow = superior vena cava, A = ascending aorta, P = main pulmonary artery, D = descending aorta.

distinguish between fat and soft tissue, and therefore can diagnose specifically a fat-containing nodule as a pulmonary hamartoma. But it cannot distinguish between soft tissue in an enlarged lymph node containing granulomatous disease or amyloid (Fig. 8) and an enlarged lymph node–containing tumor. Squamous tumors, in particular, have a relatively high incidence of enlarged nodes that do not contain tumor, while adenocarcinomas are more likely to have micrometastases to nonenlarged lymph nodes, which cannot be detected with CT (Fig. 9) (12).

Thus, although CT was initially heralded as a possible substitute for surgical staging, results have remained disappointing in terms of sensitivity and specificity in the mediastinum (Table 1). Interobserver variability also contributes to the problems in CT staging of the mediastinum, with one study showing poor agreement even among four expert chest radiologists in interpretation of CT scans for mediastinal adenopathy (13). CT is best thought of as providing a road map for definitive staging, or a way to detect the most obvious types of stage 4 disease. In one study, up to 37% of patients with nodes >2 cm in short-axis diameter did not contain metastatic disease (14). It is therefore a mistake to exclude patients from surgery based merely on enlarged mediastinal nodes on CT scans.

CT is also not very sensitive or specific in the detection of other crucial types of spread of lung cancer that can have an impact on surgical treatment. CT cannot

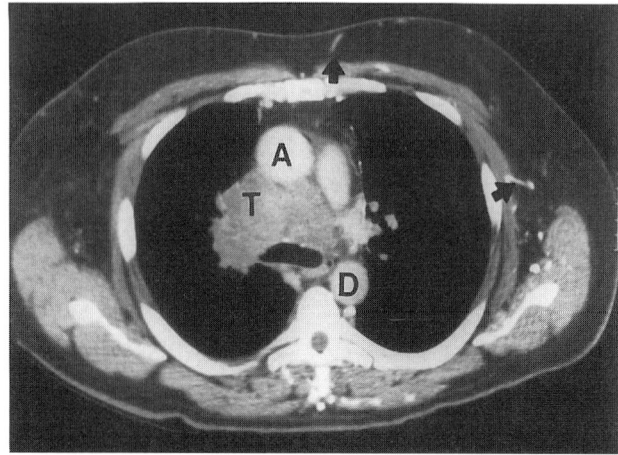

Figure 5 Use of intravenous contrast for evaluation of superior vena cava syndrome. This contrast-enhanced image in the upper mediastinum shows obliteration of the superior vena cava by a large right paratracheal tumor (T), and also demonstrates marked enhancement of dilated collateral veins (arrows), a secondary sign of vascular compression. A = ascending aorta, D = descending aorta.

reliably detect extranodal spread of tumor, or invasion by tumor of vital mediastinal structures unless the degree of invasion is quite advanced. In one study, sensitivity for locally invasive mediastinal disease was only 50%, with specificity of 89% (15). Similarly, CT can detect chest wall invasion only when it has progressed to frank bone destruction, or obvious protrusion of tumor between ribs (Fig. 10). In this same study, sensitivity for chest wall invasion was only 14%, but specificity was 99% (15). Again, since CT is an anatomical, rather than a functional, imaging method, disease must produce visible mass or displacement of normal structures in order to be detectable.

V. Intrathoracic Staging with Chest MR

When MR was initially developed, like CT, it was first used in the head. Brain and spinal imaging remain the most significant areas of usefulness of MR. However, MR offers advantages in thoracic imaging as well. MR imaging allows direct sagittal, coronal, or oblique planes to be used, and therefore can easily demonstrate lesions in the areas where CT is limited. These include the lung apices, supraclavicular areas, brachial plexus, and diaphragms (Fig. 11). In addition, contrast discrimination among various soft tissues is more dramatic in MR than in CT. MR depends for its imaging on paramagnetic properties of tissues, rather than the density of the elements present. This allows MR to detect presence of water with

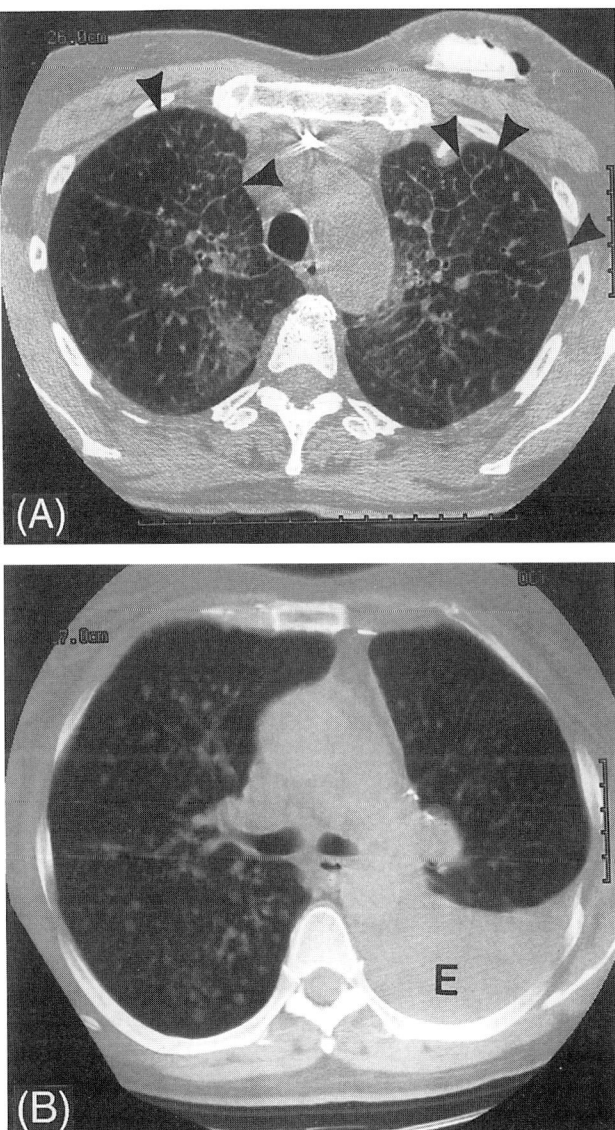

Figure 6 Use of CT scanning of the lung parenchyma. (A) Thin-section (1.5 mm), imaging of the lung reconstructed with high-resolution algorithm shows thickening of interlobular septae (arrowheads) compatible with lymphangitic tumor spread. (B) Routine 7 mm image shows miliary nodules throughout the lungs, confirmed to represent metastases from non-small-cell lung carcinoma. For lung nodules, generally 10 mm sections are preferable to thinner sections to avoid confusion with vascular structures. A moderate left pleural effusion is also present (E).

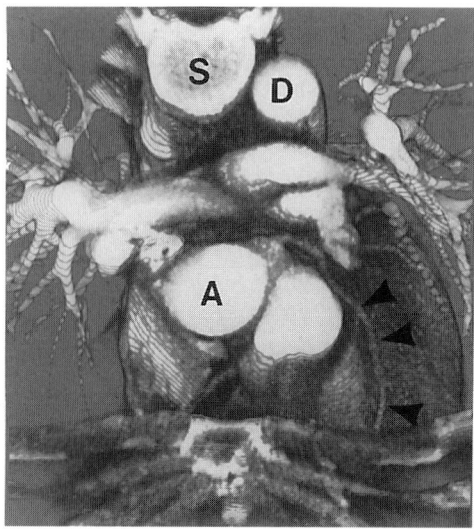

Figure 7 Electron beam (ultrafast) CT scan. Because of the very fast image acquisition time, cardiac motion does not degrade images. Thus, very detailed information about coronary arteries (arrowheads) can be obtained, and three-dimensional reconstructions such as this are possible. A = ascending aorta, S = thoracic spine, D = descending aorta. Use of this technique in evaluation of lung cancer is not generally necessary, although in cases of cardiac metastases, it may be useful. (Image courtesy of Dr. Jim Suojanen, Department of Radiology, Beth Israel Deaconess Medical Center, Boston, Massachusetts).

exquisite sensitivity. Water is increased in areas of tissue edema as well as in many tumors, and therefore is the basis for MR's ability to detect chest wall invasion with somewhat greater sensitivity than CT (Fig. 12). MR also has a definite advantage over CT in patients with allergy to iodinated contrast material, since vascular flow can be demonstrated without administration of contrast, due to the physical properties of flowing blood (Fig. 13).

However, the initial promise of a high degree of discrimination among various tissue types with MR has not been substantiated. In further examination, MR is neither sensitive nor specific in separating malignant from benign tissues in most parts of the body. While the physical basis for MR imaging is quite different from that of CT, it remains an anatomical imaging method. Thus, it is no better able to distinguish between granulomatous enlarged mediastinal nodes and mediastinal nodes filled with metastatic tumor. In addition, MR suffers from many artifacts related to motion of objects in the imaging volume, such as the heart. Also, MR has more limited spatial resolution than CT, which contributes to the poor performance of MR in staging of mediastinal disease when compared to CT. MR also cannot adequately image the lung parenchyma, since no signal is given off by air,

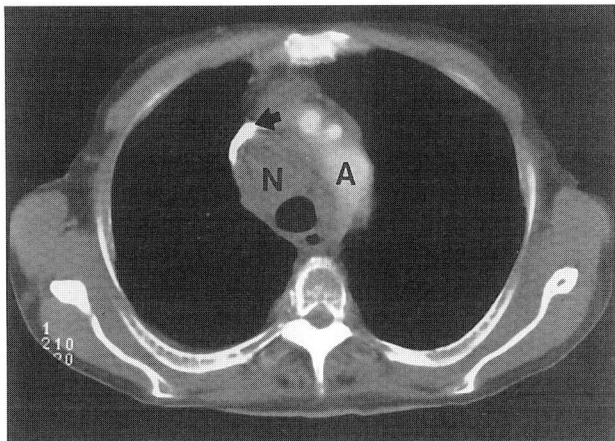

Figure 8 Enlarged mediastinal nodes do not always contain metastases. In this patient with a right lower lobe lung mass, numerous mediastinal nodes are markedly enlarged, as demonstrated on this CT image at the level of the top of the aortic arch. At mediastinoscopy, these nodes contained only amyloid, with no metastatic tumor present. A = aortic arch, arrow = superior vena cava, N = enlarged 4R mediastinal node.

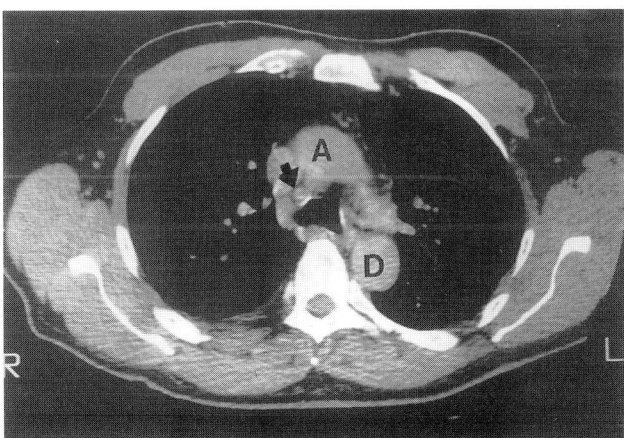

Figure 9 Non-enlarged mediastinal nodes are not always free of tumor. This CT image shows a non-enlarged right paratracheal node (arrow) in this patient with a right upper lobe lung mass. The node at surgery was 4 mm in size and contained micrometastases from the patient's primary adenocarcinoma. A = ascending aorta, D = descending aorta.

Table 1   Sensitivity and Specificity of Chest CT for Staging Mediastinal Nodes

Reference	Sensitivity %	Specificity %	Notes
Kristenson et al. (57)	72	85	Comparing CT to mediastinoscopy
Boilleau et al. (43)	66	50	Comparing CT to nuclear medicine CEA scan
Primack et al. (58)	67	58	Using long-axis measurement of nodes
Primack et al. (58)	58	86	Using short-axis measurement of nodes
Yokoi et al. (59)	62	80	Comparing CT to thallium scans
Cole et al. (60)	26	81	For N2 disease
Shea and Lillington (29)	70–90	60–90	Review of many published studies

and high spatial resolution is required to image the fine structures of the interstitium. In most comparisons of mediastinal staging by CT and MR, MR offers no advantages and may actually have slightly poorer sensitivity and specificity than CT. A comparison of technical aspects and clinical uses of plain films, CT, and MR is presented in Tables 2 and 3.

VI. Staging of Distant Metastases

The primary metastatic sites for lung cancer are the contralateral lung, adrenal glands, liver, bones, and brain. In adenocarcinomas, about 40% of patients will have brain metastases at diagnosis, one-third will have bone metastases, about 20% will have liver metastases, and 20% adrenal metastases. In squamous cell tumors, 30% will have brain metastases, 40% bone and 15% liver, with 5% adrenal metastases at diagnosis (16). The most cost-effective workup for all of these sites remains controversial. While some studies have shown that careful clinical examination and blood tests will detect most stage 4 patients, other studies have shown a significant percentage of patients without clinical signs of metastases who have distant disease detected with imaging studies.

In one study of patients with non-small-cell lung carcinoma, 15% of asymptomatic patients overall had distant metastases detected with either bone or head scans (17). Even among patients with clinical evidence of metastases, imaging studies often found other, unsuspected sites of disease. Imaging workup may be tailored to the specific type of disease present, since there is a very low likelihood of distant metastases in stage 1 squamous cell carcinoma (18). However, in this

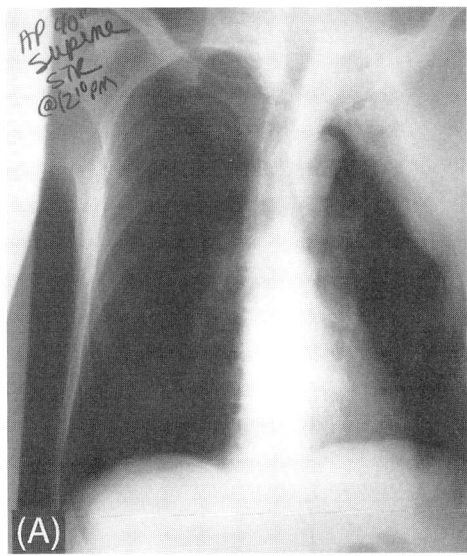

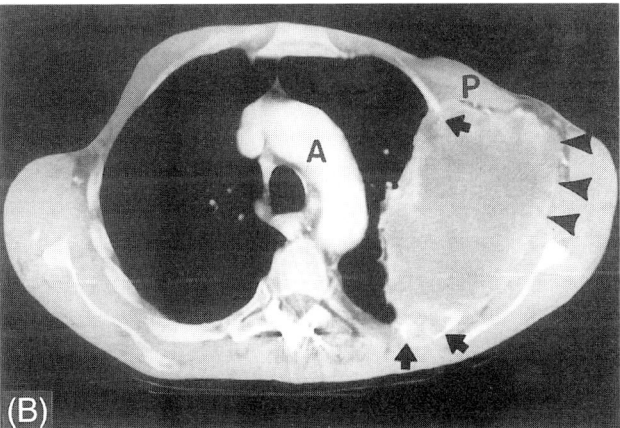

Figure 10 Chest wall invasion on chest radiograph and CT. (A) Chest radiograph shows a very large left apical mass with obvious bone destruction. The extrathoracic extent of tumor cannot be determined on plain film. (B) CT image at the level of the aortic arch (A) also shows bone destruction (arrows), as well as the large area of extension of tumor deep into the axilla (arrowheads). Tumor elevates the left pectoralis major muscle (P). CT is not very sensitive for chest wall invasion unless it is extensive, as in this case.

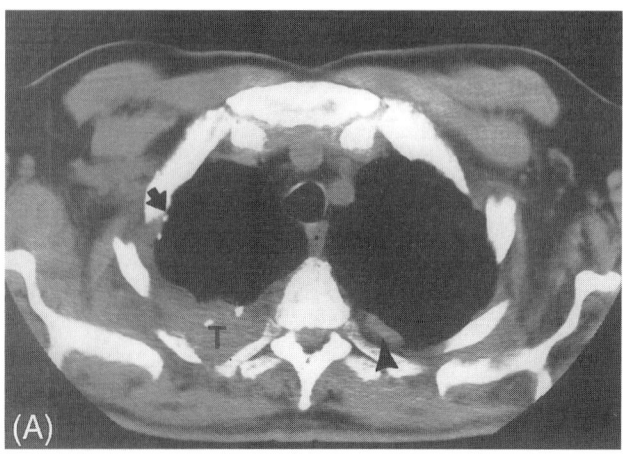

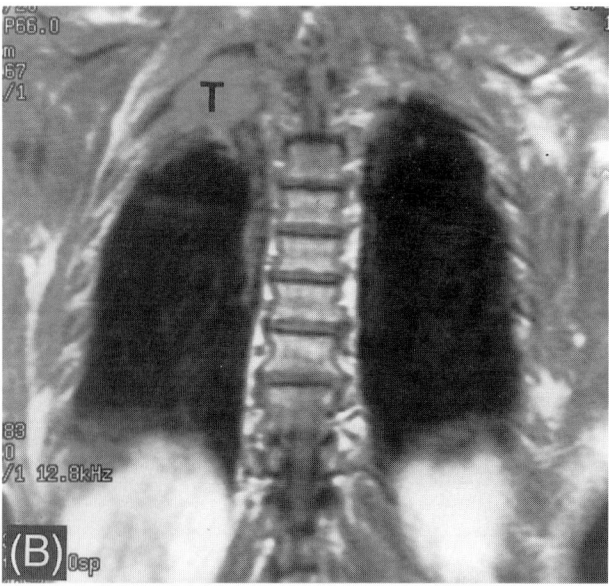

Figure 11   Because of the capability to obtain sagittal and coronal imaging planes, MR offers distinct advantages over CT in some parts of the chest such as the lung apex in Pancoast tumors. (A) CT image just below the apex shows posterior right tumor (T), with rib destruction. The patient also has calcified (arrow) and non-calcified (arrowhead) pleural plaques from asbestos exposure. (B) Coronal T1-weighted MR image clearly demonstrates the superior extent of the tumor (T), which has invaded the supraclavicular space, and invades several medial nerve roots, precluding surgery.

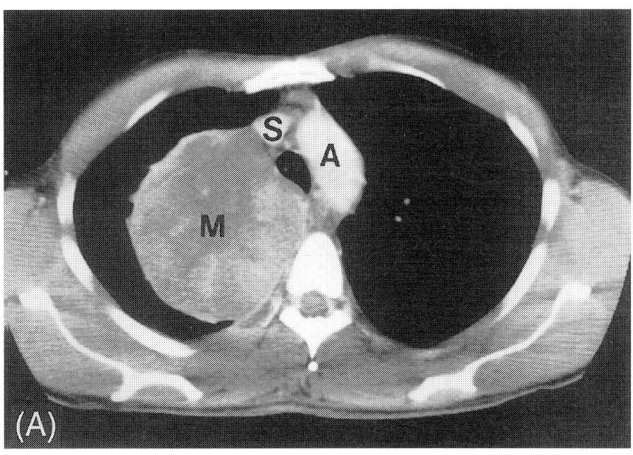

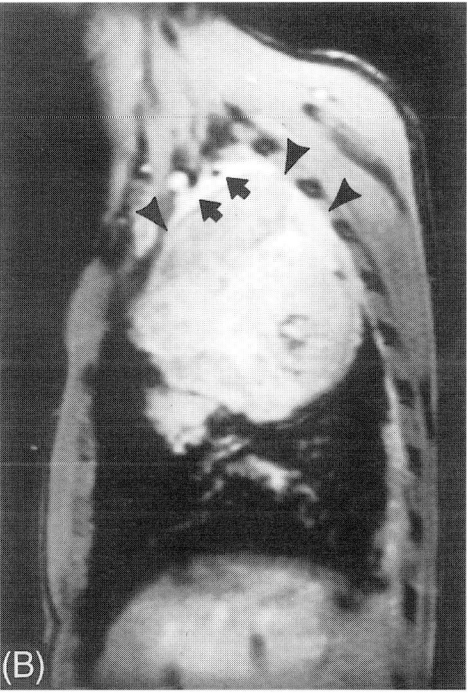

Figure 12 While MR is exquisitely sensitive in detection of edema, it is not much more sensitive and specific than CT in detection of chest wall invasion. (A) CT image shows a very large right upper lobe mass (M), that was a pulmonary blastoma on pathologic examination. The mass abuts the posterior chest wall over a wide area, but had no obvious rib destruction. A = aortic arch, S = superior vena cava. (B) Sagittal gradient echo MR imaging performed with "bright blood" technique also shows tumor abutting a wide area of the chest wall superiorly and posteriorly (arrowheads), and chest wall invasion is suggested. The subclavian vein is visible, running above the tumor and appearing white on this pulse sequence (arrows). At surgery, no invasion was present.

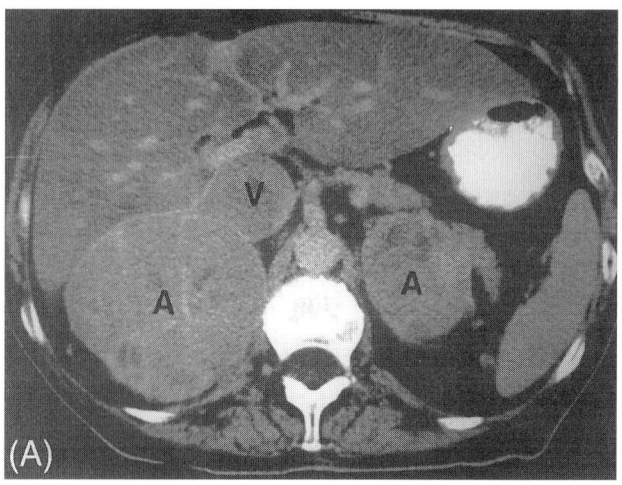

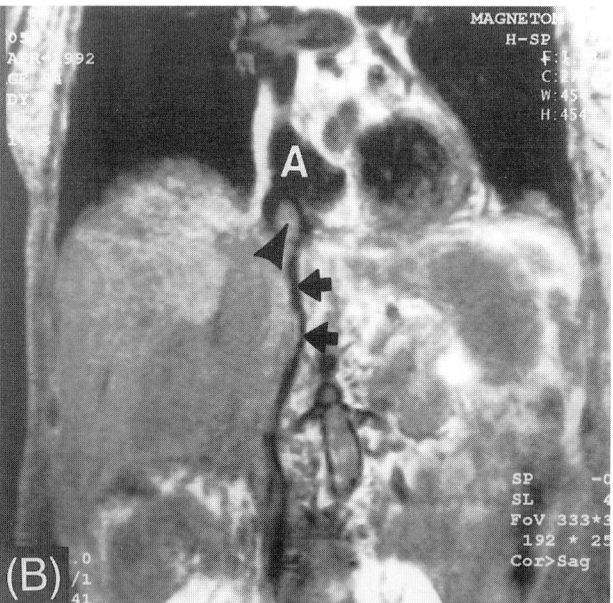

Figure 13 Use of MR in evaluation of vascular invasion. (A) CT image in the upper abdomen in a patient with non-small cell lung carcinoma and large bilateral adrenal masses [A]. The inferior vena cava (V) appears enlarged and heterogeneous, suggesting obstruction by tumor. (B) Coronal T1-weighted MR shows tumor (arrowhead) extending from the inferior vena cava into the right atrium [A]. Flow is still present in the narrowed inferior vena cava (arrows). No intravenous contrast material is needed for this study.

Table 2 Comparison of Technical Aspects of Different Imaging Methods for the Chest

	CXR	Chest CT	Chest MR
Contrast material used	None	Occasional use of IV and/or oral iodinated (slight risk of allergy)	Occasional use of IV gadolinium (very low risk of allergy)
Cost	$50	$300	$350
Radiation	0.03–0.04 cGy for PA and lateral	1–3 cGy	None—no proven ill effects of magnetic fields
Portability	Excellent	None	None
Number of images in study	Two	20–24, filmed twice at different contrast/brightness settings	20–24 per sequence, from 3 to 6 sequences
Time for study	5 min	20 min	60 minutes
Contraindications	None	Claustrophobia, contrast allergy,[a] renal failure[a]	Claustrophobia ocular implants ocular metallic foreign bodies, cochlear implants, pacemakers certain vascular clips
Causes of image degradation	Respiratory motion mildly degrades images	Respiratory motion moderately degrades images, but can redo individual images; metallic objects produce considerable artifact	Respiratory motion moderately degrades images, may degrade entire image sequence; metallic objects produce moderate artifact

[a]Contraindication for use of IV contrast.

Table 3 Comparison of Clinical Uses of Imaging Methods for the Chest

	CXR	Chest CT	Chest MR
Areas of particular utility	overall survey of chest, initial screening follow-up demonstration of collapsed lobes demonstration of fissures, especially minor fissure	Fine detail of lung parenchyma (lymphangitic tumor) mediastinal adenopathy hilar adenopathy (with IV contrast) pleural disease detection of adrenal masses	Chest wall invasion; lung apices; diaphragms; vascular structures (especially in patients with allergy to CT contrast); characterization of adrenal masses; spinal canal, leptomeningeal invasion; bone marrow infiltration
Areas of weakness	Mediastinum, adrenals fine detail of lung parenchyma	Chest wall invasion, unless bone erosion is present; vascular invasion, unless IV contrast is used	Lung parenchyma cortical bone detection of calcification within masses or nodes
Special techniques	Low kV for detection of calcification; apical lordotic or kyphotic views for apices; fluoroscopy for eliminating overlap, detection of phrenic nerve dysfunction; guidance for biopsy	Spiral/helical for single-breath examination of chest; high-resolution imaging for interstitium; thin sections for eliminating volume averaging; sagittal or coronal reconstructions; guidance for biopsy	Oblique planes for demonstrating particular anatomy; sagittal planes for diaphragms; ?guidance for biopsy with new magnet design

same study, in patients with higher-stage disease or adenocarcinoma, 21% of brain metastases and 61% of liver metastases were asymptomatic. It is clearly in the best interest of the patient to detect sites of metastatic disease before proceeding with extensive thoracic surgery, if it can be done in a cost-effective manner.

Metastatic disease within the thorax to the contralateral lung will generally be detected during routine thoracic staging with chest radiography and CT scanning. Lung metastases are present at diagnosis in 10% to 15% of cases, and are slightly more frequent in adenocarcinomas than squamous tumors (16). With excellent CT technique, incidental finding of tiny pulmonary nodules is not uncommon, even in patients with no history of malignancy. Most of these nodules represent either intrapulmonary lymph nodes or noncalcified granulomas. However, in a patient with a history of lung cancer, these tiny subpleural nodules must be taken seriously, as in one study 30% of such lesions represented malignancy (19). In another recent study of patients with nodules under 1 cm noted on chest CT, among patients with a known history of malignancy, only 18% of resected nodules were benign. Even in patients with no prior history of malignancy, only 59% of the nodules were benign (20).

Most chest CT scans will also include the adrenal glands if the scan is continued to the lowest point of the posterior costophrenic angle. If the adrenal glands are not completely examined, addition of several more slices at the bottom of the study can easily image the adrenals in most cases (Fig. 14). In a review of 173 lung cancer patients, 26 adrenal metastases were found, all in patients with other signs

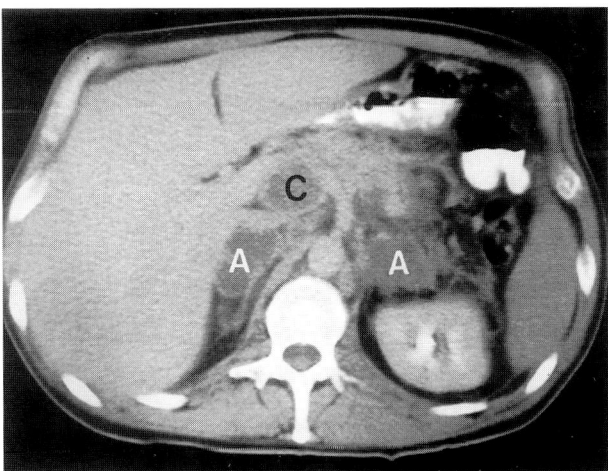

Figure 14   Use of CT in evaluating adrenal masses. Adenomas are often low attenuation due to presence of intracellular lipid. In this case, the low attenuation value of the bilateral adrenal masses is due to extensive necrosis within metastases from non-small cell lung carcinoma. A = adrenal metastases, C = necrotic celiac node metastasis.

of extensive disease (21). In another study, only 6.3% of patients with lung cancer had adrenal lesions detected with CT, and of those with adrenal metastases, all had other evidence of advanced disease (22). The authors concluded that additional imaging specifically for the adrenal was not cost-effective.

Unfortunately, benign tumors of the adrenal glands are common, being present in 3% to 5% of normal people (23). Thus, detection of an adrenal mass does not always indicate stage 4 disease. In fact, isolated adrenal masses are over two times as likely to represent adenomas than metastatic disease even in patients with a known diagnosis of lung cancer (24). CT size criteria have been proposed for distinguishing between adenomas and metastases, since the average adenoma has a diameter of about 2 cm, while the average metastasis measures 4 cm in diameter, but measurement of CT density is more accurate than size measurements (25). Adenomas contain intracellular lipid, and thus will generally have lower attenuation on CT than tumor (26).

MR can offer slightly more specificity in assessment of small adrenal masses (27), since MR can detect intracellular lipid with great sensitivity (Fig. 15). In particular, use of chemical shift imaging can detect the intracellular lipid of adenomas with even greater specificity than is possible using CT density (28). Questionable masses should probably be evaluated with percutaneous biopsy before proceeding with definitive surgical treatment of thoracic disease. In a large review of multiple studies evaluating the usefulness of CT and MR in staging lung cancer, 10% to 20% of patients had adrenal abnormalities, about one-third of which were ultimately found to represent metastatic disease (29).

The liver is another common site of metastatic disease from lung cancer. While most liver metastases will be visible after IV contrast administration, it is often useful to obtain scans both before and after contrast administration, since some relatively vascular metastases may become less evident after contrast administration (Fig. 16). Chest CT scans do not routinely include the entire liver, so if staging of the liver is required, an abdomen CT should be ordered in addition to the chest CT. MR of the liver offers no advantage in detection of metastases, since contrast material for visualizing normal liver parenchyma with MR is limited. Newer agents are being developed that may increase the sensitivity and specificity of liver MR, and in the future, this method may rival CT in usefulness. Most of these agents either are chelates of manganese (30,31) or use superparamagnetic iron oxide particles (32–34).

Detection of bone metastases from lung cancer is also an important part of staging. Nuclear medicine bone scans offer a cost-effective method for screening the entire body for evidence of bone disease, and will detect most lesions, although bone scans also have a considerable number of false-positive results. In a study of 110 patients with lung cancer, all of whom had some serum or clinical evidence suggesting bone metastasis, about one-third of the bone scans were positive, but only one-fourth of these ultimately represented metastatic disease (35).

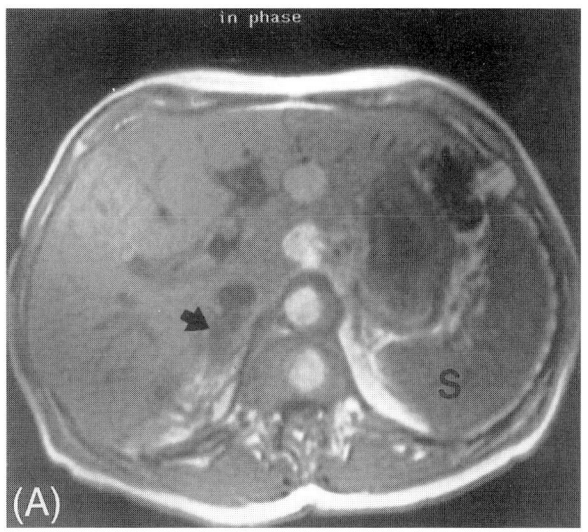

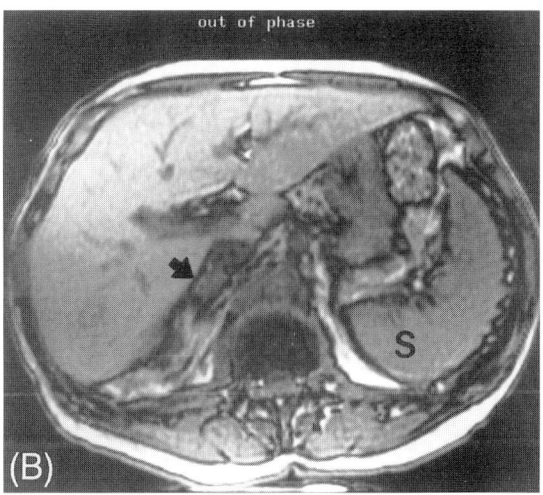

Figure 15 MR, with the ability to detect lipid in a specific manner through chemical shift imaging, may offer more sensitive and specific imaging of adrenal masses than CT. (A) small right adrenal metastasis (arrow) on in-phase sequence, shows signal similar to spleen [S]. (B) same adrenal metastasis (arrow) on out-of-phase sequence, shows signal again similar to spleen. The lack of change in signal on in-phase vs. out-of-phase imaging suggests metastases. (C) small right adrenal adenoma (arrow) on in-phase sequence, shows signal similar to liver. V = inferior vena cava. (D) same adenoma (arrow) on out-of-phase sequence, shows marked decrease in signal, now much lower than liver. V = inferior vena cava. The decrease in signal on out-of-phase imaging suggests that the mass contains lipid, and is likely an adenoma. (Images courtesy of Dr. Ramin Khorasani, Department of Radiology, Brigham and Women's Hospital, Boston, Massachusetts).

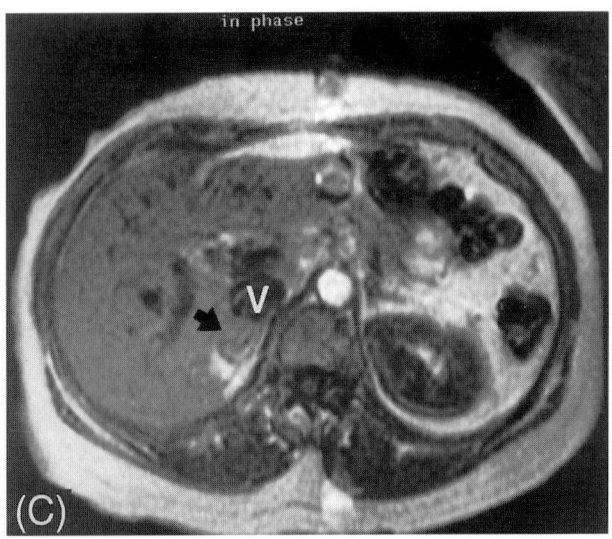

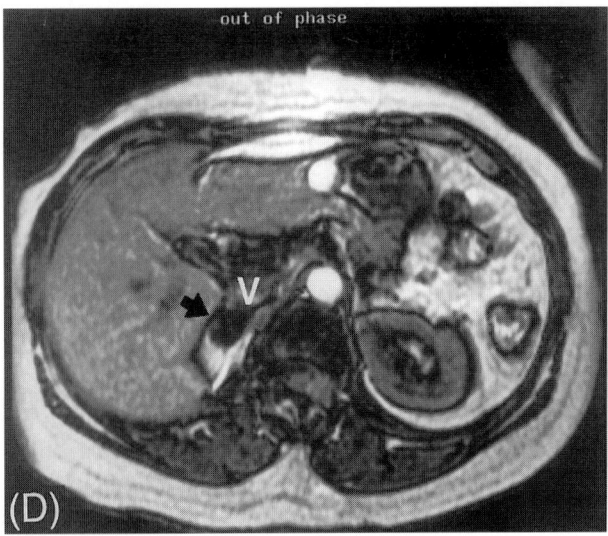

Figure 15 Continued

MR can also be useful in selected cases when findings on CT or bone scan are indeterminate, or in cases with lack of correlation of symptoms and standard imaging studies (Fig. 17). MR does not image cortical bone, since dense bone does not give off enough signal due to its low water content. MR does image the bone marrow, which can be a site of metastatic disease that may be difficult to

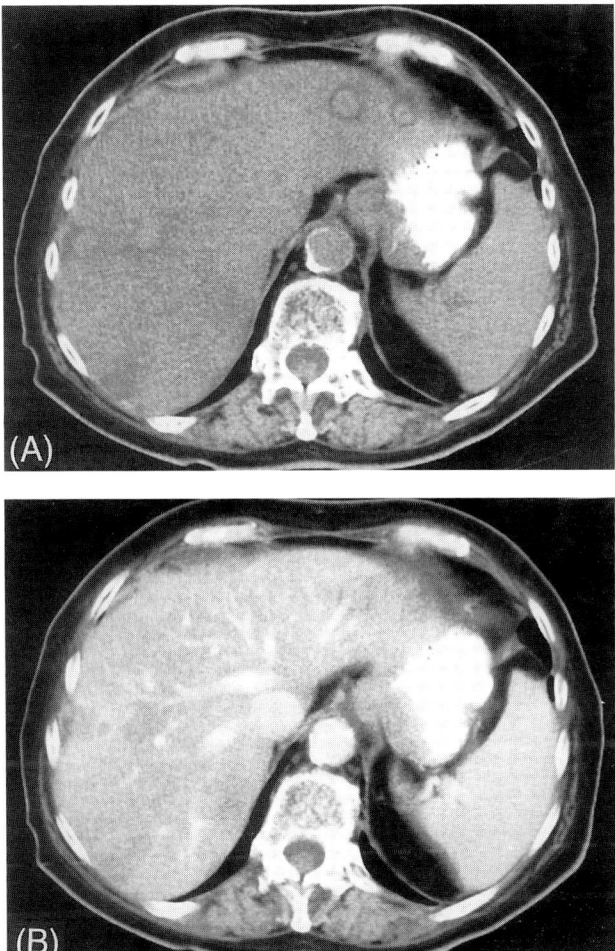

Figure 16 Problems with use of intravenous contrast in detection of liver metastases. (A) Liver metastases on this CT image are easily visible before intravenous contrast administration. (B) The metastases in this case are less evident after contrast administration. This appearance is most often seen in breast and pancreatic tumors, but can also be seen in unusually vascular lung tumors.

detect with plain films. However, bone MR must be interpreted with caution, as equivocal results are not uncommon (36).

The brain is the most common site of metastatic disease from lung cancer (37). The most sensitive and specific method of detection of these lesions is brain MR, which detects smaller lesions and a greater number of lesions, and is much

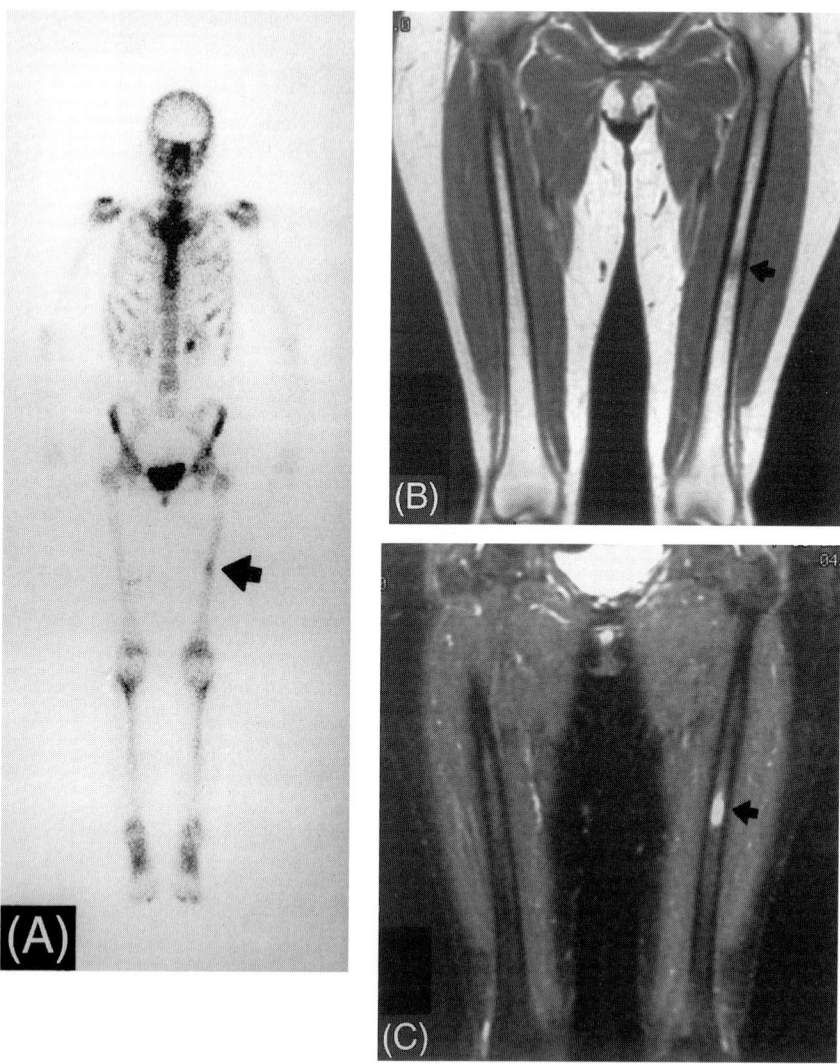

Figure 17   Use of MR in detection of bone metastases. (A) Bone scan in a patient with squamous cell lung carcinoma and no symptoms, shows a faint area of abnormal uptake in the mid-shaft of the left femur (arrow). Plain films of the area were normal. (B) T1-weighted coronal MR of the femurs shows abnormal signal in the central marrow space corresponding to the bone scan finding (arrow). (C) T2-weighted coronal MR also shows the lesion (arrow).

more sensitive than CT for infratentorial lesions (38). MR should be performed with and without gadolinium enhancement for maximizing detection rate (Fig. 18). However, head CT after contrast administration is also quite sensitive and specific, and may be more readily available in many areas. Cost-effectiveness of routine head CT or MR in asymptomatic patients with lung cancer has been questioned, but in a study of 184 patients, 64% of positive head CTs were in patients with no neurologic symptoms, and 10% of brain metastases were in patients who were otherwise operable (39).

VII. Staging with PET and Nuclear Medicine

Nuclear medicine techniques offer several theoretical advantages in staging of lung cancer over plain film, CT, or MR. The imaging agents used can be much more selective in detection of disease than other anatomical imaging methods. Nuclear medicine agents include isotopic tracers bound to monoclonal antibodies, receptor molecules, or substrates that can directly demonstrate physiological functions in tissues. Positron emission tomography (PET) is a specialized nuclear medicine technique that offers the possibility of functional imaging, as well as superior image quality due to the physical nature of the method. In PET scanning, radiotracers are used that decay via positron emission, generating two gamma rays separated by 180°, upon annihilation with electrons within tissues. This process occurs very rapidly after emission of the positron, producing very little scatter of radiation within the body, which degrades image quality in routine nuclear medicine scans. However, PET scanning is quite expensive, since specialized cameras must be used to image the very high energy gamma rays, and the isotopes for scanning must be generated in a cyclotron, and have very short half-lives.

Several monoclonal agents have shown promise in lung cancer staging. Most of these agents have only been used in small numbers of patients and therefore cannot be recommended as part of routine staging. However, in cases where other studies are equivocal, or when serum markers are elevated with no corresponding CT or MR finding, these scans can be helpful (Fig. 19). For imaging non-small-cell lung cancer, some encouraging results have been obtained with antibodies to CEA. In one study, 21/28 patients with known disease had positive scans (40); in another, sensitivity of up to 72% was demonstrated if SPECT imaging was performed (41). In a study comparing CEA scans to CT scans, similar accuracy for predicting stages 3 and 4 was noted (42). A high rate of false positives, however, has been a problem with this agent, yielding specificities as low as 12% (43). For small-cell carcinoma, somatostatin-binding agents have been used, yielding encouraging results (44); however, this agent cannot detect bone or liver metastases (45). Another monoclonal agent that binds to an antigen on both small-cell and non-small-cell carcinoma (NR-LU-10) has also been used, with results for staging of nodes similar to CT (46–48).

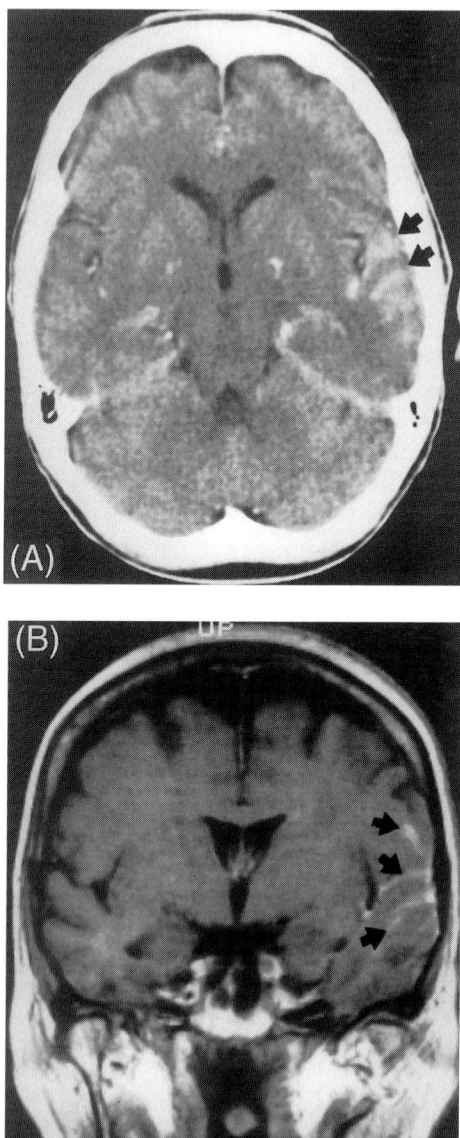

Figure 18   Use of MR in detection of brain metastases. (A) contrast-enhanced head CT in a patient with lung carcinoma and mental status changes. There is a suggestion of abnormal enhancement in the left temporal area (arrows). (B) Contrast-enhanced coronal T1-weighted MR of the head more clearly demonstrates the abnormal signal along sulci in the left temporal region (arrows), consistent with leptomeningeal spread of tumor. (Images courtesy of Dr. Liangge Hsu, Department of Radiology, Brigham and Women's Hospital, Boston, Massachusetts).

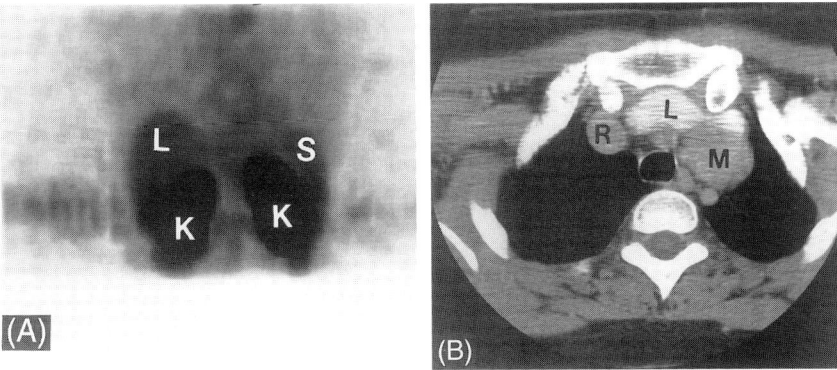

Figure 19 Use of monoclonal nuclear medicine imaging in tumor detection. (A) Patient had an elevated serum CEA, but no other clinical or laboratory abnormalities. On the CEA scan, abnormal tracer activity is seen in the upper mediastinum (arrow). Marked uptake in kidneys [K] and less marked uptake in liver [L] and spleen [S] is normal in this type of scan. (B) CT of the chest shows a mass in the upper left mediastinum that was poorly seen on chest radiograph. R = right brachiocephalic vein, L = left brachiocephalic vein, M-mass.

Most current PET scanning takes advantage of enhanced glucose uptake by a variety of tumor cells, with the contrast agent 18-fluoro-deoxy-glucose (FDG). This agent is taken up by metabolically active cells, but cannot be used within the cell as an energy source, and thus remains in the cell marking it for imaging purposes (Fig. 20). As with the new monoclonal imaging agents, many of the clinical studies of PET are limited by small patient numbers, but initial results are encouraging. Sensitivities and specificities in the 80% to 90% range have been reported (49–52). In a direct comparison of CT with PET for staging the mediastinum, PET was correct in 96% of cases, and CT in only 79% (53). PET may also play a role in follow-up of XRT changes and may be able to distinguish between fibrosis and tumor recurrence (54). Other agents besides FDG can be used for PET imaging, such as L-methyl-11C-methionine, but all suffer from lack of sensitivity for lesions <1.5 cm in diameter (55). While PET scanning remains expensive, in one decision tree analysis, use of both CT and PET in preoperative staging of lung cancer actually saved over $1000 per patient over use of CT alone (56).

VIII. Conclusion

Imaging studies have historically played a major role in detecting lung cancer, in staging of disease, and in following response to treatment. While no imaging

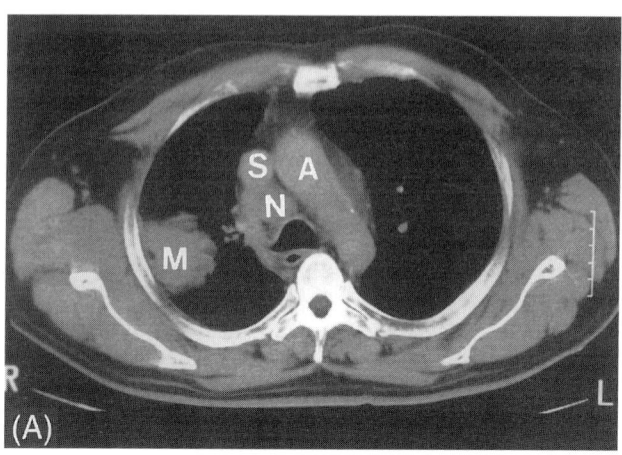

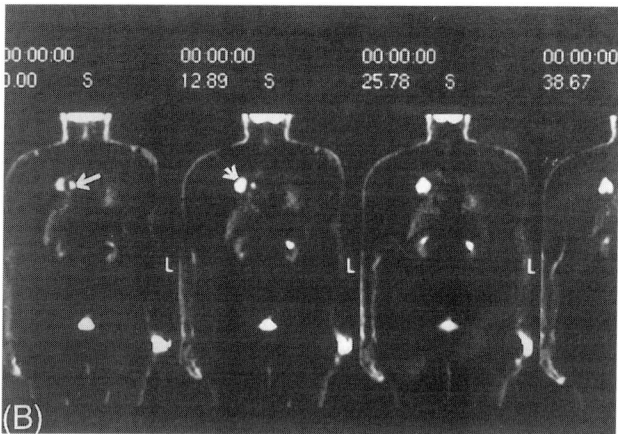

Figure 20 Use of positron emission tomography (PET) in lung cancer. (A) Chest CT image showing large lateral right upper lobe mass [M] and enlarged right paratracheal node [N]. A = aortic arch, S = superior vena cava. (B) PET scan image of the whole body using 18-fluoro-deoxyglucose, with abnormal uptake in both the lung mass (short arrow) and the node (long arrow), indicating at least stage 3A disease. (Images courtesy of Dr. Edward N. Patz, Department of Radiology, Duke University Medical Center, Durham, North Carolina).

studies can replace careful surgical and pathologic staging, standard radiologic techniques can be useful as a road map to guide the surgeon to the most appropriate staging procedure. Newer, more specific imaging agents may offer the opportunity in the future to forgo some surgical procedures in patients with advanced disease.

References

1. Greene R, Francis H, Williams MD. Father of chest radiology in North America. RadioGraphics 1991; 11:325–332.
2. Adler I. Primary Malignant Growths of the Lungs and Bronchi. New York: Longmans, Green, 1912.
3. Boring C, Squires T, Tong T. Cancer statistics, 1991. CA Cancer J 1991; 41:19–36.
4. Gurney J. Why chest radiography became routine. Radiology 1995; 195:245–246.
5. Friedland G, Thurber B. The birth of CT. AJR 1996; 167.
6. Cormack A. Representation of a function by its line integrals with some radiological applications. J Appl Physics 1963; 34.
7. Hounsfield G. Computerized transverse axial scanning (tomography). 1. Description of a system. Br J Radiol 1973; 46:1016–1022.
8. Brooks R, di Chiro G. Principles of computer assisted tomography (CAT) in radiographic and radioisotopic imaging. Phys Med Biol 1976; 21:689–732.
9. Kuhl D, Hale J, Eaton W. Transmission scanning: a useful adjunct to conventional emission scanning for accurately keying isotope deposition to radiographic anatomy. Radiology 1966; 87:278–284.
10. Bull J. History of computed tomography. In: Newton T, Potts D, eds. Radiology of the Skull and Brain: Technical Aspects of Computed Tomography. St. Louis: Mosby, 1981:3835–3852.
11. Pearson F. Staging of the mediastinum. Role of mediastinoscopy and computed tomography. Chest 1993; 103:346S–348S.
12. Izbicki J, Thetter O, Karg O, et al. Accuracy of computed tomographic scan and surgical assessment for staging of bronchial carcinoma. A prospective study. J Thorac Cardiovasc Surg 1992; 104:413–420.
13. Webb R, Sarin M, Zerhouni E, Heelan R, Glazer G, Gatsonis C. Interobserver variability in CT and MR staging of lung cancer. J Comput Assist Tomogr 1993; 17:841–846.
14. McCloud T, Bourgouin P, Greenberg R, et al. Bronchogenic carcinoma: analysis of staging in the mediastinum with CT by correlative lymph node mapping and sampling. Radiology 1992; 182:319–323.
15. White P, Adams H, Crane M, Butchart E. Preoperative staging of carcinoma of the bronchus: can computed tomographic scanning reliably identify stage III tumours. Thorax 1994; 49:951–957.
16. Quint L, Tummala S, Brisson L, et al. Distribution of distant metastases from newly diagnosed non-small cell lung cancer. Ann Thorac Surg 1996; 62:246–250.
17. Quinn D, Ostrow L, Porter D, Shelton DJ, Jackson DJ. Staging of non-small cell bronchogenic carcinoma: relationship of the clinical evaluation to organ scans. Chest 1986; 89:270–275.
18. Salvatierra A, Baamonde C, Llamas J, Cruz F, Lopez-Pujol J. Extrathoracic staging of bronchogenic carcinoma. Chest 1990; 97:1052–1058.
19. Keogan M, Tung K, Kaplan D, Goldstraw P, Hansell K. The significance of pulmonary nodules detected on CT staging for lung cancer. Clin Radiol 1993; 48:94–96.

20. Munden R, Pugatch R, Liptay M, Le L. Small pulmonary lesions detected at CT: clinical importance. Radiology 1997; 202:105–110.
21. Silvestri G, Lenz J, Harper S, Morse R, Colice G. The relationship of clinical findings to CT scan evidence of adrenal gland metastases in the staging of bronchogenic carcinoma. Chest 1992; 102:1748–1751.
22. Eggesbo H, Hansen G. Clinical impact of adrenal expansive lesions in bronchial carcinoma. Acta Radiol 1996; 37:343–347.
23. Commons R, Calloway C. Adenomas of the adrenal cortex. Arch Intern Med 1948; 81:37–41.
24. Oliver TJ, Bernadino M, Miller J, Mansour K, Greene D, Davis W. Isolated adrenal masses in non-small cell bronchogenic carcinoma. Radiology 1984; 153:217–218.
25. Korobkin M, Brodeur F, Yutzy G, et al. Differentiation of adrenal adenomas from nonadenomas using CT attenuation values. AJR 1996; 166:531–536.
26. Korobkin M, Giordano T, Brodeur F, et al. Adrenal adenomas: relationship between histologic lipid and CT and MR findings. Radiology 1996; 200:743–747.
27. Reinig J, Doppman J, Johnson A, Knop R. Adrenal masses differentiated by MR. Radiology 1986; 158:81–84.
28. Korobkin M, Lombardi T, Aisen A, et al. Characterization of adrenal masses using chemical shift and gadolinium enhanced MR imaging. Radiology 1995; 197:411–418.
29. Shea J, Lillington G. Preoperative staging of lung cancer. West J Med 1994; 161:508–509.
30. Bernardino M, Young S, Lee J, Weinreb J. Hepatic MR imaging with Mn-DPDP: safety, image quality and sensitivity. Radiology 1992; 183:53–58.
31. Slater G, Saini S, Mayo-Smith W, Sharma P, Eisenberg P, Hahn P. Mn-DPDP-enhanced MR imaging of the liver: analysis of pulse sequence performance. Clin Radiol 1996; 51:484–486.
32. Ros P, Freeny P, Harms S, et al. Hepatic MR imaging with ferumoxides: a multicenter clinical trial of the safety and efficacy in the detection of focal hepatic lesions. Radiology 1995; 196:481–488.
33. Winter TC III, Freeny PC, Nghiem HV, et al. MR imaging with IV superparamagnetic iron oxide: efficacy in the detection of focal hepatic lesions. AJR 1993; 161:1191–1198.
34. Bellin M, Zaim S, Auberton E, et al. Liver metastases: safety and efficacy of detection with superparamagnetic iron oxide in MR imaging. Radiology 1994; 193:657–663.
35. Michel F, Soler M, Imhof E, Perruchoud A. Initial staging of non-small cell lung cancer: value of routine radioisotope bone scanning. Thorax 1991; 46:469–473.
36. Milleron B, Breton CL, Carette M, Cadranel J, Akoun G. Assessment of bone marrow involvement by magnetic resonance imaging in small cell lung cancer. No significant change of staging. Chest 1994; 106:1030–1035.
37. Andrews R, Gluck D, Konchingeri R. Surgical resection of brain metastases from lung cancer. Acta Neurochirurg 1196; 138:382–389.
38. Nomoto Y, Miyamoto T, Yamaguchi Y. Brain metastasis of small cell lung carcinoma: comparison of Gd-DTPA enhanced magnetic resonance imaging and enhanced computerized tomography. Jpn J Clin Oncol 1994; 24:258–262.

39. Ferrigno D, Buccheri G. Cranial computed tomography as a part of the initial staging procedures for patients with non-small-cell lung cancer. Chest 1994; 106:1025–1029.

40. Vuillez J, Moro D, Brambilla E, et al. Immunoscintigraphy using ^{111}In-labelled F(ab′)2 fragments of anti-carcinoembryonic antigen (CEA) monoclonal antibody for staging of non-small cell lung carcinoma. Eur J Cancer 1994; 30A:1089–1092.

41. Kramer E, Noz M, Liebes L, Murthy S, Tiu S. Radioimmunodetection of non-small cell lung cancer using technetium-99m-anticarcinoembryonic antigen IMMU-4 Fab′ fragment. Preliminary results. Cancer 1994; 73:890–895.

42. Buccheri G, Biggi A, Ferrigno D, et al. Imaging lung cancer by scintigraphy with indium 111-labeled F(ab′)[2] fragments of the anticarcinoembryonic antigen monoclonal antibody FO23C5. Cancer 1992; 70:749–759.

43. Boilleau G, Pujol J, Ychou M, et al. Detection of lymph node metastases in lung cancer: comparison of ^{131}I-anti-CEA-anti-CA 19-9 immunoscintigraphy versus computed tomography. Lung Cancer 1994; 11:209–219.

44. O'Byme K, Ennis J, Freyne P, Clancy L, Prichard J, Carney K. Scintigraphic imaging of small-cell lung cancer with [^{111}In]pentetreotide, a radiolabelled somatostatin analogue. Br J Cancer 1994; 69:762–766.

45. Leitha T, Meghdadi S, Studnicka M, et al. The role of iodine-123-tyr-3-octreotide scintigraphy in the staging of small-cell lung cancer. J Nucl Med 1993; 34:1397–1402.

46. Rusch V, Macapinlac H, Heelan R, et al. NR-LU-10 monoclonal antibody scanning. A helpful new adjunct to computed tomography in evaluation non-small-cell lung cancer. J Thorac Cardiovasc Surg 1993; 106:200–204.

47. Balaban E, Walker B, Cox J, et al. Detection and staging of small cell lung carcinoma with a technetium-labeled monoclonal antibody. A comparison with standard staging methods. Clin Nucl Med 1992; 17:439–445.

48. Vansant J, Johnson D, O'Donnell D, et al. Staging lung carcinoma with a Tc-99m labeled monoclonal antibody. Clin Nucl Med 1992; 17:431–438.

49. Patz E, Goodman P. Positron emission tomography imaging of the thorax. Radiol Clin North Am 1994; 32:811–823.

50. Patz E, Lowe V, Goodman P, Herndon J. Thoracic nodal staging with PET imaging with 18FDG in patients with bronchogenic carcinoma. Chest 1995; 108:1617–1621.

51. Wahl R, Quint L, Greenough R, Meyer C, White R, Orringer M. Staging of mediastinal non-small cell cancer with FDG PET, CT and fusion images: preliminary prospective evaluation. Radiology 1994; 191:371–377.

52. Bury T, Paulus P, Dowlati A, et al. Staging of the mediastinum: value of positron emission tomography imaging in non-small cell lung cancer. Eur Respir J 1996; 9:2560–2564.

53. Steinert H, Hauser M, Allemann F, et al. Non-small cell lung cancer: nodal staging with FDG PET versus CT with correlative lymph node mapping and sampling. Radiology 1997; 202:441–446.

54. Ichaya Y, Kuwabara Y, Sasaki M, et al. A clinical evaluation of FDG-PET to assess the response in radiation therapy for bronchogenic carcinoma. Ann Nucl Med 1996; 10:193–200.

55. Inoue T, Kim E, Wong F, et al. Y Comparison of fluorine-18-fluorodeoxyglucose and

carbon-11-methionine PET in detection of malignant tumors. J Nucl Med 1996; 37:1472–1476.

56. Gambhir S, Hoh C, Phelps M, Madar I, Maddahi J. Decision tree sensitivity analysis for cost-effectiveness of FDG-PET in the staging and management of non-small-cell lung carcinoma. J Nucl Med 1996; 37:1428–1436.

57. Kristensen S, Aaby C, Nielsen S. Mediastinal staging of lung cancer. Is mediastinoscopy still essential? Dan Med Bull 1995; 42:192–194.

58. Primack S, Lee K, Logan P, Miller R, Muller N. Bronchogenic carcinoma: utility of CT in the evaluation of patients with suspected lesions. Radiology 1994; 193:795–800.

59. Yokoi K, Okuyama A, Mori K, et al. Mediastinal lymph node metastasis from lung cancer: evaluation with TI-201 SPECT—comparison with CT. Radiology 1994; 192:813–817.

60. Cole P, Roszkowski A, Firouz-Abadi A, Dare A. Computerized tomography does not predict N2 disease in patients with lung cancer. Aust N Z J Med 1993; 23:688–691.

4

Non-Small-Cell Lung Cancer Surgical Staging

RAJA M. FLORES

Brigham and Women's Hospital
Harvard Medical School
Boston, Massachusetts

JOSÉ J. NORBERTO

Ohio State University Medical Center
Columbus, Ohio

MICHAEL T. JAKLITSCH

Brigham and Women's Hospital
Harvard Medical School
Boston, Massachusetts

DAVID J. SUGARBAKER

Brigham and Women's Hospital
Dana-Farber Cancer Institute
Harvard Medical School
Boston, Massachusetts

I. Introduction

Lung cancer is the leading cause of cancer death in the United States. Cancer statistics for 1997 estimate 178,100 new cases and 160,400 deaths (1). Unfortunately, two-thirds of newly diagnosed lung cancers present with advanced locoregional disease or distant metastasis (2). The extent of disease at presentation, the "stage," will dictate the specific treatment measures: chemotherapy, radiotherapy, surgery, or combination therapy. Surgical staging is therefore the foundation of patient management and clinical research.

Accurate staging permits surgeons to stratify patients into homogeneous groups by prognosis. Treatment options for patients within these specific groups may be compared and outcomes assessed in a controlled setting. The utility of staging depends on its accurate assessment of the extent of disease as well as universal application and reproducibility among treatment centers. Tumor size and gross metastatic disease are easily determined and standardized. The difficulty arises in the evaluation of mediastinal lymph nodes. A variety of diagnostic techniques are currently used to determine nodal status. Some centers use computed tomography (CT) scan alone while others routinely use mediastinoscopy to surgically assess lymph nodes. In addition, several lymph node mapping systems exist, which leaves classifications unstandardized and confounds study results. There is a need to confirm a universal standard in both the role of diagnostic techniques and the use of an exact mapping system for classification of the nodes based on anatomic location.

Accurate staging makes evaluation, treatment, and comparison of different treatment modalities possible. Its value and importance have grown with the ever-increasing availability of new techniques that improve its accuracy. We believe mediastinoscopy and surgical preresectional staging of disease are essential to determine the need for thoracotomy and the possible role of neoadjuvant therapy. In addition, postoperative pathologic staging determines if adjuvant therapy is required. In this chapter we discuss the recent revisions to the international staging system for lung cancer and nodal classification, present the case for use of mediastinoscopy in appropriate patients, and justify systematic lymph node evaluation at the time of curative resection.

II. History

The international staging system for lung cancer has gradually evolved. By 1973, Ishikawa published a staging system that was the standard in Japan until the 1980s (3). In 1985, the Japanese Cancer Committee (JCC), the first American Joint Committee for Cancer (AJCC), and the Union Internationale Contra Cancer (UICC) formed a universal TNM staging system with four stages which accurately stratified 5-year patient survival (4). This new system became the standard for all patients. However, it lacked accuracy in defining certain subsets of patients with locally advanced disease. In 1997, revisions were made in the international lung cancer staging system to provide greater specificity for identifying patient groups with similar prognoses and treatment options with the least disruption of the already established staging system (5).

III. TNM Classification Revisions in 1997
A. Primary Tumor (T)

In the new staging system, the majority of the TNM descriptors remain the same (Table 1) (5). Two additions were made with regard to the primary tumor. First, satellite tumor nodules in the primary tumor lobe of the lung are classified as T4. The second change was separate metastatic tumor nodules in the ipsilateral non-primary tumor lobes of the lung are designated M1 (5). These two changes more accurately stratify long-term survival.

Table 1   TNM Descriptors from the Revisions to the International Staging System for Lung Cancer

---

Primary tumor (T)

TX   Primary tumor cannot be assessed or tumor proven, by the presence of malignant cells in sputum or bronchial washings but not visualized by imaging or bronchoscopy

T0   No evidence of primary tumor

Tis   Carcinoma in situ

T1   Tumor ≤3 cm in greatest dimension, surrounded by lung or visceral pleura, without bronchoscopic evidence of invasion more proximal than the lobar bronchus[a] (i.e., not in the main bronchus)

T2   Tumor with any of the following features of size or extent:
>3 cm in greatest dimension
Involves main bronchus, ≥2 cm distal to the carina
Invades the visceral pleura
Associated with atelectasis or obstructive pneumonitis that extends to the hilar region but does not involve the entire lung

T3   Tumor of any size that directly invades any of the following: chest wall (including superior sulcus tumors), diaphragm, mediastinal pleura, parietal pericardium; or tumor in the main bronchus < 2 cm distal to the carina, but without involvement of the carina; or associated atelectasis or obstructive pneumonitis of the entire lung

T4   Tumor of any size that invades any of the following: mediastinum, heart, great vessels, trachea, esophagus, vertebral body, carina; or tumor with a malignant pleural or pericardial effusion,[b] or with satellite tumor nodule(s) within the ipsilateral primary-tumor lobe of the lung

Regional lymph nodes (N)

NX   Regional lymph nodes cannot be assessed

N0   No regional lymph node metastasis

N1   Metastasis to ipsilateral peribronchial and/or ipsilateral hilar lymph nodes, and intrapulmonary nodes involved by direct extension of the primary tumor

N2   Metastasis to ipsilateral mediastinal and/or subcarinal lymph node(s)

N3   Metastasis to contralateral mediastinal, contralateral hilar, ipsilateral or contralateral scalene, or supraclavicular lymph node(s)

Distant metastasis (M)

MX   Presence of distant metastasis cannot be assessed

M0   No distant metastasis

M1   Distant disease present[c]

---

[a]The uncommon superficial tumor of any size with its invasive component limited to the bronchial wall, which may extend proximal to the main bronchus, is also classified T1.

[b]Most pleural effusions associated with lung cancer are due to tumor. However, there are a few patients in whom multiple cytopathologic examinations of pleural fluid show no tumor. In these cases, the fluid is nonbloody and is not an exudate. When these elements and clinical judgment dictate that the effusion is not related to the tumor, the effusion should be excluded as a staging element and the patient's disease should be staged T1, T2, or T3. Pericardial effusion is classified according to the same rules.

[c]Separate metastatic tumor nodule(s) in the ipsilateral nonprimary-turmor lobe(s) of the lung also are classified M1.

Source: Ref. 5.

B. Regional Lymph Nodes (N)

Lymph node mapping was developed to mark disease progression and patient prognosis by assessing nodal metastasis. Mapping provided invaluable information for the lung cancer staging system and influenced the development of new surgical staging techniques. The prognostic implications of lymph nodes in the surgical specimen was first appreciated by Churchill and published in 1950 (6). In that series, patients with positive lymph nodes in the specimen had poorer prognosis than patients who had negative lymph nodes—a 5-year survival of 0% versus 34%, respectively. The findings were duplicated by other investigators in the 1950s and '60s (7,8). The findings quickly stimulated changes in surgical strategies. Radical excision of mediastinal lymph nodes at the time of resection became common practice (9,10).

The lymphatic system appears to be the earliest method of tumor spread in the disease course. Therefore, the prognostic significance of the status of the lymph nodes cannot be overemphasized. The lymphatic channels of the lung parallel the bronchoarterial branching pattern, and lymph nodes are located at branch points. The lymph nodes of the segmental and lobar bronchi receive the lymphatic drainage from the smaller peripheral areas. The lymphatics of the right upper lobe drain toward the superior mediastinum. The lymphatics of the left upper lobe run along the aorta in the anterior mediastinum and the left mainstem bronchus into the superior mediastinum. The lower lobe lymphatics drain to the posterior mediastinum and eventually into the subcarinal lymph nodes (11) (Fig. 1) (12).

The need for a reproducible universal method of lymph node mapping led to a unification of the American Joint Committee on Cancer (AJCC) schema based on the work of Naruke (13) and the schema by the American Thoracic Society and the North American Lung Cancer Study Group. The new lymph node schema (14) designates lymph nodes within the mediastinal pleural reflection as N2 nodes and labels them with single-digit numbers. All lymph node stations distal to the mediastinal pleural reflection within the visceral pleural envelope are N1 nodes and are labeled with double-digit numbers (Fig. 2; Table 2) (14). This resolved a classification difference between the previous two systems that led to confusion in the interpretation of study results (14).

C. Distant Metastasis (M)

The extent of metastasis is classified as the presence (M1) or absence (M0) of distant disease (Tables 1, 3) (14). Separate metastatic tumor nodules in the ipsilateral nonprimary tumor lobes of the lung are the newest addition to the M1 descriptor.

D. Staging Categories

The current international staging system, which includes the revisions published in 1997, classifies patients into seven subsets according to the anatomic character-

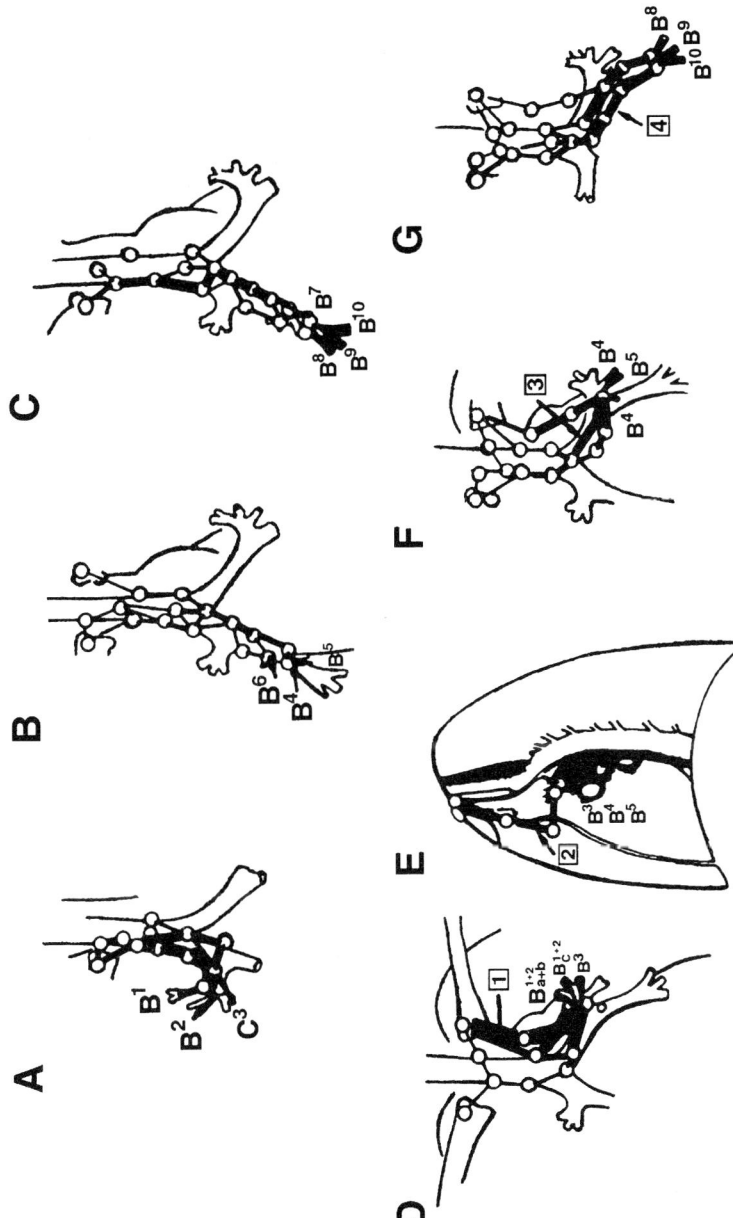

Figure 1 Illustrations of drainage to lymph nodes from the lung: (A) right upper lobe, (B) right middle lobe and superior segment of right lower lobe, (C) right lower lobe, (D) route 1 from the left lung, (E) route 2 from the left lung, (F) route 3 from the left lung, (G) route 4 from the left lung. (From Ref. 12.) July, 1986 Jichi Medical School.

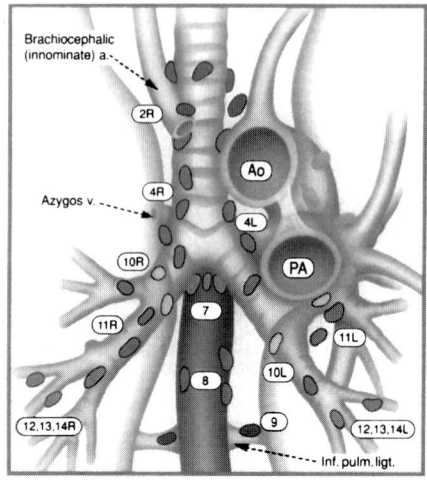

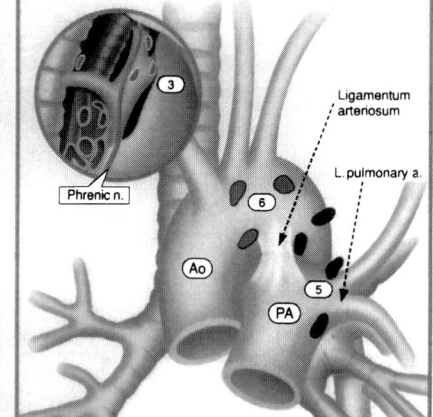

Superior Mediastinal Nodes

● **1** Highest Mediastinal

● **2** Upper Paratracheal

● **3** Pre-vascular and Retrotracheal

● **4** Lower Paratracheal
   (including Azygos Nodes)

   N_2 = single digit, ipsilateral
   N_3 = single digit, contralateral or supraclavicular

Aortic Nodes

● **5** Subaortic (A-P window)

● **6** Para-aortic (ascending
   aorta or phrenic)

Inferior Mediastinal Nodes

● **7** Subcarinal

● **8** Paraesophageal
   (below carina)

● **9** Pulmonary Ligament

N_1 Nodes

○ **10** Hilar

● **11** Interlobar

● **12** Lobar

● **13** Segmental

● **14** Subsegmental

Figure 2 Regional lymph node stations for lung cancer staging which illustrates the use of anatomic landmarks to identify lymph node stations within the mediastinal pleural reflection as N2 nodes and all lymph node stations distal to the mediastinal pleural reflection and within the visceral pleura as N1 nodes. (From Refs. 13, 14, 50.)

istics of their disease (Table 3). Stage IA (T1N0M0) is resectable disease with a tumor size ≤3 cm and no lymph node involvement. The surgical-pathologic survival rate for patients with this stage disease is 67% at 5 years. There is a statistically significant difference between the survival rates of patients with stage IA disease and that of patients with stage IB disease.

Table 2 Lymph Node Map Definitions

Nodal station	Anatomic landmarks
N2 nodes—All N2 nodes lie within the mediastinal pleural envelope	
1 Highest mediastinal nodes	Nodes lying above a horizontal line at the upper rim of the brachiocephalic (left innominate) vein where it ascends to the left, crossing in front of the trachea at its midline.
2 Upper paratracheal nodes	Nodes lying above a horizontal line drawn tangential to the upper margin of the aortic arch and below the inferior boundary of No. 1 nodes.
3 Prevascular and retrotracheal nodes	Prevascular and retrotracheal nodes may be designated 3A and 3P; midline nodes are considered to be ipsilateral.
4 Lower paratracheal nodes	The lower paratracheal nodes on the right lie to the right of the midline of the trachea between a horizontal line drawn tangential to the upper margin of the aortic arch and a line extending across the right main bronchus at the upper margin of the upper lobe bronchus, and contained within the mediastinal pleural envelope; the lower paratracheal nodes on the left lie to the left of the midline of the trachea between a horizontal line drawn tangential to the upper margin of the aortic arch and a line extending across the left main bronchus at the level of the upper margin of the left upper lobe bronchus, medial to the ligamentum arteriosum and contained within the mediastinal pleural envelope. Researchers may wish to designate the lower paratracheal nodes at No. 4s (superior) and No. 4i (inferior) subsets for study purposes; the No. 4s nodes may be defined by a horizontal line extending across the trachea and drawn tangential to the cephalic border of the azygos vein; the No. 4i nodes may be defined by the lower boundary of No. 4s and the lower boundary of No. 4, as described above.
5 Subaortic (aortopulmonary window)	Subaortic nodes are lateral to the ligamentum arteriosum or the aorta or left pulmonary artery and proximal to the first branch of the left pulmonary artery and lie within the mediastinal pleural envelope.
6 Para-aortic nodes (ascending aorta or phrenic)	Nodes lying anterior and lateral to the ascending aorta and the aortic arch or the innominate artery, beneath a line tangential to the upper margin of the aortic arch.
7 Subcarinal nodes	Nodes lying caudal to the carina of the trachea, but not associated with the lower lobe bronchi or arteries within the lung.
8 Paraesophageal nodes (below carina)	Nodes lying adjacent to the wall of the esophagus and to the right or left of the midline, excluding subcarinal nodes.
9 Pulmonary ligament nodes	Nodes lying within the pulmonary ligament, including those in the posterior wall and lower part of the inferior pulmonary vein.

Table 2 Continued

N1 nodes—All N1 nodes lie distal to the mediastinal pleural reflection and within the visceral pleura	
10 Hilar nodes	The proximal lobar nodes, distal to the mediastinal pleural reflection and the nodes adjacent to the bronchus intermedius on the right; radiographically, the hilar shadow may be created by enlargement of both hilar and interlobar nodes.
11 Interlobar nodes	Nodes lying between the lobar bronchi.
12 Lobar nodes	Nodes adjacent to the distal lobar bronchi.
13 Segmental nodes	Nodes adjacent to the segmental bronchi.
14 Subsegmental nodes	Nodes around the subsegmental bronchi.

Source: Ref. 14.

Stage IB (T2N0M0) is resectable disease with tumor >3 cm and no lymph node involvement. The 5-year survival rate seen for patients staged surgical-pathologically with this disease is 57% (5).

Stage IIA (T1N1M0) is disease with tumor ≤3 cm with lymph node involvement in the ipsilateral peribronchial and/or ipsilateral hilar nodes and intrapulmonary nodes. Surgical-pathologic staging of these tumors has shown patient survival of 55% at 5 years.

Stage IIB (T2N1M0, T3N0M0) is disease with tumor >3 cm and lymph node involvement in the ipsilateral peribronchial and /or ipsilateral hilar nodes, and intrapulmonary nodes, or no nodal involvement with tumor of any size which invades the chest wall or diaphragm, pleura, or pericardium or tumors in the mainstem bronchus <2 cm distal to the carina. Disease status of T3N0M0 was originally staged as IIIA, but has been reassigned to stage IIB because of improved patient survival when compared to other stages of IIIA. Surgical-pathological staging of this disease demonstrates patient survival of 39% at 5 years.

Stage IIIA (T3N1M0, T1N2M0, T2N2M0, T3N2M0) is disease with tumor of any size and evidence of invasion of the chest wall, diaphragm, pleura, or pericardium and lymph node involvement of the ipsilateral peribronchial and/or ipsilateral hilar nodes and intrapulmonary node. Stage IIIA is also a tumor of any size with evidence of ipsilateral mediastinal and/or subcarinal lymph node involvement. The survival rate for patients with IIIA disease is 23% at 5 years.

Stage IIIB (T4N0M0, T4N1M0, T4N2M0, T1N3M0, T2N3M0, T3N3M0, T4N3M0) is tumor of any size invading major structures such as the heart, great vessels, trachea, esophagus, mediastinum, vertebral body, or carina. Stage IIIB is also tumor with either malignant pleural or pericardial effusion, or tumor that has

Table 3 Stage Grouping—TNM Subsets[a]

Stage	TNM subset
0	Carcinoma in situ
IA	T1N0M0
IB	T2N0M0
IIA	T1N1M0
IIB	T2N1M0
	T3N0M0
IIIA	T3N1M0
	T1N2M0
	T2N2M0
	T3N2M0
IIIB	T4N0M0
	T4N1M0
	T4N2M0
	T1N3M0
	T2N3M0
	T3N3M0
	T4N3M0
IV	Any T any N M1

[a]Staging is not relevant for occult carcinoma, designated TXNOMO.
Source: Ref. 5.

metastasized to contralateral mediastinal or hilar lymph nodes or to ipsilateral scalene or supraclavicular nodes. This stage disease is considered unresectable. Treatment is chemotherapeutic with or without radiation therapy for control or palliation.

Stage IV (any T any N with M1) (14) is tumor of any size with distant metastases. Standard treatment is palliative, and patient survival rarely reaches 5 years.

The new, revised lung cancer staging system was validated with a database of 5319 patients treated for primary lung cancer. It may be applied to patients with squamous cell carcinoma, small cell carcinoma, large cell carcinoma, adenocarcinoma (including bronchoalveolar carcinoma), or undifferentiated carcinomas (14).

E. Clinical Staging Versus Surgical-pathological Staging

Preresectional staging inconsistencies are related to the extent of preresectional evaluation of the patient. Evaluation varies from institution to institution and from surgeon to surgeon. Clinical staging usually involves a complete history, physical exam, and CT assessment of the primary tumor and mediastinal lymph nodes. Mediastinal lymph node involvement is assessed based on nodal size and suspicious characteristics without histologic confirmation. When patients are studied more extensively, where surgical-pathological staging is done, the chances of finding additional disease (i.e., lymph nodal involvement) are greater.

Preresectional surgical staging classifies a greater number of patients into advanced stages and a lower number of patients into earlier stages. The effect of inaccurate downstaging will be minimized (15). The end result is better statistical survival estimates at each stage of disease. This has been described as the Will Rogers Phenomenon (16). Clinical staging without surgical staging often results in unknowingly categorizing disease into an earlier stage than actual fact. This can lead to reports of poor survival in patients falsely classified into stage groups with better prognosis. The issues between the two evaluation practices are these:

1. Because there is inaccurate downstaging, patients do not receive appropriate treatment for the actual stage of their disease.
2. The inconsistencies of patients categorized into the same stage confound ability to draw firm conclusions from studies and reports.
3. The individual surgeon cannot, because of (2) above, draw standardized information from the literature to use for his or her own patient population.

At the present time, there is no standard recommendation for preresectional evaluation, and practice varies.

Nodal involvement is such a powerful prognosticator that surgeons should be encouraged to perform surgical lymph node sampling as a standard of practice to accurately stage all patients, as is done in breast cancer surgery (15). The role of mediastinal lymph node resection as an effective method of obtaining better tumor control in the resection of early stage lung cancer has yet to be established. Two recent publications have emphasized the role of systematic mediastinal lymph node evaluation in the detection of occult mediastinal disease, since both CT and intraoperative inspection of grossly normal-appearing lymph nodes failed to identify patients with microscopic positive disease (17,18). Of 575 patients with clinical stage I disease who underwent lobectomy and systematic mediastinal lymphadenectomy, 79 (14%) had positive mediastinal lymph nodes by pathologic evaluation (17). Until well-designed clinical trials better define the impact of mediastinal lymphadenectomy on patient outcome and survival, at least selective ipsilateral mediastinal lymph node sampling should be performed in all cases to accurately and pathologically stage each patient (19).

F. Preoperative Staging

Once the diagnosis of lung cancer has been made, the next step in patient treatment should focus on determining the extent of disease. Clinical staging involves history, physical exam, blood chemistry, and radiological evaluation. Patient history should focus on risk factors for lung cancer and concomitant malignancy. It is also important to evaluate weight loss because of its known association with metastatic disease. The physical exam focuses on the identification of suspicious lymph nodes and the presence of any chest wall lesions. Abnormalities in blood chemistry, such as calcium or alkaline phosphatase, may suggest metastatic disease.

The initial radiological evaluation should include posteroanterior and lateral chest x-rays to evaluate the size of the lesion, synchronous lesions, mediastinal adenopathy, or pleural effusion. Chest and upper abdomen CT is the next radiological exam (Chap. 3 describes radiological staging). CT is very helpful in the evaluation of the primary tumor, mediastinum, liver, and adrenal glands. However, resectional therapy should not be based solely on the CT scan for several reasons. There is evidence that adenocarcinoma of the lung, which has become the most common subtype, frequently metastasizes to the mediastinal lymph nodes without demonstrating radiological evidence of disease. Cybulsky and colleagues (20) demonstrated that 60% of patients with adenocarcinoma subtype who showed negative N2 nodes on CT scan were found to have N2 disease at resection. They also observed a survival disadvantage in those patients N2-negative by CT scan who were found to be N2-positive on surgical resection (6% vs. 13.5%, 5-year survival) (20). The false-negative rate of CT scan to predict mediastinal lymph node metastasis varies from 5% to 39% (21).

Magnetic resonance imaging (MRI) has not offered any advantage over CT scan except in the evaluation of tumor invasion to the vertebral body. Recent data suggest that positron emission tomographic (PET) imaging may have a role in lung cancer staging. Patz et al. (22) reported a sensitivity and specificity in the range of 92% and 100% in the evaluation of mediastinal lymph nodes. However, this technology has not been compared with mediastinoscopy in a prospective and randomized setting.

Based on this evidence, we do not recommend basing the resectional therapy only on radiological findings. We believe that surgical staging is the most accurate and reproducible method of preresectional staging available at this time and that it should be performed in all patients undergoing surgery for lung cancer.

IV. Procedures of Surgical-Pathological Staging

A. Bronchoscopy

Bronchoscopy is a helpful procedure in the diagnosis and staging of lung cancer. It can not only provide tissue for pathologic diagnosis, but also determine the distance between the tumor and the carina. This determination is important in designating the T category (Table 1) and it also assists in surgical planning, especially if sleeve resection is contemplated.

B. Cervical Mediastinoscopy

In 1954, Harken at the Peter Bent Brigham (23) introduced a Jackson laryngoscope into the superior mediastinum through a supraclavicular incision. His technique allowed sampling of ipsilateral mediastinal lymph nodes. Soon after, Carlens (24) modified Harkens' technique and developed the current cervical mediastinoscopy. Through this approach, he was able to biopsy bilateral mediastinal lymph nodes.

Cervical mediastinoscopy has become the traditional method for mediastinal staging because of its superb specificity and sensitivity (100% and 93%, respectively) (25). It can be performed with negligible morbidity and mortality (< 1%). The prognostic significance of preresectional mediastinoscopy has been well documented by Pearson and the Toronto group (26). They demonstrated that patients with mediastinoscopically proven N2 disease had a poorer prognosis than patients with negative N2 (15% vs. 41% 5-year survival, respectively) (26).

The preresectional diagnosis of N2/N3 disease is the main goal of the surgical staging procedures. There is evidence that a subgroup of patients with N2 disease may benefit from neoadjuvant therapy (27–32). For instance, identifying patients with N2 disease preoperatively would maximize the therapeutic benefit of neoadjuvant chemotherapy and surgical resection. If one does not believe in giving neoadjuvant therapy for N2 disease, then a positive mediastinoscopy would avoid futile thoracotomy. Patients with contralateral adenopathy (N3 disease) are for practical purposes considered unresectable; however, a subgroup of patients with microscopic N2 disease who responded to neoadjuvant therapy and subsequently underwent surgery has been reported (29).

The current indications for mediastinoscopy could be classified as absolute or relative (Table 4) (33). The absolute indication for mediastinoscopy is the finding of enlarged lymph nodes by CT scan. It has been demonstrated that most of the enlarged lymph nodes are malignant. Lymph nodes >1.5 cm by CT scan are benign in only 20% to 45% of the cases (34–36).

The relative indications for mediastinoscopy refer to special situations in which the preresectional CT scan is negative for enlarged lymph nodes (Table 4) (33). Independent of size, lesions classified as central are associated with positive mediastinal lymph nodes. According to Kirsh et al. (37), central tumors were found to have positive lymph nodes in 39% of the cases. Meanwhile, peripheral tumors were found to have positive N2 nodes in 24% of the cases.

Histologic subtype has to be considered in the decision process to perform mediastinoscopy. In a series reported by Jolly et al., small-cell carcinoma was associated with N2 disease in 65% of the cases, large-cell carcinoma in 46%, adenocarcinoma in 35%, and squamous cell carcinoma in 19% (38). As mentioned previously, Cybulsky also demonstrated a strong association between adenocarcinoma subtype and N2 disease. We believe that the presence of adenocarcinoma, large-cell, or small-cell histology in the preoperative biopsy demands the performance of mediastinoscopy.

Table 4 Absolute and Relative Indications for Mediastinoscopy

Absolute
    Mediastinal lymph node involvement (>1.5 cm)
Relative
    T2 or T3 primary lesion
    Intent to use neoadjuvant therapy
    Adenocarcinoma or large-cell tumors
    Multiple primary lesions
    Vocal cord paralysis
    Central location

Source: Ref. 33.

Mediastinoscopy is also indicated in patients with multiple synchronous lesions. In this setting, the main goal is to rule out metastatic disease. The prognosis in cases of multiple primaries is determined by the tumor with the higher stage (39). Positive mediastinal lymph nodes in patients with multiple parenchymal lesions suggest metastatic disease instead of multiple primaries. Hoarseness in a lung cancer patient is also a relative indication for mediastinoscopy. The development of hoarseness suggests involvement of the subaortic lymph nodes, and this leads to paresis of the ipsilateral vocal cords.

The intention to use multimodality therapy should be supported by surgical staging because CT mediastinal staging has significant false-negative or false-positive rates. Trials evaluating multimodality therapy should not be based on CT scan alone because this would add a significant number of confounding variables.

C. Cervical Mediastinoscopy: Surgical Technique

This procedure is performed through a small collar incision 2 cm above the sternal notch. The initial dissection is similar to tracheostomy. The median raphe is incised and the strap muscles are spread. Once the trachea is visualized, the pretracheal plane is followed caudally. Digital blunt dissection is performed in this pretracheal plane and carried out toward the mediastinum (Fig. 3) (33). A digital examination of the mediastinum is performed, searching for enlarged and hard nodes. It is recommended to perform this examination following a routine and systematic approach. The right paratracheal, subcarinal, and then left paratracheal spaces are palpated in a sequential fashion. It is also important to palpate the subinnominate space and sweep down the nodes into the right paratracheal space (Fig. 4) (33). The mediastinoscope is introduced following the trachea as a road map. This instrument allows biopsy of the different nodal stations, as presented in Figure 5 (33). The importance of accurate labeling of the nodal stations is obvious.

Cervical mediastinoscopy does not allow access to the subaortic or aortopulmonary window nodes. These nodal stations need to be evaluated routinely in

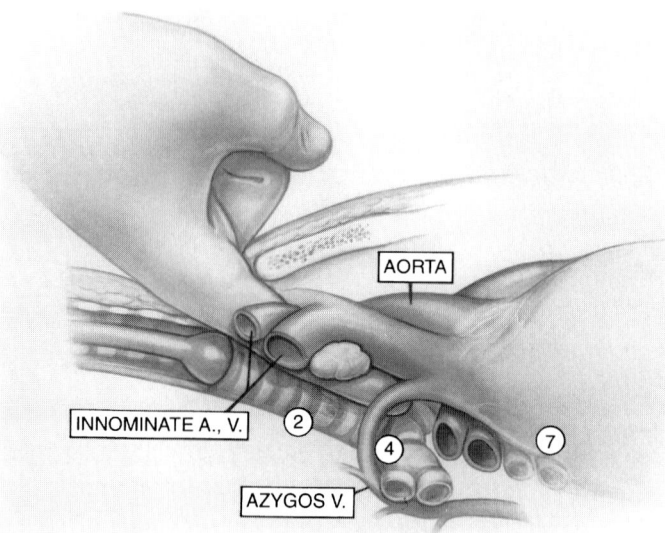

Figure 3 Surgeon's finger in the mediastinum to palpate adenopathy. Nodal stations are numbered. (From Ref. 33.)

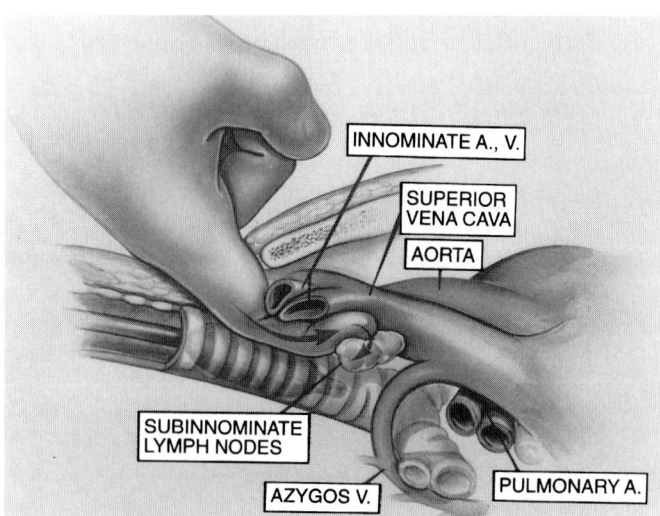

Figure 4 Surgeon's finger pushing down the nodes away from the innominate artery for biopsy. (From Ref. 33.)

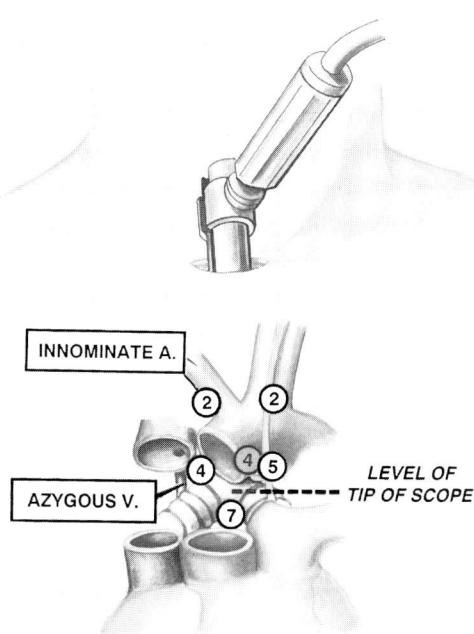

Figure 5 Mediastinoscope in mediastinum for open biopsy with numbered nodal stations. (From Ref. 33.)

left upper lobe lesions. The Chamberlain procedure, extended cervical mediastinoscopy, or VATS, is available for the evaluation of the subaortic nodes and AP window.

D. Anterior Mediastinoscopy (Chamberlain Procedure)

The inability to reach the lymph nodes at the aortopulmonary (AP) window prompted the development of other techniques, including the Chamberlain procedure (40) and extended cervical mediastinoscopy (41), to sample lymph nodes in the AP window region.

The Procedure: In the original description, the procedure was carried out through a parasternal incision at the level of the second intercostal space and removing the second cartilage. The procedure is also performed through a transverse incision lateral to the sternal border at the second intercostal space. This approach does not remove the second cartilage as originally described. After the skin incision is performed (3 to 4 cm), the dissection is carried down sharply until the pectoralis major is visualized. The fibers of this muscle are separated until the intercostal muscle is exposed. The intercostal muscle is separated from the superior border of the second cartilage using cautery. The mediastinal pleura is bluntly dissected down to the AP window.

During the procedure, care should be taken to avoid entering the pleural space. At this point the mediastinoscope is used to visualize the subaortic space and AP window, and graspers are used to sample the desired lymph nodes. One must be cognizant of the proximity of the phrenic nerve, vagus nerve, internal thoracic vessels, left main pulmonary artery, superior pulmonary vein, and aorta to avoid injury to these structures.

E. Extended Cervical Mediastinoscopy

This procedure was described by Ginsberg in 1987 (41). It is carried out through the same cervical incision used for routine mediastinoscopy. Using digital dissection the tissue between the innominate and carotid artery is opened. This maneuver allows the introduction of the mediastinoscope anterior to the aortic arch reaching to the AP window and the subaortic space. The same anatomic structures at risk in mediastinotomy are at risk in extended cervical mediastinoscopy. The procedure is difficult to perform, and many surgeons opt to perform anterior mediastinoscopy instead.

F. Scalene or Supraclavicular Lymph Node Biopsy

In 1949, scalene fat pad biopsy was described by Daniels (42). Although he found the technique useful in the diagnosis of lung cancer, biopsy of nonpalpable scalene or supraclavicular nodes is not routinely advocated. The diagnostic yield of this procedure in patients with routine lung cancer and nonpalpable lymph nodes is very low (43). However, in patients with palpable lymph nodes the diagnostic yield is approximately 90% (44).

G. Video-Assisted Thoracoscopic Surgery (VATS) and Closed Thoracoscopy

The improvement in video-optics has produced a remarkable enthusiasm for endoscopic techniques by the thoracic surgery community. Minimally invasive techniques can be performed as pure thoracoscopy (Figure 6) (33) or as a VATS procedure (Fig. 7) (33). The difference between these two approaches is whether or not a utility incision is used.

Closed thoracoscopy utilizes thoracoscopic ports to perform biopsies of pleural masses and treatment of pleural effusions. It has also been used to obtain biopsy of mediastinal lymph nodes. Figure 6 demonstrates the placement of ports in a routine thoracoscopic procedure. The use of a utility incision <8 cm increases the versatility of minimally invasive procedures. VATS has been used in diagnostic, therapeutic, and mixed procedures (Figure 7) (45–49).

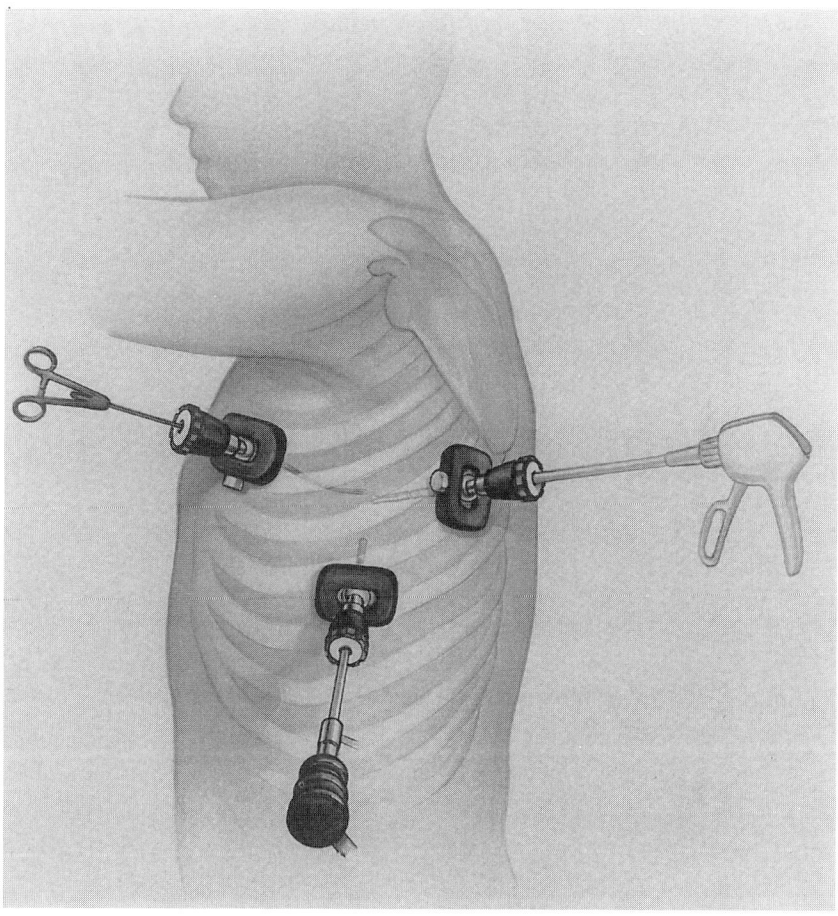

Figure 6   Thoracoscopic procedure using three intercostal ports. Note: camera on the thoracoscope and two working ports. (From Ref. 33.)

The role of VATS in the current approach to staging has not been determined despite its well-known versatility. Cervical mediastinoscopy occupies an undisputed central role in surgical staging. The digital evaluation of the mediastinum is an advantage of cervical mediastinoscopy. Nevertheless, our experience at Brigham and Women's Hospital suggests that VATS exploration of the mediastinum in cases of suspected AP window or subaortic nodes may be superior to Chamberlain's procedure. Our experience has not been studied in prospective trials. We believe that VATS may play a role in preresectional restaging after induction therapy. Albain et al. (29) demonstrated that patients with persistent N2 disease after induction therapy had poorer prognosis than N2-negative patients. In a

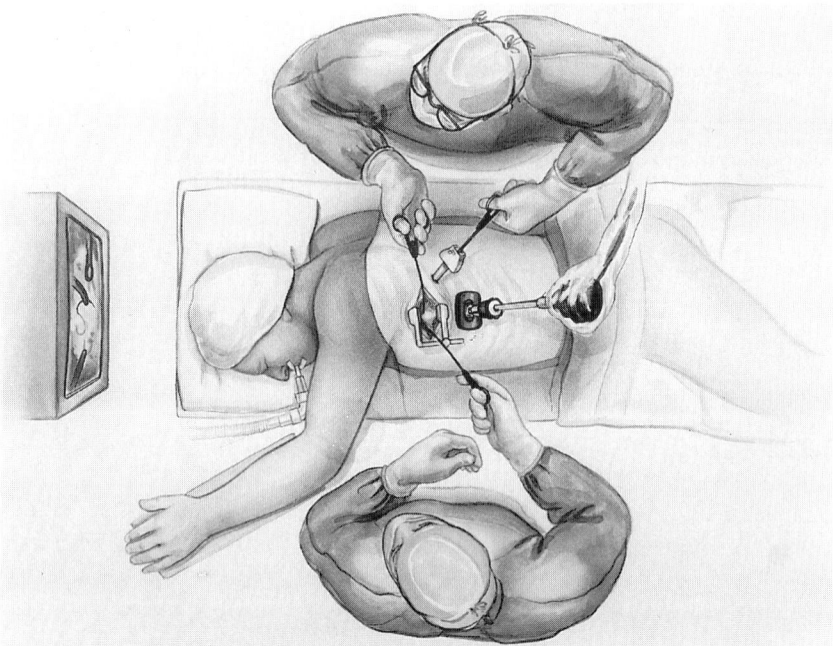

Figure 7 A video-assisted, left-sided thoracoscopic procedure. Two surgeons are seen working thoracoscopic instruments through the utility incisions of <8 cm. (From Ref. 33.)

long-term follow-up of a cohort that underwent multimodality therapy in CALGB trial 8935 (30), we have found a substantial survival difference in patients with N2-negative and N2-positive disease after induction therapy (median survival 43.6 mo vs. 16.9 mo). We propose that VATS preresectional restaging could stratify these two different subgroups of patients and avoid thoracotomy in those patients who may benefit from further chemoradiotherapy.

V. Summary

Lung cancer constitutes a major health problem worldwide. One of the major advances in lung cancer therapy is the development of an efficient staging system. This staging system permits a more objective and consistent evaluation of traditional as well as new therapeutic modalities. Mediastinal lymph node evaluation plays a central role in the current staging system. Radiological evaluation should be considered as complementary to and not in lieu of surgical preresectional staging. A standard and universally accepted algorithm of surgical staging must be developed and implemented upon which well-designed clinical trials may be based. This will ensure accuracy and consistency in results obtained from different treatment modalities. Only then can sound conclusions be made concerning different treatments for specific stages of lung cancer. The role of new techniques such as VATS, PET scanning, and the analysis of biologic markers remains undetermined in the current staging process and requires further investigation.

Acknowledgments

The authors thank Mary S. Visciano for editorial assistance.

References

1. Parker SL, Tong T, Bolden S, Wingo PA. Cancer statistics, 1997. CA 1996; 47:5–27.
2. Parker SL, Tong T, Bolden S, et al. Cancer statistics, 1996. CA 1996; 46(1):5–29.
3. Ishikawa S. Staging system on TNM classification for lung cancer. Jpn J Clin Oncol 1973; 3:19.
4. Mountain CF. A new international staging system for lung cancer. Chest 1986; 89(suppl):225S–233S.
5. Mountain CF. Revisions in the international system for staging lung cancer. Chest 1997; 111:1710–1717.
6. Churchill ED, Sweet RH, Soutter L, Scannell JG. The surgical management of carcinoma of the lung: a study of the cases treated at the Massachusetts General Hospital from 1930 to 1950. J Thorac Surg 1950; 20:349–365.
7. Adams R. Carcinoma of the lung: factors affecting survival after resection of cancer of the lung. J Thorac Surg 1948; 17:306–322.
8. Overholt RH, Schmidt IC. Survival in primary carcinoma of the lung. N Engl J Med 1949; 240:491–497.
9. Cahan WG, Watson WL, Pool JL. Radical pneumonectomy. J Thorac Surg 1951; 22:449–473.
10. Cahan WG. Radical lobectomy. J Thorac Cardiovasc Surg 1960; 39:555–572.
11. Ginsberg RJ, Vokes EE, Raben A. Non-small cell lung cancer. In: DeVita VT Jr, Hellman S, Rosenberg SA, eds. Cancer Principles and Practice of Oncology. 5th ed. Philadelphia: Lippincott-Raven, 1997:858–911.
12. Hata E, Miyamoto H, Kohiyama R, Tanaka M, Sakao Y, Harada R. Resection of N2/N3 mediastinal disease. In: Motta G, ed. Lung Cancer Frontiers in Science and Treatment. Genoa: Grafica, 1994:431–444.
13. Naruke T, Suemasu K, Ishikawa S. Lymph node mapping and curability at various

levels of metastasis in resected lung cancer. J Thorac Cardiovasc Surg 1978; 76:832–839.

14. Mountain CF, Dresler CM. Regional lymph node classification for lung cancer staging. Chest 1997; 111:1718–1723.

15. Jett JR. What's new in staging lung cancer? Chest 1997; 111:1486–1487.

16. Feinstein AR, Sosin DM, Wells CK. The Will Rogers Phenomenon: stage migration and new diagnostic techniques as a source of misleading statistics for survival in cancer. N Engl J Med 1985; 312:1604–1608.

17. Takizawa T et al. Mediastinal lymph node metastasis in patients with clinical stage I peripheral non-small cell lung cancer. J Thorac Cardiovasc Surg 1997; 113:248–252.

18. Oda M et al. The role of mediastinal lymph node dissection for clinical stage I non-small cell lung cancer. Lung Cancer 1997; 18(suppl 1):97.

19. Holmes EC. General principles of surgical quality control. Chest 1994; 106(suppl): 334S–336S.

20. Cybulsky IJ, Lanza LA, Ryan MB, Putnam JB Jr, McMurtrey MM, Roth JA. Prognostic significance of computed tomography in resected N2 lung cancer. Ann Thorac Surg 1992; 54:533–537.

21. Hosking MP, Mongan PD, Peterson RE. Removal of a large intrathoracic tumor in a child: neurogenic motor-evoked potential monitoring of spinal cord integrity and anesthetic management. Anesth Analg 1992; 74:460–463.

22. Patz EF Jr, Shaffer K, Piwnica-Worms DR, et al. Malignant pleural mesothelioma: value of CT and MR imaging in predicting resectability. AJR Am J Roentgenol 1992; 159:961–966.

23. Harken DE, Black H, Clauss R, Farrand RE. A simple cervicomediastinal exploration for tissue diagnosis of intrathoracic disease. With comments on the recognition of inoperable carcinoma of the lung. N Engl J Med 1954; 251:1041–1044.

24. Carlens E. Mediastinoscopy: a method for inspection and tissue biopsy in the superior mediastinum. Dis Chest 1959; 36:343–352.

25. Coughlin M, Deslauriers J, Beaulieu M, et al. Role of mediastinoscopy in pretreatment staging of patients with primary lung cancer. Ann Thorac Surg 1985; 40:556–560.

26. Pearson FG, DeLarue NC, Ilves R, Todd TRJ, Cooper JD. Significance of positive superior mediastinal nodes identified at mediastinoscopy in patients with resectable cancer of the lung. J Thorac Cardiovasc Surg 1982; 83:1–11.

27. Rosell R, Gomez-Codina J, Camps C, et al. A randomized trial comparing preoperative chemotherapy plus surgery with surgery alone in patients with non-small-cell lung cancer. N Engl J Med 1994; 330:153–158.

28. Samuel C, Bird DR, Burton JL. Hyperpigmentation after sympathectomy. Clin Exp Dermatol 1980; 5:349–350.

29. Albain KS, Rusch VW, Crowley JJ, et al. Concurrent cisplatin/etoposide plus chest radiotherapy followed by surgery for stages IIIA (N2) and IIIB non-small-cell lung cancer: mature results of Southwest Oncology Group phase II study 8805. J Clin Oncol 1995; 13:1880–1892.

30. Sugarbaker DJ, Herndon J, Kohman LJ, Krasna MJ, Green MR. Results of Cancer and Leukemia Group B protocol 8935. A multiinstitutional phase II trimodality trial

for stage IIIA (N2) non-small-cell lung cancer. Cancer and Leukemia Group B Thoracic Surgery Group. J Thorac Cardiovasc Surg 1995; 109:473–483; discus.

31. Kirn DH, Lynch TJ, Mentzer SJ, et al. Multimodality therapy of patients with stage IIIA, N2 non-small-cell lung cancer. Impact of preoperative chemotherapy on resectability and downstaging. J Thorac Cardiovasc Surg 1993; 106:696–702.

32. Pass HI, Pogrebniak HW, Steinberg SM, Mulshine J, Minna J. Randomized trial of neoadjuvant therapy for lung cancer: interim analysis. Ann Thorac Surg 1992; 53:992–998.

33. Sugarbaker DJ, Strauss GM. Advances in surgical staging and therapy of non-small cell lung cancer. Semin Oncol 1993; 20:163–172.

34. Faling LJ, Pugatch RD, Jung Legg Y, et al. Computed tomographic scanning of the mediastinum in the staging of bronchogenic carcinoma. Am Rev Respir Dis 1981; 124:690–695.

35. Underwood GH Jr, Hooper RG, Axelbaum SP, Goodwin DW. Computed tomographic scanning of the thorax in the staging of bronchogenic carcinoma. N Engl J Med 1979; 300:777–778.

36. Lewis JW Jr, Madrazo BL, Gross SC, et al. The value of radiographic and computed tomography in the staging of lung carcinoma. Ann Thorac Surg 1982; 34:553–558.

37. Kirsh MM, Sloan H. Mediastinal metastases in bronchogenic carcinoma: influence of postoperative irradiation, cell type, and location. Ann Thorac Surg 1982; 33:459–463.

38. Jolly PC, Hutchinson CH, Detterbeck F, Guyton SW, Hofer B, Anderson RP. Routine computed tomographic scans, selective mediastinoscopy, and other factors in evaluation of lung cancer. J Thorac Cardiovasc Surg 1991; 102:266–270; discus.

39. Deschamps C, Pairolero PC, Trastek VF, Payne WS. Multiple primary lung cancers: results of surgical treatment. J Thorac Cardiovasc Surg 1990; 99:769–778.

40. McNeill TM, Chamberlain JM. Diagnostic anterior mediastinotomy. Ann Thorac Surg 1966; 2:532–539.

41. Ginsberg RJ, Rice TW, Goldberg M, Waters PF, Schmocker BJ. Extended cervical mediastinoscopy: a single staging procedure for bronchogenic carcinoma of the left upper lobe. J Thorac Cardiovasc Surg 1987; 94:673–678.

42. Daniels AC. A method of biopsy useful in diagnosing certain intrathoracic diseases. Dis Chest 1949; 16:360–367.

43. Brantigan JW, Brantigan CO, Brantigan OC. Biopsy of nonpalpable scalene lymph nodes in carcinoma of the lung. Am Rev Respir Dis 1974; 107:962.

44. Ferguson MK. Diagnosing and staging of non-small cell lung cancer. Hematol Oncol Clin North Am 1990; 4:1053–1068.

45. DeCamp MM Jr, Jaklitsch MT, Mentzer SJ, Harpole DH Jr, Sugarbaker DJ. The safety and versatility of video-thoracoscopy: a prospective analysis of 895 consecutive cases [see comments]. J Am Coll Surg 1995; 181:113–120.

46. Jaklitsch MT, DeCamp MM Jr, Liptay MJ, et al. Video-assisted thoracic surgery in the elderly. A review of 307 cases. Chest 1996; 110:751–758.

47. Mack MJ, Aronoff RJ, Acuff TE, Douthit MB, Bowman RT, Ryan WH. Present role of thoracoscopy in the diagnosis and treatment of diseases of the chest. Ann Thorac Surg 1992; 54:403–409.

48. Landreneau RJ, Mack MJ, Hazelrigg SR, et al. Video-assisted thoracic surgery: basic

technical concepts and intercostal approach strategies. Ann Thorac Surg 1992; 54: 800–807.

49.   Landreneau RJ, Hazelrigg SR, Mack MJ, et al. Thoracoscopic mediastinal lymph node sampling: useful for mediastinal lymph node stations inaccessible by cervical mediastinoscopy. J Thorac Cardiovasc Surg 1993; 106:554–558.

50.   Tisi GM, Friedman PJ, Peters RM, et al. Clinical staging of primary lung cancer. Am Rev Respir Dis 1983; 127:659–664.

Part Two

NON-SMALL-CELL LUNG CANCER

5

Role of Video-Assisted Thoracic Surgery in the Diagnosis and Treatment of Non-Small-Cell Lung Cancer

STEVEN J. MENTZER

Harvard Medical School
Brigham and Women's Hospital
Boston, Massachusetts

I.   Introduction

Recent advances in video optics and endoscopic instrumentation have led to changes in surgical approaches to diagnosis, staging, and treatment of non-small-cell cancer (NSCLC) of the lung. The most important illustration of these advances has been the practice of thoracoscopy. Thoracoscopy was initially described more than 70 years ago as a procedure for the lysis of intrathoracic adhesions and the drainage of pleural effusions (6,7). The poor optics and illumination techniques available at that time limited the procedure to the pleural space. In the past decade, advances in video optics and fiber-optic illumination has improved visualization of the intrathoracic cavity. The improved exposure has led to the development of a broad range of endoscopic instrumentation. Thoracoscopy is now applied in almost all areas of thoracic surgery.

Thoracoscopes are constructed at a variety of angles, permitting visualization of the entire hemithorax through a single access port. The currently available endoscopic instruments can fit through 8- to 12-mm ports in the chest wall. In

Supported in part by NIH grant HL47078.

addition to grasping endoscopic instrumentation, endoscopic staplers have been developed for stapling the lung parenchyma, bronchus, and vessels. Staplers currently in use range in length from 30 to 60 mm. In most cases, the 30- to 60-mm staplers are used for the lung parenchyma and 30- to 45-mm staplers are used for the pulmonary vessels. The recent development of reticulating staplers has minimized the need for additional access ports.

As with the development of any new area in surgery, the expanded repertoire has been accompanied by confusing terminology (10). VATS has been used to describe "video-assisted thoracoscopic surgery." VATS has also been used to describe "video-assisted thoracic surgery." MIVTS, or minimally invasive video-assisted thoracic surgery, reflects a variety of surgical approaches and instruments designed to minimize morbidity. As experience with the thoracoscope and endoscopic instruments grows, there is less formal distinction between the various forms of thoracoscopy and standard thoracic surgery. The thoracoscope and endoscopic instruments are being used in procedures involving standard thoracotomy (3). Similarly, standard thoracotomy instrumentation is being adapted to increase the repertoire of thoracoscopy. The result is expanded clinical options for the staging and treatment of patients with NSCLC.

II. Operative Principles

Video-assisted thoracic procedures generally require general anesthesia to control movement and breathing. General anesthesia also provides a convenient opportunity for bronchoscopy. For most patients, general anesthesia involves the placement of a double-lumen endotracheal tube. Double-lumen endotracheal tube permits ventilation of a single lung and deflation of the contralateral lung. The deflation of the ipsilateral lung results in improved visualization of the hemithorax.

The introduction of the thoracoscope into the hemithorax typically involves the use of an "access port." The port is usually 8 to 12 mm and permits the introduction of the thoracoscope and/or endoscopic instrumentation. After the application of an intercostal rib block for preemptive analgesia, the initial access port is placed in the seventh interspace anterior axillary line. This interspace is chosen in most patients because it is a wider intercostal space and its location low in the chest provides maximum flexibility. In addition, there is a lower chance of adhesions near the diaphragm and heart because of the movement in this area. The incision is made wide enough to admit an 8-mm thoracoscopy port. Using a 30° thoracoscope, this access port provides a panoramic view of the chest, including the diaphragm, hilum, mediastinum, chest wall, and superior sulcus. At the conclusion of routine thoracoscopic explorations of the chest, standard chest tubes are used to facilitate evacuation of pleural air during lung reinflation. In most cases, the chest tubes are removed in the operating room or in the recovery room. Patients are usually admitted for an overnight hospital stay.

III. Pleural Disease

Most pleural masses or malignant pleural effusions are diagnosed by cytology from thoracentesis or needle aspirates. The occasional malignant pleural process is recalcitrant to cytologic diagnosis. This pleural disease may be readily diagnosed with thoracoscopic exploration and biopsy. Thoracoscopy permits examination of the pleural space and directed pleural biopsies. An exploration of the pleural space occasionally demonstrates a discrete mass or pleural studding. In malignant lung processes with a prominent lymphatic component, pleural studding may be visualized on discrete areas of the visceral and parietal pleural surfaces. The areas of malignant studding are frequently limited to the area of the diseased lobe. A disease such as diffuse bronchoalveolar carcinoma may present with this localized pleural disease. The identification of pleural disease can provide a definitive diagnosis of stage IIIB carcinoma. In the case of malignant mesothelioma or lymphoma, pleural biopsy may be useful to obtain sufficient diagnostic material for a definite histologic diagnosis.

The interoperative diagnosis of malignant pleural disease can also be important therapeutically. In patients with large and persistent pleural effusions, thoracoscopy can provide a definitive intraoperative diagnosis. In these patients, immediate pleurodesis using talc can be performed. Intraoperative talc pleurodesis has several advantages. When the pleural fluid is evacuated under direct vision, there is no dilution effect and the talc powder can be evenly distributed over the pleural surfaces. Visualization of the hemithorax also permits optimal tube placement to facilitate reinflation to maximize drainage of any potential recurrent effusion. The use of general anesthesia also allows aggressive reinflation of the lung with positive pressure ventilation. Potential areas of lung "entrapment" can be assessed under positive pressure ventilation. In cases of tumor entrapment, a realistic assessment of the benefits of prolonged tube drainage can also be made. Doxycycline has been associated with extraordinary pleuritic discomfort and is rarely used in our institution. Bleomycin has also been associated with effective pleurodesis, but is used less frequently because of cost considerations.

IV. Solitary Nodule

Coin lesions in the lung are common presentations for patients with a thoracic malignancy. Coin lesions are defined as spherical lesions, <3 cm in diameter, present in the outer one-third of the lung. The relative risk that these nodules represent cancer varies with age and smoking history. When considering all patients, most coin lesions do not represent lung cancer (14,30).

Transthoracic needle biopsy has been advocated as a procedure of choice in patients with coin lesions (24). Transthoracic needle biopsy provides a diagnosis of malignancy in most cases of cancer. The morbidity of transthoracic needle biopsy is small with a <10% chance of pneumothorax in normal patients and a slightly higher risk in patients with emphysema (1,2,15,29,32). There are two basic limitations of transthoracic needle biopsy. First, transthoracic needle biopsies rarely are able to positively establish a benign diagnosis. Second, there is a small, but tangible, false-negative rate with transthoracic needle biopsies.

An alternative to transthoracic needle biopsies is thoracoscopic resection (3,12,13). A thoracoscopic resection of a solitary pulmonary nodule has the distinct advantage of avoiding a false-benign diagnosis. In contrast to transthoracic needle biopsy, thoracoscopy can positively establish a diagnosis of benign disease. The disadvantage of thoracoscopic resection is that it requires general anesthesia and an overnight stay in the hospital. The postoperative pain syndrome 10 days after thoracic surgery is associated with anterior numbness in the intercostal nerve distribution of the anterior thoracoscopy port. In addition, there is occasional focal incisional discomfort. In most patients, however, there is no respiratory limitation. The average visual analog scale pain score is 1.5 out of a possible 10 ten days after the surgery (Mentzer et al., in preparation).

Peripheral nodules in the lung can be resected safely even in high-risk patients. Thoracoscopy in elderly patients was studied in our institution (8). The morbidity of thoracoscopic resection was primarily limited to atrial arrhythmias. Chest wall discomfort may be decreased in patients with small stature and kyphosis because of the decreased intercostal space.

V. Surgical Staging

In addition to providing a tissue diagnosis, thoracoscopy can contribute to surgical staging (18). Frozen-section diagnosis of malignancy at the time of operation can provide an opportunity for aggressive surgical staging of the ipsilateral hemithorax. For example, a patient with a right upper lobe nodule that proves to be a NSCLC on frozen section can have simultaneous hilar and right peritracheal lymph node staging. The visceral and parietal pleura can be examined for studding. Any pleural fluid can be sent for cytologic evaluation. Since the first site of N2 nodal disease in a patient with a right upper lobe nodule is the right peritracheal lymph nodes (21), the area cephalad to the azygos vein (level 4R) can be readily assessed using the thoracoscope (25). Biopsies of the right lower (level 4R) and upper (2R) provides excellent staging of the lymphatic drainage of a right upper lobe nodule (22,28). A disadvantage of thoracoscopic staging, when compared to conventional cervical mediastinoscopy, is that it cannot effectively evaluate contralateral lymph node disease. This clinical situation would only be of concern in the event of so-called skip metastases (26). Skip metastases are felt to be unlikely in right-sided disease.

The pattern spread for right lower lobe lesions is generally the subcarinal space (22). The first site of N2 metastases is the peribronchial sump nodes that primarily drain to the subcarinal (level 7) lymph nodes (16,17). Metastases in the level 7 lymph nodes are generally followed by secondary metastases to the right lower peritracheal lymph nodes (level 4R) and upper right peritracheal lymph nodes (level 2R) (22). Although the peribronchial sump nodes are generally inaccessible to thoracoscopic biopsy, the lateral subcarinal (level 7) lymph nodes can be biopsied thoracoscopically. In most cases, level 7 lymph nodes can be biopsied on the medial border of the bronchus intermedius. Deeper lymph nodes in the subcarinal space are less accessible using thoracoscopy. Thoracoscopic dissection of the subcarinal space is limited by the presence of bronchial arteries that may result in late bleeding complications.

The lymph node drainage of left upper lobe nodules is to the aortopulmonary (AP) window (27). Lymph nodes in the AP window (level 5) are juxtaposed to the pulmonary artery. These lymph nodes may be large in the absence of metastases and generally require a histologic biopsy. A secondary site of left upper lobe nodule lymphatic drainage is the preaortic (level 6) lymph nodes (23). These lymph nodes are found at the base of innominate artery straddling the vagus and phrenic nerves. Both level 5 and level 6 lymph nodes are typically staged by anterior mediastinoscopy (also known as a Chamberlain procedure) (11). Anterior mediastinoscopy is typically performed within the mediastinal pleura (9). The mediastinoscope is advanced in the anatomic plain between the mediastinal structures and the mediastinal pleura. In many cases, the view of the AP window is limited by mediastinal fat. Transpleural mediastinoscopy is also possible, but the view of the AP window is limited by the mediastinal pleura. In most cases, the transpleural visualization of the AP window lymph nodes is best achieved by thoracoscopy.

An additional advantage of mediastinal staging by thoracoscopy is the improved view of the posterior hilum. Anterior mediastinotomy provides sampling of the typical level 5 and level 6 lymph nodes (17). Left lung cancers can also metastasize along the mainstem bronchus in the posterior mediastinum. This area is frequently inaccessible by mediastinoscopy as the posterior mediastinum may be several centimeters beyond the length of the typical mediastinoscope. The disadvantage of thoracoscopic staging of left upper lobe tumors is that the left-sided lymphatic development can be limited (25,26). Atrophic lymphatics along the trachea result in a significantly higher incidence of skip metastases to right-sided lymph nodes. Thoracoscopic evaluation of the left hilum and AP window does not evaluate this potential site of spread. Because of this limitation of thoracoscopy, cervical mediastinoscopy is commonly used to complement a thoracoscopic staging of the left hilar lymph nodes.

Left lower lobe nodules, similar to right lower lobe lesions, commonly metastasize to the subcarinal space (19,20,22). The presence of a lower lobe nodule presents comparable issues to those encountered in the right lower lobe. Thoracoscopic staging of the subcarinal space can be limited. In most lower lobe cancers, cervical mediastinoscopy provides a better sampling of the subcarinal space than does thoracoscopy.

VI. Anatomic Resections

An advantage of thoracoscopy in the evaluation of a peripheral lung lesion is that a definitive diagnosis can be obtained. In many cases, the histologic diagnosis of malignancy can facilitate a definitive resection during the same anesthetic. In patients in whom the diagnosis is ambiguous or further staging evaluation is required, definitive treatment can be deferred. Thoracoscopy provides flexibility in the decision to proceed with a definitive resection or wait for permanent histopathology because of the limited morbidity and short length of stay required for the procedure.

Definitive resections of lung cancers can include anatomic resections, such as segmentectomy or lobectomy. Recent evidence suggests that anatomic resections such as lobectomy have a lower local recurrence rate than wedge resection. Ginsberg and Rubinstein have shown that local recurrences are 2.5-fold higher in nonanatomic resections (5). Although mortality differences are small in this limited sample, anatomic resections are preferred in patients who have sufficient pulmonary function to tolerate an anatomic resection.

Anatomic resections can be performed with a video-assisted surgical technique. The differences between standard lobectomy and a thoracoscopic lobectomy have become less distinct in recent years. Thoracoscopic instruments have become commonplace in the resection of a lobe of the lung, even when performed through a standard thoracotomy. The improved visualization and smaller instruments have resulted in smaller incisions and less morbidity. The blurred distinction between standard and thoracoscopic instrumentation has led to some confusion regarding the precise nomenclature used to describe a lobectomy in which video optics and thoracoscopic instrumentation are used. We have used the term video-assisted thoracic surgery, or VATS, lobectomy to describe an anatomic resection that incorporates the thoracoscope and thoracoscopic instrumentation.

In most cases, the thoracoscope is used at the beginning of an operation to evaluate the hemithorax and the mediastinal lymph nodes. At the outset of the operation, the exploration of the chest is performed with two to three access ports. In any given case, given the completeness of the fissures and the location of the pulmonary arteries, the size of the incision, and the instruments used will vary. For example, the removal of an average adult lobe requires a 40-mm incision. In many cases, this incision is made at the outset of the operation and can be used to facilitate dissection of the vascular structures. In most upper lobectomies, the incision is placed on the lateral chest wall at the level of the axillary hair line. This level permits a view of the superior hilum and the early branches of the pulmonary artery. The incision for lower lobectomies is generally placed laterally over the major fissure to facilitate exposure of the pulmonary artery in the major fissure. A similar incision is used for middle lobectomies, although the incision is displaced slightly more anteriorly.

A common criticism of thoracoscopic lobectomies is that the hospital stay is determined by the air leak and not the size of the incision. In the early days of thoracoscopic instrumentation, instruments were limited in their ability to dissect complete fissures without a substantial air leak. The incomplete fissure has become less of an obstacle with the development of improved staplers such as the 60-mm endoscopic stapler.

Right lower lobectomies are performed with the larger incision over the major fissure. The 40-mm incision is typically placed anterior to the latissimus dorsi muscle. The incision is generally placed in the rib spaces, limiting the injury to the serratus anterior muscle. The sparing of both latissimus dorsi and serratus anterior muscle significantly limits postoperative muscle pain.

Left upper lobectomies are also performed through an axillary incision. The axillary incision provides a clear view of the initial branches of the proximal pulmonary artery. We do not use this approach for hilar tumors because of the limited length of extra pericardial pulmonary artery required for proximal vascular control. Left lower lobectomies are performed similar to right lower lobectomies.

A concern with thoracoscopic lobectomies is that the oncologic objectives of the procedure not be compromised by the small incisions. In general, thoracoscopic procedures are generally limited to patients with N0 disease. The thoracoscope facilitates exposure of the segmental (level 11) lymph nodes. Biopsies of the level 11 lymph nodes can provide intraoperative staging that can accurately classify patients as stage I or stage II. In patients with segmental nodal disease, an expanded incision is generally preferred to facilitate extensive mediastinal lymph node dissection and more accurate N2 staging. Another area in which thoracoscopic procedures are limited is the area of hilar tumors. Because of the necessity for safe proximal vascular control, thoracoscopic access ports can limit the vascular instruments used to control the hilum. We generally prefer wider exposure in hilar (T3) tumors.

A potential problem with thoracoscopic or video-assisted lobectomies is the problem of tumor implantation. Walsh and Nesbitt (31) and Downey et al. (4) have reported tumor implants in the area of the thoracoscopic incision. We routinely place the resected lung in an endoscopic bag before removing any nodule or lobe from the field. In our first 890 thoracoscopic resections, we had no episodes of tumor implantation (3).

VATS lobectomy has resulted in comparable operating times to open lobectomy. The video-assisted approach requires a slightly longer dissection time, especially in a teaching institution. This increased time in dissection is compensated by a faster closure. Despite the comparable operating times, VATS lobectomy may cost more at the present time because of the novelty of endoscopic instruments. In general, endoscopic instrumentation is more expensive and the staplers are uniquely designed for thoracoscopic application. We anticipate that operative costs will fall as VATS lobectomy becomes more commonplace.

In our initial series of VATS lobectomy, the initial length of hospital stay, as well as the duration of chest tubes, was no different whether the procedure was performed open or thoracoscopically. We anticipate that the length of hospital stay may decrease with time. Roberts has reported a decreased hospital stay (J. Roberts, in preparation). Perhaps more importantly, normal activities are resumed faster. This is the result of the limited muscular injury and the rapid mobilization of patients after surgery.

The morbidity of VATS lobectomy is less than with open thoracotomy procedures. The typical pain profile after a thoracoscopic surgery is characterized by localized bruising (S. Mentzer, in preparation). The intensity of the pain correlates with the size of the patient, suggesting the possibility that narrow interspaces are more readily bruised by the 10- to 12-mm thoracoscope. In addition, most patients report anterior numbness in the distribution of the terminal portion of the intercostal nerve. This is felt to be due to intercostal nerve trauma. Patients who have had thoracoscopic procedures, however, report much less latissimus dorsi muscle pain. In many patients with posterolateral thoracotomies, latissimus dorsi pain can be the dominant component of their postoperative morbidity.

The minimized chest wall muscular injury suggests improved postoperative function. Although we have not documented a significant difference in postoperative complications (8) less pain in the latissimus dorsi muscle would most likely result in less splinting of the chest wall and improved postoperative respiratory function. Limited postoperative pain may have some advantage in elderly patients or patients with compromised respiratory function.

References

1. Charig MJ, Stutley JE, Padley SP, Hansell DM. The value of negative needle biopsy in suspected operable lung cancer. Clin Radiol 1991; 44:147–149.
2. Collins CD, Breatnach E, Nath PH. Percutaneous needle biopsy of lung nodules following failed bronchoscopic biopsy. Eur J Radiol 1992; 15:49–53.
3. DeCamp MM Jr, Jaklitsch MT, Mentzer SJ, Harpole DH Jr, Sugarbaker DJ. The

safety and versatility of video-thoracoscopy: a prospective analysis of 895 consecutive cases. J Am Coll Surg 1995; 181:113–120.

4. Downey RJ, McCormack P, LoCicero J III. Dissemination of malignant tumors after video-assisted thoracic surgery: a report of twenty-one cases. Video-Assisted Thoracic Surgery Study Group. J Thorac Cardiovasc Surg 1996; 111:954–960.

5. Ginsberg RJ, Rubinstein LV. Randomized trial of lobectomy versus limited resection for T1 N0 non-small cell lung cancer. Lung Cancer Study Group. Ann Thorac Surg 1995; 60:615–622; discussion 622–623.

6. Jacobaeus HC. The cauterization of adhesions in pneumothorax treatment of tuberculosis. Surg Gynecol Obstet 1921; 33:493–500.

7. Jacobaeus HC. The practical importance of thoracoscopy in surgery of the chest. Surg Gynecol Obstet 1922; 34:289–296.

8. Jaklitsch MT, DeCamp MM Jr, Liptay MJ, et al. Video-assisted thoracic surgery in the elderly. A review of 307 cases. Chest 1996; 110:751–758.

9. Jolly PC. Anterior mediastinoscopy for evaluation of mediastinal metastases of cancer of the left lung. South Med J 1982; 75:1487–1490.

10. McKneally MF, Lewis RJ, Anderson RJ, et al. Statement of the AATS/STS Joint Committee on Thoracoscopy and Video Assisted Thoracic Surgery. J Thorac Cardiovasc Surg 1992; 104:1.

11. McNeill TM, Chamberlain JM. Diagnostic anterior mediastinotomy. Ann Thorac Surg 1966; 2:532–539.

12. Mentzer SJ. Mediastinoscopy, thoracoscopy, and video-assisted thoracic surgery in the diagnosis and staging of lung cancer. Hematol Oncol Clin North Am 1997; 11:435–447.

13. Mentzer SJ, DeCamp MM, Harpole DH Jr, Sugarbaker DJ. Thoracoscopy and video-assisted thoracic surgery in the treatment of lung cancer. Chest 1995; 107:298S–301S.

14. Miller DL, Allen MS, Deschamps C, Trastek VF, Pairolero PC. Video-assisted thoracic surgical procedure: management of a solitary pulmonary nodule. Mayo Clin Proc 1992; 67:462–464.

15. Morcos SK. The value of negative needle biopsy in suspected operable lung cancer. Clin Radiol 1992; 45:68.

16. Mountain CF. Revisions in the International System for Staging Lung Cancer. Chest 1997; 111:1710–1717.

17. Mountain CF, Dresler CM. Regional lymph node classification for lung cancer staging. Chest 1997; 111:1718–1723.

18. Naruke T, Asamura H, Kondo H, Tsuchiya R, Suemasu K. Thoracoscopy for staging of lung cancer. Ann Thorac Surg 1993; 56:661–663.

19. Naruke T, Suemasu K, Ishikawa S. Lymph node mapping and curability at various levels of metastasis in resected lung cancer. J Thorac Cardiovasc Surg 1978; 76:832–839.

20. Naruke T, Suemasu K, Ishikawa S. Surgical treatment for lung cancer with metastasis to mediastinal lymph nodes. J Thorac Cardiovasc Surg 1976; 71:279–285.

21. Nohl-Oser HC. The evolution and present status of mediastinoscopy. Endoscopy 1979; 11:1–4.

22. Nohl-Oser HC. An investigation of the anatomy of the lymphatic drainage of the lungs as shown by the lymphatic spread of bronchial carcinoma. Ann R Coll Surg Engl 1972; 51:157–176.

23. Patterson GA, Piazza D, Pearson FG, et al. Significance of metastatic disease in subaortic lymph nodes. Ann Thorac Surg 1987; 43:155–159.

24. Penketh AR, Robinson AA, Barker V, Flower CD. Use of percutaneous needle biopsy in the investigation of solitary pulmonary nodules. Thorax 1987; 42:967–971.

25. Riquet M, Dupont P, Hidden G, Debesse B. Mediastinal lymphatic pathways of the azygos and aortic arches: injection based on segments of the adult lung. Surg Radiol Anat 1991; 13:149–152.

26. Riquet M, Hidden G, Debesse B. Direct lymphatic drainage of lung segments to the mediastinal nodes. An anatomic study on 260 adults. J Thorac Cardiovasc Surg 1989; 97:623–632.

27. Rouviere H. Anatomie des Lymphatiques de L'Homme. Paris: Libraires de L'Academie de Medicine, 1932.

28. Sarin CL, Nohl-Oser HC. Mediastinoscopy: a clinical evaluation of 400 consecutive cases. Thorax 1969; 24:585–588.

29. Sokolowski JW Jr, Burgher LW, Jones FL Jr, Patterson JR, Selecky PA. Guidelines for percutaneous transthoracic needle biopsy. This position paper of the American Thoracic Society was adopted by the ATS Board of Directors, June 1988. Am Rev Respir Dis 1989; 140:255–256.

30. Swensen SJ, Jett JR, Payne WS, Viggiano RW, Pairolero PC, Trastek VF. An integrated approach to evaluation of the solitary pulmonary nodule. Mayo Clin Proc 1990; 65:173–186.

31. Walsh GL, Nesbitt JC. Tumor implants after thoracoscopic resection of a metastatic sarcoma. Ann Thorac Surg 1995; 59:215–216.

32. Zakowski MF, Gatscha RM, Zaman MB. Negative predictive value of pulmonary fine needle aspiration cytology. Acta Cytol 1992; 36:283–286.

6

Non-Small-Cell Lung Cancer: Surgery for Stage I and II Disease

MALCOLM M. DeCAMP, JR. and RAJA M. FLORES

Harvard Medical School
Brigham and Women's Hospital
Boston, Massachusetts

I. Introduction

Perhaps the greatest challenge in the treatment of non-small-cell lung cancer (NSCLC) is identifying patients at a period in their disease course when resection has the greatest chance of resulting in cure. Of all patients who initially present with lung cancer, 55% are found to have distant metastasis, 30% to have regional spread, and only 15% have tumor confined to the lung amenable to curative resection (1). The reasons for the low percentage of patients presenting with "early" disease, stage I and II, are that most of these patients are asymptomatic and routine screening of patients at risk is not encouraged. Usually stage I and II disease patients are identified by incidental findings on chest radiographs obtained during evaluation of other medical problems or as part of a preoperative, preprocedure, or employment insurance screening routine. Early-stage lesions are usually asymptomatic because of their peripheral location; however, when located centrally in the bronchial tree, some may produce hemoptysis, cough, or a postobstructive pneumonia. Vigilant surveillance of patients at risk and improved methods of early detection are needed in order to identify more early staged patients when resection offers the greatest chance of cure.

Anatomic resection is the treatment of choice for stage I and II NSCLC. The most common procedure performed is lobectomy. However, bilobectomy or even pneumonectomy may be required depending on the precise location of the tumor. Lesser resections such as segmentectomy or wedge resection may be performed as a compromise procedure in patients with poor lung function. Lobectomy is regarded as the minimally acceptable procedure resecting an adequate amount of parenchyma and associated intrapulmonary lymph nodes in patients with sufficient pulmonary reserve; lesser resections are associated with a higher local recurrence rate.

II. Diagnosis: The Solitary Pulmonary Nodule

Early-stage NSCLC most commonly presents as an asymptomatic, radiographically defined abnormality. The solitary pulmonary nodule (SPN) is usually defined as a well-circumscribed, round lesion <3 cm in diameter surrounded by lung parenchyma without bronchial obstruction. The definition of an SPN does not differentiate between a benign or malignant origin, and the burden of proof usually falls upon the clinician. Other presenting patterns may be less well defined densities or infiltrates that fail to respond or incompletely respond to therapy for pulmonary infections. Most patients are asymptomatic and lesions are identified incidentally on routine chest radiographs and computed tomography (CT). CT may be helpful in determining certain benign lesions. For example, a lesion with a popcornlike calcification is highly suggestive of a hamartoma. However, CT, per se, does not rule out carcinoma, and additional means are necessary to obtain a definitive diagnosis.

When patients are found to have an SPN or residual radiographic abnormality after treatment, an aggressive diagnostic workup should be embarked upon to determine if the nodule is malignant. In assessing an SPN, one must take into account patient history; risk factors such as smoking, pulmonary function, or medical comorbidities; and the availability and comparison of previous radiologic examinations. The consequences of observing or resecting a potential cancer and the risk: benefit ratio of the diagnostic procedure chosen must be considered. Methods of diagnosing an SPN include needle aspiration, transbronchial biopsy, thoracoscopic lung biopsy and open lung biopsy. Each diagnostic procedure has associated morbidity and differing diagnostic yields. The potential complications of the diagnostic procedure must be weighed against the influence of surgical intervention on the natural history of the disease process. For example, if one believes that surgery has no direct effect on overall survival, then the added risks of a diagnositic procedure are unnecessary. However, most physicians believe that surgery offers the best potential for cure in patients with stage I and II disease. If a patient has the potential to tolerate a curative surgical procedure (i.e., lobectomy or pneumonectomy), most clinicians would pursue an invasive diagnostic procedure to determine if an SPN is malignant.

The advent of video-assisted thoracic surgery (VATS) has obviated the need for thoracotomy in many cases. A VATS procedure is a thoracoscopic approach with the addition of an 8-cm utility incision without the use of major muscle transection, rib resection, or a rib spreader. We have reported on 360 nodulectomies using the VATS method. Of these procedures, 147 (40%) were benign and 213 (60%) were malignant (2). However, if diagnosis cannot be made via VATS, then one must proceed to a standard thoracotomy.

III. Staging
A. Remote Metastatic Survey

Lung cancer has the proclivity to metastasize to the brain, liver, adrenal glands, and skeletal system. In patients with early-stage disease, the routine use of CT scan to evaluate the presence of brain lesions is debatable and is not clearly supported in the literature. Surgeons do agree that patients with neurologic signs and symptoms should undergo CNS imaging with either contrast-enhanced head CT or MRI. However, controversy exists over the routine use of head CT in asymptomatic patients from a cost effectiveness viewpoint (3). The sensitivity of multiorgan scanning for metastatic disease in patients with lung cancer without systemic symptoms has been reported as low as 0.78% (4). Recently, Ferrigno et al. performed a retrospective study of 184 patients with lung cancer (5). Of the 25 patients with positive head CT scans, 16 were asymptomatic. In addition, 10% of patients with brain metastasis were found to have resectable lesions. Based on their results, they conclude that routine head CT scanning is appropriate and cost-effective in staging patients with lung cancer. We do not routinely obtain head CT scans on asymptomatic patients with small peripheral lesions. However, patients with central tumors, large tumors, or any hint of symptomatology will undergo head CT evaluation.

A complete chest CT evaluation should routinely include the upper abdomen in order to identify metastasis to the contralateral lung, liver, and adrenal glands. Identification of distant metastasis is usually a contraindication to surgery. Adrenal metastasis is noted in approximately 15% of lung cancer patients (6). However, the finding of a solitary adrenal mass requires histologic confirmation via fine-needle aspiration. Since 3% to 5% of the general population have a benign cortical adenoma as an incidental finding, its presence would not preclude curative resection (7).

Skeletal metastasis should be identified prior to subjecting patients to curative surgery. Most patients with bony metastasis present with pain, point tenderness, elevated serum calcium, and increased alkaline phosphatase. Michel et al. performed a prospective study of 110 patients with clinical indicators of skeletal metastasis (8). The relationship of positive clinical indicators to positive bone-scan results demonstrated a sensitivity of 100% for identifying metastatic lesions in patients with clinical indicators but a specificity of 54%. They concluded that bone-scan studies obtained during the initial clinical evaluation of patients with NSCLC should be limited to symptomatic patients. The high rate of false-positive bone-scan results reduces its utility as a routine preoperative procedure and may subject many patients to an array of unnecessary additional examinations. Until a more specific test is identified, bone scans should be limited to symptomatic patients with otherwise clinical stage I and II NSCLC.

Positron emission tomography (PET) has emerged as an exciting new imaging modality useful in evaluating distant metastases in patients with lung cancer. PET allows for the identification of areas of intense glucose uptake (metabolically active tumor) throughout the body with a single scan (9). Cost as well as limited scanner availability has hindered its widespread application. Resolution of smaller (<1 cm) foci of abnormal activity remains a technical shortcoming.

B. Locoregional Staging

In patients with early-stage lung cancer, CT is performed routinely to assess resectability, tumor size, involvement of surrounding structures, and metastatic disease. Locoregional lymph node staging helps to identify patients who would not benefit from immediate surgical resection. The specific role of CT scanning in the evaluation of mediastinal lymph nodes and the role of routine mediastinoscopy for early-stage lung cancer are controversial and extensively reviewed (see chapters on Radiology and Staging). Accurate surgical staging of the mediastinum whether by mediastinoscopy or lymphadenectomy at the time of resection is vital when evaluating outcomes from different centers or trials. As neoadjuvant approaches for earlier-stage NSCLC are found to be feasible and/or efficacious, preresectional surgical/pathologic staging will become even more critical.

The sensitivity and specificity of CT scan and MRI in the detection of mediastinal disease varies from study to study. A literature review performed by members of the Lung Cancer Study Group found the sensitivity range from 70% to 90% and the specificity range from 60% to 90% (10). When CT scan or MRI failed to demonstrate enlarged lymph nodes, the risk of identifying a positive N2 node at surgery was 15%. Lymph nodes between 2 and 4 cm defined by CT scan were without evidence of metastasis 37% of the time and found to be hyperplastic (11). Many factors may account for the discrepancies between studies. These include variables such as type of scanner, differences in image acquisition technique, small lymph nodes at an early stage of tumor invasion, large lymph nodes without tumor involvement, and differing radiologist opinions as to what constitutes a suspicious node. Therefore, patients with normal-size lymph nodes cannot be definitively diagnosed as having early-stage disease, and patients with enlarged lymph nodes should not automatically be classified as inoperable.

PET scanning has also been utilized to assess for metabolically active metastatic disease in the mediastinum. Scott and co-workers found this imaging technique to be both sensitive and specific in evaluating N2 and N3 disease is patients with new or suspected lung cancer (12). More recently, PET has been used in a semiquantitative fashion to look at specific metabolic pathways in the primary tumor (13). Investigators from Duke University demonstrated prognostic significance for PET when the amount of fluorodeoxyglucose uptake in the primary lung tumor was measured in 155 patients with NSCLC. Standard uptake ratios of >10 (adjusted for the dose injected and the patient's weight) predicted decreased survival independent of tumor size or stage (14).

CT or MRI and perhaps PET should be used as a road map to guide mediastinoscopy rather than in lieu of surgery. CT scan and MRI may identify enlarged or suspicious nodes and help direct surgical sampling. CT scan may also identify calcified lymph nodes so that extra caution may be exercised when performing biopsy. CT scan and MRI are also useful in identifying anatomic variations which may increase the risk of complication in performing surgery such as anomalous vessels and cardiac abnormalities (15).

IV. Defining Early-Stage Disease

A. Stage I

1. IA

The newly revised staging system makes its largest changes in the subset groupings of stage I and stage II disease (16). Stage I lung cancer has been subdivided into stage IA (T1N0M0) and stage IB (T2N0M0) because of the statistically significant difference in survival at 5 years between patients with small (T1) and those with larger, central, or pleural invasive tumors (T2) (Figs. 1–3) (17,18). In Mountain's series, patients with stage IA lesions enjoyed a 67% 5-year survival whereas stage IB patients had only a 57% 5-year survival (16). These refinements provide for a more precise staging system that permits a more accurate prediction of survival and a better-defined and reproducible means of comparing results from different institutions.

T1N0M0 lesions are small (<3 cm), peripheral tumors completely surrounded by lung without metastases or pleural invasion. Many of these stage IA cancers present as asymptomatic SPNs. In a patient with a suspicious nodule found on chest radiogaph, a complete history and physical and a thorough search for previous chest radiographs are essential for appropriate management. If the stability of such a lesion remains in doubt, other diagnostic procedures such as fine-needle aspiration and transbronchial bronchoscopy under flourocoscopic guidance may be helpful. The lack of a definitive diagnosis should not deter the timely performance of surgery as a diagnostic and potentially therapeutic maneu-

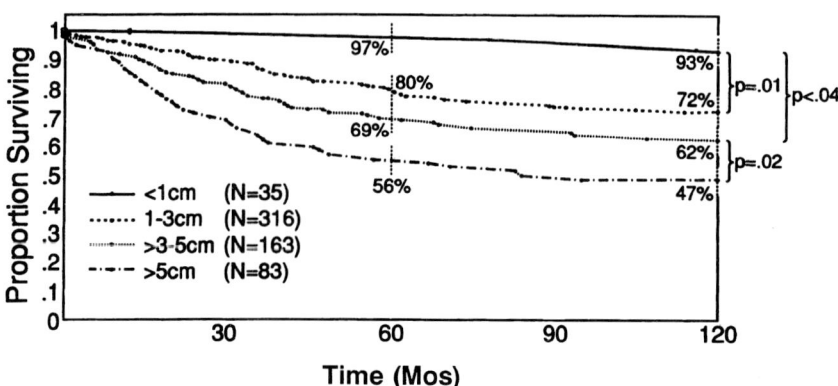

Figure 1 Survival by tumor size in centimeters in patients with negative lymph nodes. (From Ref. 17.)

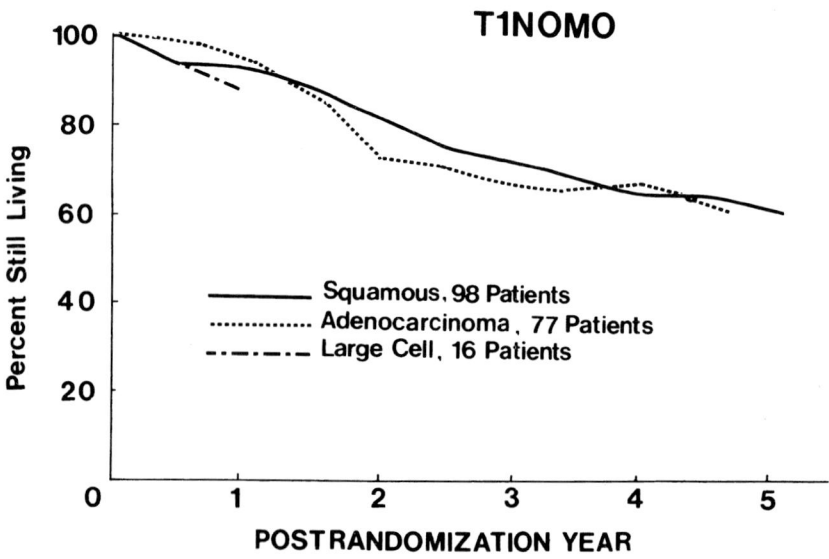

Figure 2 Survival curves of patients with T1N0M0 disease by cell type. (From Ref. 18.)

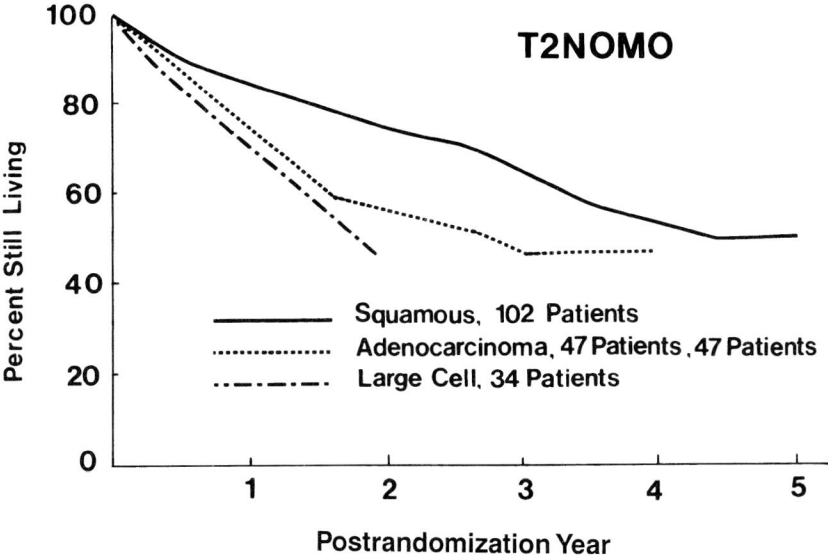

Figure 3 Survival curves of patients with T2N0M0 disease by cell type. (From Ref. 18.)

ver, especially in a patient with any significant smoking history. The surgical options for approaching these lesions will be discussed later in this chapter.

2. IB

The revised staging system defines a higher-risk stage I subpopulation (IB disease) appropriate for adjuvant or even neoadjuvant clinical trials. T2N0M0 lesions are larger than 3 cm and confined to the pulmonary parenchyma, are lesions invading the visceral pleura regardless of size, or are lesions within a lobar bronchus or in the main stem bronchus at least 2 cm distal to the carina. Lobectomy is the procedure of choice in these cases. However, wedge resection or segmentectomy may be performed in patients with compromised pulmonary function who are unable to tolerate lobectomy. Lesions traversing the major fissure require pneumonectomy. When faced with proximal bronchial lesions, one should always consider the possibility of performing a bronchoplastic or sleeve resection because the reimplanted lobe functions normally and contributes significantly to preservation of overall pulmonary function without compromising surgical oncologic standards.

The common denominator in stage I disease is N0 status. Node-negative disease must be confirmed by systematic surgical evaluation of the mediastinum either by preresectional mediastinoscopy or intraoperative nodal dissection to exclude occult N2 disease. Rigorous pathologic review of resected parenchyma is necessary to exclude N1 disease.

B. Stage II

1. IIA

The new staging system subdivides stage II into stage IIA, T1N1M0 with survival of 55% at 5 years; and IIB, T2N1M0 and T3N0M0 with survival of 39% at 5 years (16). Surgical resection is the current primary treatment of choice for patients with disease in this stage. Surgery for stage II cancer involves an en bloc resection of the primary tumor with hilar, interlobar, lobar, and segmental lymph nodes and a systematic dissection of the mediastinal lymph nodes to exclude unsuspected N2 disease. Surgery followed by adjuvant radiotherapy for patients with N1 nodal involvement has been shown to decrease locoregional recurrence at best, but over-all survival is unchanged when compared to surgery alone (19).

2. IIB

In patients with T3N0M0 lesions, resection of involved tissues including the bony chest wall, diaphragm, or soft tissues of the mediastinum with the primary tumor is the accepted standard of care (20,21). If a tumor invades chest wall, diaphragm, pericardium, superior sulcus, or mediastinum, resection should be performed en bloc to avoid the potential for tumor spillage. Such en bloc removal provides the greatest chance of cure because the major factor impacting survival is complete resection. Radiation therapy has traditionally been used prior to resection in chest wall-invasive, clinically node-negative tumors. The strategy has been to enhance resectability and decrease the risk of intraoperative tumor dissemination. Because of the relative paucity of such T3N0 patients, no large, randomized trials validating the efficacy of the approach have been done. An intergroup Phase II feasibility trial of induction chemoradiation for superior sulcus tumors (non-N2) has completed accrual but has yet to be reported.

C. Occult Lung Carcinoma

An occult lung cancer is not radiologically apparent and places patients with it in a special category. They may be considered Tx or Tis from the standpoint of the staging system. They comprise 1% of patients presenting with lung cancer (22,23). The diagnosis is usually made by sputum cytology or bronchoscopy in patients who have presented with hemoptysis or persistent cough and a normal chest radiograph. Fluorescene bronchoscopy has been helpful in locating the abnormal epithelium and allowing for directed biopsy to assess for true invasion (24). Most lesions are centrally located, and if a discrete invasive lesion can be defined, surgical treatment usually requires lobectomy or pneumonectomy. Due to the anatomic location and small tumor size of these lesions, sleeve resections are often performed to preserve lung function. Surgical treatment is curative in this subset of patients. Martini reports no recurrences after resection for such lesions with follow-up periods of >20 years (25). The risk of developing a new primary lung cancer may be as high as 45% (25). For patients with positive cytology but no defined primary lesion, careful follow-up with surveillance bronchoscopy and contrast-enhanced CT imaging every 4 to 6 months is encouraged.

V. Approach to Resection

Surgery is generally considered the standard treatment for patients with stage I and II NSCLC. Most physicians agree that surgery offers the best chance of cure in patients with early disease. The National Screening Study compared 5-year survival in patients with an early diagnosis of lung cancer undergoing surgery versus survival of patients with similar disease undergoing alternative treatment. There were no survivors at 5 years without surgical intervention (26). Although alternative treatments have been given with curative intent, the results have proven inferior to surgical resection. In patients with operable lung cancer treated by radiotherapy alone, 5-year survival rates of 6% have been reported (27). The outcome of patients with early-stage NSCLC treated by chemotherapy alone is unknown.

Complete resection is the ultimate goal of surgery for bronchogenic carcinoma. For early-stage disease, it remains one of the factors most closely linked with prolonged survival. The exact amount of lung tissue to be removed in order to provide the maximal chance of cure has been debated. The various procedures used to resect lung cancers include lobectomy, sleeve lobectomy, bilobectomy, pneumonectomy, segmentectomy, and wedge resection.

A. Standard Anatomic Resection

1. Lobectomy

An anatomic lobectomy is performed for lesions arising within the boundaries of a discrete lung lobe. It requires the meticulous dissection of the branch pulmonary arteries to the lobe and the draining pulmonary veins. Hilar and lobar nodes and associated lymphatics are stripped along the lobar bronchus toward the parenchyma being resected to allow for their en bloc removal with the tumor.

Lobectomy is the smallest excisional procedure recommended for cancer patients with acceptable postoperative pulmonary reserve and disease limited to a single lobe. A predicted postoperative FEV_1 of ≥ 0.8 L is generally viewed as adequate to allow lobectomy (28). Patients with spirometric values less than this may be considered on an individual basis. Formal preoperative cardiopulmonary exercise testing may allow better perioperative risk assessment in the otherwise severely obstructed or restricted pulmonary patient (29). The absolute low end of acceptable pulmonary function is unclear and depends on a variety of factors including the size and location of the mass, which lobe is to be resected, and the lifestyle, motivation, and overall physiologic reserve of the patient.

2. Sleeve Lobectomy

Bronchoplastic resections were introduced into the therapeutic arsenal for lung cancer in the 1950s (30). The operations involve resecting an entire lung lobe with a circumferential portion of the main bronchus with subsequent anastomosis of the distal airway to the more proximal main stem bronchus. They were initially utilized and are still advocated for patients with central, clinically node-negative lesions whose spirometric reserve would not tolerate pneumonectomy. By reconnecting seemingly unaffected distal lung parenchyma, the surgeon achieves the oncologic goal of anatomic lobar resection while maintaining adequate ventilatory capacity for the patient. Any of the five lung lobes are amenable to sleeve resection, though upper lobectomies (right > left) dominate most clinical series. Over the past 20 years, nearly 2000 sleeve lobectomies have been reported, with operative mortalities ranging between 0% and 11% (average 5.6%). Actual 5-year survival reported for this heterogeneous, mostly clinically staged group of patients ranges from 17% to 64% (31). Refinements in operative technique and anesthetic management now make bronchoplastic resections the procedure of choice when anatomically feasible for any proximal lesion. Sleeve resections are routinely associated with lower death and complication rates as compared to the operative mortality and morbidity reported in most pneumonectomy series.

3. Bilobectomy

Bilobectomy may be performed on the right lung by removing either the right upper and middle lobes (5/10 segments) or the right lower and middle lobes (7/10 segments). Traditionally, this was not considered a compromise procedure because it obeyed the oncologic principle of complete resection of all parenchymal segments and associated draining lymphatics of the lobes involved with tumor. Patients with both stage I and II tumor have undergone this procedure. However, Massard et al. reported a higher local recurrence rate following bilobectomy than was seen following pneumonectomy in patients with stage I disease. No such difference was demonstrated in patients with stage II disease (32). More retrospective studies are necessary to determine the validity of this study and the necessity of a prospective randomized trial.

4. Pneumonectomy

Pneumonectomy is the complete excision of an entire lung including ligation and division of either the right or left main pulmonary artery, both ipsilateral pulmonary veins as they enter the left atrium, and the main bronchus flush with the main carina. This can be accomplished either outside the pericardium or if tumor/nodal bulk dictates from within the pericardial sac. Patient disease settings which may require a pneumonectomy include proximal involvement of the right or left main pulmonary artery; tumor or lymph node encasement of the pulmonary artery within the fissure; tumor involvement of upper and lower lobes of the lung; or extensive involvement of the main stem bronchi when a sleeve resection is not possible. Pneumonectomy generally carries a higher risk of perioperative death and complication than do lesser lung cancer resections. The Lung Cancer Study Group clearly demonstrated the higher mortality for pneumonectomy over lobectomy across multiple experienced centers (33). Harpole and colleagues from Brigham and Women's Hospital (Boston) showed pneumonectomy to be an independent predictor for postoperative complications and extended hospital stay (34).

The complete extent of lung involvement with tumor can always be misjudged preoperatively. Therefore, most patients undergoing thoracotomy for lung cancer should be assessed for their suitability for or tolerability of pneumonectomy. The evaluation usually requires pulmonary function testing to demonstrate a predicted postoperative FEV_1 of at least 0.8 L (28). Preoperative bronchoscopy, quantitative radionucleide ventilation-perfusion lung scanning, and formal cardiopulmonary exercise testing may also help define a patient's ability to tolerate pneumonectomy (29).

B. Lesser and Nonanatomic Resections

In patients with N1 or N0 disease, complete resection can be performed without removing the entire involved lobe. The Lung Cancer Study Group performed a randomized trial comparing lobectomy to lesser resections in treating T1N0 NSCLC lesions. The limited resection patient group had a 50% increase in the rate of death from cancer and a threefold increase in the locoregional recurrence rate when compared to the lobectomy group (35). The lesser resection cohort also experienced a 30% increase in the mortality rate from all causes. This surprising difference cannot be linked to comorbidities in the segment/wedge group because the randomized schema of the trial should have distributed these factors evenly between the two treatment groups.

1. Segmentectomy

Segmentectomy is usually reserved for patients with poor pulmonary function. The procedure allows removal of the lymphatic channels and lymph nodes of the discrete bronchopulmonary segment draining the tumor bed. As such, segmentectomy represents a middle ground, preserving the principles of resecting the draining lymph structures but allowing preservation of some portion of the involved lobe. A proper segmentectomy involves the complete dissection, ligation, and division of the segmental branch(es) of the PA, draining PV branches, and segmental bronchi. It is possible to resect each of the 19 bronchopulmonary segments, though composite resections of one to four segments are common. Prior to segmentectomy, a complete bronchoscopic examination must be performed. The segmental bronchial anatomy and changes in the mucosa must be thoroughly assessed. If extrinsic compression or a visible tumor is identified within the segmental bronchus, then segmentectomy is contraindicated. The Lung Cancer Study Group reported a recurrence rate per person-year of 0.020 for lobectomy and 0.044 for segmental resection (35). However, when segmentectomy was compared to nonanatomic resection (rate per person-year of 0.086), there appeared to be a lower rate of local recurrence with segmentectomy (35).

Warren and colleagues reported their results of segmentectomy versus lobectomy in 169 patients with lung cancer (36). When tumors of all sizes were considered, a statistically significant improvement in survival was observed in patients undergoing lobectomy when compared to survival of patients who underwent segmental resection ($P = .035$). In this retrospective study, the survival difference was attributed to the observation that patients with marginal cardiopulmonary reserve were more likely to undergo a segmental resection and more likely to die of causes other than cancer in 5 years. There was no statistically significant difference observed in survival when lobectomy was compared to segmental resection in patients with tumors of <3 cm. It is possible that this observation resulted from an adequate surgical removal of the lymphatic drainage and a lower predilection for smaller diameter tumors to involve lymphatic channels. The Warren study did demonstrate an increase in the rate of locoregional recurrence after segmentectomy 15/66 (22.7%) when compared to lobectomy 5/103 (4.9%); however, no P value was reported (36).

2. Wedge or Nonanatomic Resection

A nonanatomic resection is commonly referred to as a wedge resection. The procedure is usually performed on patients with poor lung function unable to tolerate lobectomy. The resection removes a particular lesion with 2 cm (varies if the lung is inflated or atelectatic) of surrounding normal lung tissue to obtain a negative resection margin. The surrounding lung parenchyma is excised, usually with stapling devices, with minimal regard for anatomic detail or lymphatic drainage. The procedure may be performed utilizing a VATS technique facilitated by endoscopic staplers or by standard thoracotomy using conventional instruments and staplers.

Wedge resection must be considered a compromise procedure, regardless of the size or stage of the tumor. The Lung Cancer Study Group performed a prospective randomized trial in which segmentectomy and wedge resection were compared to lobectomy. When limited resection (segmentectomy and wedge) was compared to lobectomy, a statistically significant increase in recurrence rate was observed in the limited resection group of patients (35). The threefold increase in locoregional recurrence when limited resection was compared to lobectomy was associated with a two-sided *P* value of .008 (37). When lobectomy was compared to wedge resection alone, a locoregional recurrence rate per person-year of 0.020 for lobectomy was observed, and a 0.086 recurrence per person-year for wedge resection. There was marginal difference in survival ($P = .08$) demonstrated when lobectomy was compared to limited resection (35).

Older published series report results from uncontrolled studies and are confounded by the addition of postoperative radiotherapy. Surgery plus radiotherapy is currently being evaluated in a Phase II Cancer and Leukemia Group B (CALGB)-led intergroup study to determine the feasibility of treating high-risk patients with cardiopulmonary dysfunction and T1 peripheral NSCLC by VATS with adjuvant radiotherapy. All patients in this protocol undergo video-assisted wedge resection. Those who have a complete resection receive local radiotherapy to 56 Gy (cone down). Patients who have an incomplete resection (positive microscopic margins) receive local radiotherapy to 66 Gy. Secondary objectives of this protocol include identification of locoregional recurrence, feasibility of complete resection and ipsilateral lymph node sampling, rate of conversion to open thoracotomy, and complications associated with radiotherapy after VATS.

C. Route of Resection

1. Thoracotomies

a. Anterior

An anterolateral thoracotomy is performed with the patient in the 30° to 40° forward decubitus position. The incision is made over the fourth or fifth interspace in the inframammary crease extending from the midaxillary line to the sternum. The pectoralis muscle must be divided to gain access to the interspace. Exposure of the posterior hilum and hemithorax is limited compared to a posterolateral thoracotomy. However, exposure is excellent for performing a right middle lobectomy or lingulectomy, and improved cardiopulmonary function can be expected with this approach (38).

b. Lateral or Posterolateral

In lung cancer surgery, a posterolateral thoracotomy is the most frequently used approach, offering excellent exposure. The patient is placed in the lateral decubitus position. The incision is placed several centimeters below the tip of the scapula. The latissimus dorsi muscle and serratus anterior muscle are divided. This approach provides optimal exposure of the mediastinum, chest wall, diaphragm, lung, and hilar stuctures (38). If greater exposure is necessary, the lower portion of the trapezius and the rhomboid muscle may be divided in the posterior aspect of the wound. The thorax is entered through the fourth or fifth intercostal space to adequately dissect the hilum. Ribs can either be completely resected or shingled, or the costotransverse ligament can be divided from within the thorax. Each of these maneuvers enhances exposure and minimizes the risk of painful rib fracture.

c. Muscle-Sparing Incisions

A muscle-sparing thoracotomy can be performed through a posterolateral, transverse axillary or vertical incision. Hilar exposure via the fourth or fifth interspace is usually adequate. The posterior or lateral approaches usually involve division of the latissimus dorsi muscle while preserving the integrity of the serratus anterior muscle; the tranverse or verticle axillary incisions allow both muscles to be spared (39,40). The theoretical benefits of the latter are less pain and improved early pulmonary function. Lateral or serratus-sparing incisions can always be extended or converted to a formal thoracotomy to enhance exposure. In contrast, axillary incisions are not easily extended and should be reserved for the resection of smaller or less bulky tumors. Carefully constructed comparative trials of standard thoracotomy to these muscle-sparing techniques are lacking in the literature.

d. Median Sternotomy

A median sternotomy is also a muscle-sparing incision which provides bilateral access to the pleural space and anterior hila. It is most frequently performed to address bilateral pulmonary lesions though some surgeons use the approach routinely in their treatment of resectable bronchogenic carcinoma. Patients often report less postoperative pain than experienced after thoracotomy, presumably because very little muscle is divided. However, the access allowed by median sternotomy provides poor exposure of the left lower lobe, either posterior hilum, and posterior pleural space. Difficulty is also encountered with this procedure when excising posterior mediastinal lymph nodes (41,42).

2. Video-Assisted Thoracic Surgery (VATS)

This contemporary approach utilizes several advances in modern technology including xenon light sources, fiber optics, and chip camera technology to provide a magnified view of the pleural space similar if not superior to that afforded by standard thoracotomy. The VATS procedure is usually performed under video-endoscopic visualization through three seperately placed port sites and an optional 6- to 8-cm "access" thoracotomy without rib resection or retraction. In addition to wedge resections, major resections, including lobectomy (43,44), have been performed with this method. However, many of the presumed advantages of the VATS approach remain unproven in the treatment of lung cancer, and controlled trials are necessary to define its role. The only prospective randomized trial compared VATS to muscle-sparing thoracotomy in the treatment of clinical stage I NSCLC. The small sample size (n = 55) limited the ability to detect any difference in outcome between the treatment groups. There were no statistical differences in operative time, mortality, morbidity, or hospital length of stay based on the incision used. Cancer-related survival has not been reported (40).

D. Mediastinal Nodal Dissection Versus Sampling

The efficacy and role of mediastinal lymph node resection to achieve better local control in early-stage lung cancer have yet to be established. Two recent publications have emphasized the role of systematic mediastinal lymph node evaluation in the detection of occult mediastinal disease. Both CT and intraoperative inspection of grossly normal-appearing lymph nodes have failed to identify patients with microscopic positive disease (45,46). Of 575 patients with clinical stage I disease who underwent lobectomy and systematic mediastinal lymphadenectomy, 79 (14%) had positive mediastinal lymph nodes (45). Until well-designed clinical trials better define the impact of mediastinal lymphadenectomy on patient outcome and survival, at least selective ipsilateral mediastinal lymph node sampling should be performed in all cases to accurately and pathologically stage each patient (47).

VI. Surgical Results

Over the past 40 years, the 5-year survival for patients undergoing surgical resection for lung cancer has improved from 23% to 40% (48). (Table 1) (33,48,49). The improvement in the 5-year survival rate is attributed to better patient selection and improved stage classification rather than advancement in surgical technique. Patients are undergoing more extensive preresectional staging with radiologic scanning and mediastinoscopy. This preoperative evaluation identifies patients with advanced-stage disease, i.e., mediastinal involvement or distant metastasis. It avoids unnecessary surgery on patients who have poorer prognosis. As a result, contemporary studies evaluating patients operated on for stage I or II disease are not confounded by the inclusion of patients with pathologic stage III disease who have been understaged by clinical criteria.

One of the largest studies investigating the 30-day operative mortality for

Table 1 Five-Year Survival Following Surgery for Lung Cancer Report Since 1960

Report year	5-Year survival	Operative mortality
1960	23%	10%
1998	40%	2%

Source: Refs. 33, 48, 49.

thoracotomy in lung cancer comes from Wada and his colleagues in Japan (49). Their series includes 7099 patients. Overall operative mortality was 1.3%. There was a statistically significant difference in mortality between pneumonectomy, 19 of 586 patients (3.2%), and lobectomy, 67 of 5609 patients (1.2%), ($P < .01$). However, the difference in mortality seen between lobectomy and lesser resection, 7 of 904 patients (0.8%), was not significantly different.

In 1995, the Lung Cancer Study Group published their results of a multi-institutional trial comparing lobectomy versus limited resection for T1 NSCLC in an effort to identify the optimal oncologic procedure (35). Of the 247 patients who were eligible for analysis, 30 of the 122 limited-resection patients and 21 of the 125 lobectomy patients died of cancer—24.6% versus 16.8%, respectively. However, this was not a statistically significant difference. Recurrences occurred in 38 of 122 patients with limited resections and in 23 of 125 patients with lobectomies—31% versus 18.4%, respectively. The most significant finding in this study was the three-times higher locoregional recurrence seen with limited resection versus lobectomy, 21 of 122 patients, 17.2%; and 8 of 125, 6.4% ($P = .008$ two-sided).

Although this study clearly shows a statistically significant increase in recurrence rate when limited resection is compared to lobectomy, it does not definitively demonstrate that patients undergoing limited resection have a significantly greater chance of death (35). According to the database of 5319 patients used for the new international staging system, patients undergoing surgery with surgical-pathologic stage IA disease, tumor ≤3 cm, had a 5-year survival rate of 67% (Table 2) (16). Patients with surgical-pathologic stage IB disease, tumor >3 cm, had a significantly lower 5-year survival, 57%. This survival discrepancy is based solely on the significant influence of tumor size. In addition, survival is directly proportional to tumor size regardless of the 3-cm cutoff designation between the stage IA and

Table 2 Five-Year Survival (%) of Patients With Surgical/Pathologic Stage I and II Lesions

Stage	TNM subset	Survival (%)				
		12 mo.	24 mo.	36 mo.	48 mo.	60 mo.
IA	T1N0M0	94	86	80	73	67
IB	T2N0M0	87	76	67	62	57
IIA	T1N1M0	89	70	64	61	55
IIB	T2N1M0	78	56	47	42	39
	T3N0M0	76	55	47	40	38

Source: Ref. 16.

IB subsets (Fig. 1) (17). The smaller the primary tumor, the better the prognosis. Patients with tumors <1 cm had the best prognosis, and those whose tumors were >5 cm had the worst prognosis.

When tumor size was stratified based on squamous cell, adenocarcinoma, and large-cell histologic type, there appeared to be no significant difference, especially in patients with T1 lesions (Fig. 2) (18). However, when patients with T2 lesions were stratified based on histologic type, an improved survival trend was observed for patients with squamous cell cancer (Fig. 3) (18)

Patients undergoing surgical resection with surgical-pathologic stage IIA disease had a 5-year survival rate of 55%, and patients with surgical-pathologic stage IIB disease had a 5-year survival rate of 39% (Table 2). The previous staging system grouped patients with T1 or T2 tumors into stage II disease based on the involvement of N1 lymph nodes. In addition, patients with T3 tumors without lymph node involvement are now classified into stage IIB as well because of similar survival outcomes.

Stage II patients have been somewhat difficult to stage because of the variability in survival. The number of involved N1 nodes and the location of the N1 nodes (lobar versus hilar) vary among stage II patients; however, the difference in survival has not been considered significant enough to designate patients into distinct categories by the new staging system. Despite this, Yano and colleagues found that survival associated with lobar N1 disease (64.5%) was significantly better than survival of patients with N1 hilar disease (39.7%; $P = .014$) (Fig. 4) (50). Also, the pattern of distant metastasis observed in this study showed hilar N1 disease to behave similarly to N2 disease, whereas lobar N1 disease had a postresection course similar to that of N0 disease (50). Martini and colleagues looked at the number of lymph nodes involved as a measure of survival (Fig. 5) (51). They found that stage II patients with a single positive lymph node had a 5-year survival of 45% and patients with multiple lymph node involvement had a survival of 31% ($P = .016$) (51). These findings may explain the ambiguity in categorizing this subset of patients into one stage category, and future stage modifications should focus on this distinction.

The most recent additions to the stage IIB category are T3 tumors without lymph node involvement. T3N0 patients were downstaged from IIIA to IIB because the attendant 5-year patient survival of 38% was superior to and distinct from the outcome seen with stage IIIA patients with N2 disease. Stage IIB includes tumors of the superior sulcus. Ginsberg et al. compared survival in patients with this stage disease undergoing lobectomy with chest wall resection with that of patients undergoing wedge and chest wall resection (52). They showed that patients undergoing lobectomy and chest wall resection had a 65% 5-year survival, whereas patients undergoing wedge and chest wall resection had only a 30% 5-year survival ($P = .039$; Fig. 6) (52). As with all earlier stages of lung can-

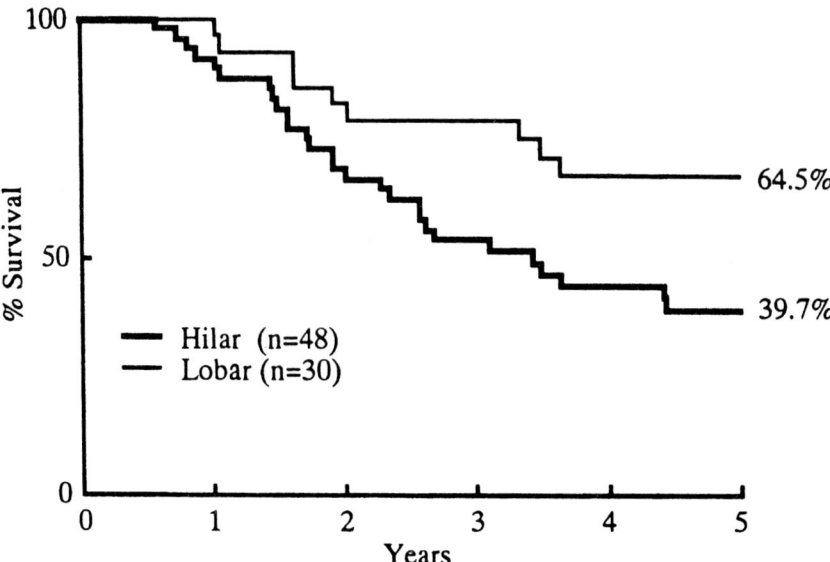

Figure 4 Survival curves after resection for patients with N1 disease according to the level of involved N1 nodes. Lobar node metastasis versus hilar node metastasis: $P = .014$. (From Ref. 50.)

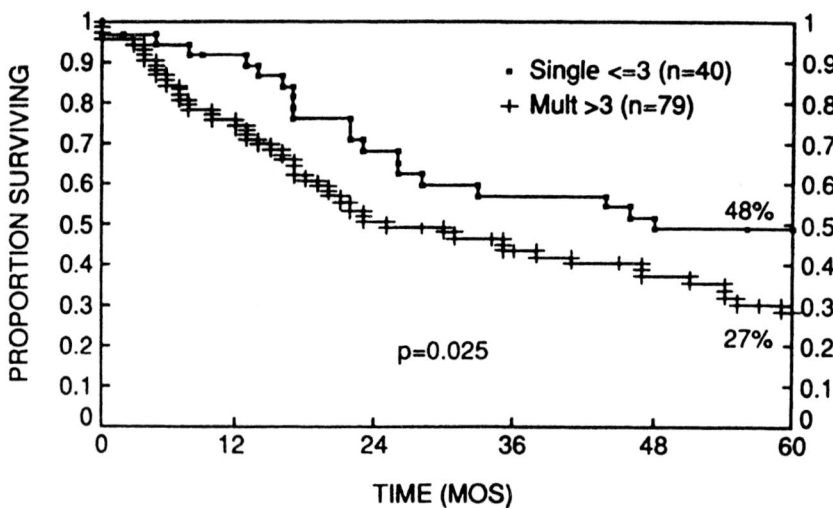

Figure 5 Survival from resection of stage II lung cancer by tumor size (in cm) and number of involved N1 nodes (mult = multiple). (From Ref. 51.)

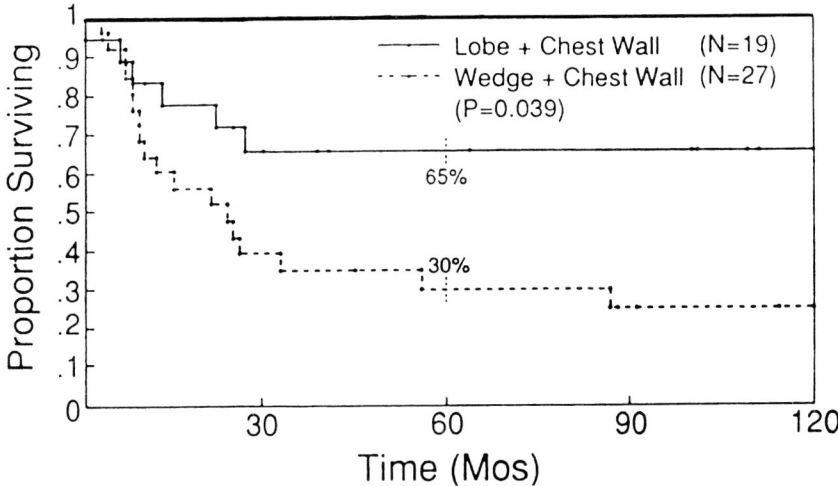

Figure 6 Survival curves comparing outcomes for patients who underwent lobectomy plus en bloc chest wall resection and patients who underwent wedge resection plus en bloc chest wall resection. (From Ref. 52.)

cer, complete resection is emphasized in stage IIB patients and should include en bloc resection of the involved chest wall with the entire involved lung lobe.

VII. Summary

Better and more efficient methods of identifying asymptomatic patients with stage I and II lung cancer are needed. When patients are identified with an SPN, an aggressive diagnostic algorithm should be followed to determine the presence of a malignancy. The principal goal of surgical therapy is to obtain a complete resection while preserving enough pulmonary function to maintain normal daily living. In patients with preserved pulmonary function, an anatomic lobectomy with a careful hilar and mediastinal lymph node evaluation remains the standard procedure for the treatment of patients with clinical stage I and II disease. This operation is most likely to result in and will best document complete resection. A complete resection offers the lowest risk of locoregional recurrence and the best chance of cure. Patients with impaired pulmonary function may undergo lesser resection as a compromise procedure. When a lesser procedure is performed, a segmentectomy is preferred over a wedge resection because of a more complete lymphatic resection. Future controlled trials will be necessary to resolve the issues of thoracotomy versus VATS and lymphadenectomy versus nodal sampling as well as to define the roles for adjuvant therapy and neoadjuvant therapy in patients with stage I and II disease.

References

1. Weisenburger TH. Definitive radiotherapy and combined modality therapy for inoperable non-small cell lung cancer. In: Roth JA, Ruckdeschel JC, Weisenburger TH, eds. Thoracic Oncology. Philadelphia: Harcourt Brace & Company, 1995:164–180.
2. DeCamp MM, Jaklitsch MT, Mentzer SJ, Harpole DH, Sugarbaker DJ. The safety and versatility of video-thoracoscopy; a prospective analysis of 895 consecutive cases. J Am Coll Surg 1995; 181:113–120.
3. Shields T. Screening, diagnosis, and staging of non-small cell lung cancer and consideration of unusual primary tumors of the lung. Curr Opin Oncol 1992; 4:299–307.
4. Ramsdell JW, Peters RM, Taylor AT, et al. Multiorgan scans for staging lung cancer. J Thorac Cardiovasc Surg 1977; 73:653–659.
5. Ferrigno D, Buccheri G. Cranial computed tomography as a part of the initial staging procedures for patients with non-small cell lung cancer. Chest 1994; 106:1025–1029.
6. Cromartie RS, Parker EF, May JE, et al. Carcinoma of the lung: a clinical review. Ann Thorac Surg 1980; 30:30–35.
7. Allard P, Yankaskas BC, Fletcher RH, et al. Sensitivity and specificity of computed tomography for the detection of adrenal metastatic lesions among 91 autopsied lung cancer patients. Cancer 1990; 66:457–462.
8. Michel F, Soler M, Imhof E, Perruchoud AP. Initial staging of non-small cell lung cancer: value of routine radioisotope bone scanning. Thorax 1991; 46:469–473.
9. Valk PE, Pounds TR, Hopkins DM, et al. Staging non-small cell lung cancer by whole body positron emission tomographic imaging. Ann Thorac Surg 1995; 60:1573–1582.
10. Shea J, Lillington G. Preoperative staging of lung cancer. West J Med 1994; 161:508–509.
11. McCloud T, Bourgouin P, Greenberg R, et al. Bronchogenic carcinoma: analysis of staging in the mediastinum with CT by correlative lymph node mapping and sampling. Radiology 1992; 182:319–323.
12. Scott WJ, Schwabe JL, Gupta NC, Dewan NA, Reeb SD, Sugimoto JT. Positron emission tomography of lung tumors and mediastinal lymph nodes using [18F]fluorodeoxyglucose. Ann Thorac Surg 1994; 58:698–703.
13. Younes M, Brown RW, Stephenson M, Gondo M, Cagle PT. Overexpression of Glut1 and Glut3 in stage I nonsmall cell lung cancer is associated with poor survival. Cancer 1997; 80:1046–1051.
14. Ahuja V, Coleman RE, Herndon J, Patz EF Jr. The prognostic significance of fluorodexyglucose positron emission tomography imaging for patients with nonsmall cell lung carcinoma. Cancer 1998; 83:918–924.
15. Shaffer K. Radiologic evaluation in lung cancer. Chest 1997; 112:235S–238S.
16. Mountain CF. Revisions in the international system for staging lung cancer. Chest 1997; 111:1710–1717.
17. Martini N, Bains MS, Burt ME, et al. Incidence of local recurrence and second pri-

mary tumors in resected stage I lung cancer. J Thorac Cardiovasc Surg 1995; 109:120–129.

18. Shields TW. Natural history of patients after resection of a bronchial carcinoma. Surg Clin North Am 1981; 61:1279.

19. Martini N, Burt ME, Bains MS, et al. Survival after resection of stage II non-small cell lung cancer. Ann Thorac Surg 1992; 54:460.

20. van Raemdonck DE, Schneider A, Ginsberg RJ. Surgical treatment for higher stage non-small cell lung cancer: a collective review. Ann Thorac Surg 1992; 54:999–1013.

21. Luketich JD, van Raemdonck DE, Ginsberg RJ. Extended resection for higher stage non-small cell lung cancer. World J Surg 1993; 17:719–728.

22. Flehinger BJ, Kimmel M, Melamed MR. The effect of surgical treatment on survival from early lung cancer. Implications for screening. Chest 1992; 101:1013–1018.

23. Cortese DA, Pairolero PC, Bergstralh EJ, et al. Roentgenographically occult lung cancer: a ten year experience. J Thorac Cardiovasc Surg 1983; 86:373–380.

24. Lam S, Kennedy T, Unger M, Miller YE, Gelmont D, Rusch V, Gipe B, Howard D, LeRiche JC, Coldman A, Grazdar AF. Localization of bronchial intraepithelial neoplastic lesions by fluorescence bronchoscopy. Chest 1998; 113:696–702.

25. Martini N, Ginsberg RJ. Treatment of stage I and II disease. In: Aisner J, Arriagada R, Green MR, Martini N, Perry MC, eds. Comprehensive Textbook of Thoracic Oncology. Baltimore: Williams & Wilkins, 1996:338–350.

26. Flehinger BJ, Melamed MR. Current status of screening for lung cancer. Chest Surg Clin North Am 1994; 4:1–15.

27. Cooper JD, Pearson FG, Todd TRJ, et al. Radiotherapy alone for patients with operable carcinoma of the lung. Chest 1985; 87:289–292.

28. Kearney DJ, Lee TH, Reilly JJ, DeCamp MM, Sugarbaker DJ. Assessment of operative risk in patients undergoing lung resection. Importance of predicted pulmonary function. Chest 1994; 104:753–758.

29. Reilly JJ. Preparing for pulmonary resection. Preoperative evaluation of patients. Chest 1997; 112:2065–2085.

30. Johnston JB, Jones PH. The treatment of bronchial carcinoma by lobectomy and sleeve resection of the main bronchus. Thorax 1959; 14:48–54.

31. Kittle CF. Atypical resections of the lung: bronchoplasties, sleeve resections and segmentectomies—their evolution and present status. Curr Prob Surg 1989; 26:89–109.

32. Massard G, Dabbagh A, Dumont P, et al. Are bilobectomies acceptable procedures? Ann Thorac Surg 1995; 60:640–645.

33. Ginsberg RJ, Hill LD, Eagan RT, Thomas P, Mountain CF, Deslauriers J, et al. Modern thirty-day operative mortality for surgical resection in lung cancer. J Thorac Cardiovasc Surg 1983; 86:654–657.

34. Harpole DH Jr, Liptay MJ, DeCamp MM Jr, Mentzer SJ, Swanson SJ, Sugarbaker DJ. Prospective analysis of pneumonectomy and risk factors for major morbidity and cardiac dysrhythmias. Ann Thorac Surtg 1996; 61:977–982.

35. Ginsberg RJ, Rubinstein LV. Randomized trial of lobectomy versus limited resection for T1N0 non-small cell lung cancer. Ann Thorac Surg 1995; 60:615–623.

36. Warren WH, Faber LP. Segmentectomy versus lobectomy in patients with stage I pulmonary carcinma: five year survival and patterns of intrathoracic recurrence. J Thorac Cardiovasc Surg 1994; 107:1087–1094.

37. Ginsberg RJ. Resection of non-small cell lung cancer: How much and by what route. Chest 1997; 112:203S–205S.
38. Fry WA. Thoracic incisions. In: Shields TW, ed. General Thoracic Surgery. Malvern, PA: Williams & Wilkins, 1994: 381–390.
39. Ginsberg RJ. Alternative (muscle-sparing) incisions in thoracic surgery. Ann Thorac Surg 1993; 56:752–754.
40. Kirby TJ, Mack MJ, Landreneau RJ, Rice TW. Lobectomy—video-assisted thoracic surgery versus muscle-sparing thoracotomy: a randomized trial. J Thorac Cardiovasc Surg 1995; 109:997–1002.
41. Watanabe Y, Ichihashi T, Iwa T. Median sternotomy as an approach for pulmonary surgery. J Thorac Cardiovasc Surg 1988; 36:227–231.
42. Cooper JD, Nelems JM, Pearson FG, et al. Extended indications for median sternotomy in patients requiring pulmonary resections. Ann Thorac Surg 1978; 26:413.
43. Giudicelli R, Thomas P, Lonjon T, et al. Comparative study of lobectomy through conventional thoracotomy and video-assisted thoracoscopy. Ann Thorac Surg 1994; 58:712–718.
44. McKenna RJ Jr. Lobectomy by video-assisted thoracic surgery with mediastinal node sampling for lung cancer. J Thorac Cardiovasc Surg 1994; 107:879–882.
45. Takizawa T, Terashima M, Koike T, et al. Mediastinal lymph node metastasis in patients with clinical stage I peripheral non-small lung cancer. J Thorac Cardiovasc Surg 1997; 113:248–252.
46. Oda M, Murakami S, Hayashi Y, et al. The role of mediastinal lymph node dissection for clinical stage I non-small cell lung cancer. Lung Cancer 1997; 18(suppl 1):97.
47. Holmes EC. General principles of surgical quality control. Chest 1994; 106(suppl): 334S–336S.
48. Pearson FG. Lung cancer: the past 25 years. Chest 1986; 89:200S–205S.
49. Wada H, Nakamura T, Nakamoto K, Maeda M, Watanabe Y. Thirty-day operative mortality for thoracotomy in lung cancer. J Thorac Cardiovasc Surg 1998; 115:70–73.
50. Yano T, Yokoyama H, Inoue T, Asoh H, Tayama K, Ichinose Y. Surgical results and prognostic factors of pathologic N1 disease in non-small cell carcinoma of the lung. Significance of N1 level: lobar or hilar. J Thorac Cardiovasc Surg 1994; 107:1398–1402.
51. Martini N, Burt ME, Bains MS, McCormack PM, Rusch VW, Ginsberg RJ. Survival after resection of stage II non-small cell lung cancer. Ann Thorac Surg 1992; 54:460–466.
52. Ginsberg RJ, Martini N, Zaman M, et al. Influence of surgical resection and brachytherapy in the management of superior sulcus tumor. Ann Thorac Surg 1994; 57:1440–1445.

7

Randomized Trials in Stages I and II Non-Small-Cell Lung Cancer

VICTORIA J. DORR and MICHAEL C. PERRY

University of Missouri
Ellis Fischel Cancer Center
Columbia, Missouri

I. Introduction

In 1998, lung cancer is expected to affect 171,500 people in the United States and to result in the death of 160,100 individuals (1). Of these cases, 75% to 85% will be identified as non-small-cell lung cancer (NSCLC) (2). The overall 5-year survival for patients diagnosed with NSCLC is 14%. The best 5-year survival rates are seen in patients with a diagnosis made while tumors are still amenable to complete surgical resection. Patients with stage I disease have a 5-year survival rate of 42%, and stage II patients have a 5-year survival of 22%. Unfortunately, fewer than 30% of lung cancers present at an early enough stage that surgery is an option. Even with complete surgical resection, over 50% will relapse within 5 years (2). The majority of these relapses occur at distant sites or at local and distant sites simultaneously (3). In 1985 the American Joint Committee on Cancer, the Union International Contra Cancer, and the Japanese Cancer Committee agreed to a worldwide staging system based on the anatomic location(s) and extent of lung cancer. This was updated in 1997. Table 1 presents TNM (tumor node, metastasis) staging and survival for NSCLC. Stage for stage, patients with adenocarcinoma fare worse than those with squamous histology (4,5).

In light of such unsatisfactory outcomes with surgery alone, other modalities have been evaluated as adjuvant therapy with the goal of improving overall

Table 1 TNM Staging and Survival in NSCLC

Stage	Definition	Overall 5-year survival (%)	Adenocarcinoma (%)	Squamous cell (%)
T1	<3 cm in diameter, not more proximal than lobar bronchus, and surrounded by lung or visceral pleura			
T2	>3 cm in diameter, or invades to mainstem bronchus 2 cm distal to carina, or invades visceral pleura, or partial lung atelectasis			
T3	Any size, invading chest wall, diaphragm, mediastinal pleura, parietal pericardium, or <2 cm from carina, or entire lung atelectasis			
T4	Invades mediastinum, heart, great vessels, trachea, esophagus, vertebral body, carina, or malignant pleural effusion			
N1	Ipsilateral peribronchial and/or ipsilateral hilar nodes			
N2	Ipsilateral mediastinal or subcarinal nodes			
N3	Contralateral mediastinal, hilar or scalene nodes, or any supraclavicular nodes			
M1	Any distant metastasis			
Stage IA	T1N0	76	69	83
B	T2N0	57	57	64
Stage IIA	T1N1	53	52	75
B	T2N1, T3N0	38	25	53
Stage IIIA	T1–3N2	15.1		
	T3N1	39		
Stage IIIB	T4 any N	8.2		
	any T N3	0		
Stage IV	M1	0		

Source: Refs. 4, 5.

and relapse-free survival. In patients with advanced NSCLC, acceptable responses to both chemotherapy and radiation have been seen, forming the basis for their use in an adjuvant setting. Intuitively one would expect an even greater benefit by using effective agents in an adjuvant setting when metastatic disease is at a microscopic level. The role of adjuvant radiation, chemotherapy, and immunotherapy will be reviewed to determine if there is sufficient basis to broadly recommend adjuvant therapy in non-small-cell lung cancer.

II. Radiation Therapy

Despite aggressive surgery, local recurrences remain high. In an autopsy series of patients who died within 30 days of curative resection of NSCLC, 40% of patients had persistent local disease (6). Adjuvant radiation, then, could conceivably benefit patients by helping to treat this residual local disease and thus favorably impact upon survival.

A. Preoperative Radiotherapy

Preoperative radiotherapy for NSCLC was first reported in 1955 (7). The rationale for preoperative radiation is that some tumors thought to be resectable by clinical staging are found to be unresectable at the time of surgery. By using radiation prior to surgery, it was thought that the resection rate might be improved. Shields (8), however, demonstrated no benefit with preoperative radiation for stage I and II NSCLC. Complete necrosis of the tumor occurred in 27% of patients who received radiation, but there was no benefit in the resection rate. At 4 years, survival favored the surgery-alone arm (21% with surgery alone vs. 14% in the combined modality arm). Future investigations with preoperative adjuvant radiotherapy may want to focus on marginally resectable tumors where there may be a role either for adjuvant radiation or chemoradiation preoperatively, similar to the therapy currently used for stage III tumors.

B. Postoperative Radiotherapy

More data are available on the use of radiation therapy after complete resection. Gebitekin et al. (9) treated 40 stage I–III patients who had positive bronchial resection margins with adjuvant radiation. Recurrences occurred in 72.5% of patients, of which 59% were local recurrences. The 5-year overall survival was 21.6% and was not improved by the addition of radiation therapy. Surprisingly, in this study only patients with stage IIIa disease had a decreased survival if the stump margins were positive.

To date, no study of postoperative adjuvant radiotherapy has demonstrated a benefit in terms of overall survival. Several papers have demonstrated a survival benefit in node-positive disease, but only upon subset analysis. A retrospective study by Kirsh and Sloan (10) demonstrated a survival benefit only in N2 squamous cell carcinoma (21% with surgery and radiation vs. 6% with surgery alone). Choi et al. (11), on the other hand, demonstrated a benefit only in node-positive adenocarcinoma patients (43% with surgery and radiation vs. 8% with surgery alone). Finally, Green et al. (12) demonstrated a benefit in both N1 and N2 adeno-carcinoma and squamous cell carcinoma with adjuvant radiotherapy. While the above studies do not clearly identify a subset of patients who will benefit from radiation, they do point out the confusion that can be caused by subset analysis.

Several studies have demonstrated a benefit in local control with adjuvant radiation therapy. The Lung Cancer Study Group (LCSG) protocol 773 found in 230 patients with stage II (defined as T2N1) or stage III (any T3 or any N2 disease) a benefit in terms of a reduction in the local recurrence rate with radiation to 50 Gy (3% vs. 41% in the nonradiated group ($P = <.0001$)). However, no benefit was seen in overall survival (13). Van Houtte et al. (14), similarly, demonstrated a reduction in local recurrences from 15% to 3% with adjuvant radiation with no effect on over-all survival. More recently, Smolle-Juettner et al. (15) demonstrated a decrease in local recurrences from 17% to 5% with adjuvant radiation therapy ($P = <.01$), but again with no effect on overall survival. Martini et al. (16), on the other hand, found postoperative radiation therapy to be the most significant factor related to poor out-come after resection ($P = .0005$). Table 2 summarizes the adjuvant radiation expe-rience.

To date, there is no evidence that demonstrates a clear statistical improve-ment in survival with the addition of adjuvant radiation. On the other hand, local control may be improved with the use of adjuvant therapy after complete resec-tion. This forms the basis for the frequent use in the United States of adjuvant radi-ation. Limitations to adjuvant radiation include the amount of disease and subse-quent amount of chest tissue requiring treatment, and the tolerance of normal tissue to radiation. Newer treatment schedules, better radiation techniques, or the combination of radiation with radiosensitizing agents may result in a significant difference in future trials.

III. Chemotherapy

Improvement in local control with radiation therapy did not subsequently translate into an improvement in overall survival, presumably because of a lack of activity on distant metastases. In the previously mentioned autopsy series of patients who had undergone curative resection and died within 30 days, 17% of squamous cell tumors and 40% of adenocarcinomas had already developed distant metastasis (6). Chemotherapy, thus, is an ideal agent to consider for adjuvant therapy, as it may be able to affect both local and distant recurrences. Additionally, adjuvant chemother-apy has already been of proven benefit in other solid tumors, including breast can-cer and colon cancer.

Table 3 represents the adjuvant chemotherapy trials reported to date in

Table 2 Adjuvant Radiation Therapy (XRT) in Resected NSCLC[a]

Reference	Stage/# treated	Treatment	Overall survival	Comments
Bangma, 1971 (17)	T1–2N0 77	XRT vs. observation	No difference	
Green, 1975 (12)	Stage II–III 137	50–60 Gy XRT vs. Observation	Squamous cell: 21% XRT vs. 6% Adenocarcinoma: 50% XRT vs. 14%	Significant benefit seen in node-positive adenocarcinoma or squamous
Warram, 1975 (18)	Resectable 568	Preop XRT 40–50 Gy vs. control	14% vs. 16% (NS)	
Choi, 1980 (11)	Stage II–III 92	XRT 40–60 Gy vs. control	Squamous cell: 33% vs. 33% Adenocarcinoma: 43% XRT vs. 8%	Significant benefit only in node-positive adenocarcinoma
Van Houtte, 1980 (14)	Stage II–III 76	XRT vs. control	No difference	3% local recurrence XRT vs. 15%
Kirsh, 1981 (10)	Stage II–III 184	XRT vs. control	Squamous cell: 34% XRT vs. 0% Adenocarcinoma: 12% vs. 0%	Benefit significant only in N2 squamous cell Retrospective
Weisenberger, 1986 (13)	Stage II–III 230	50 Gy XRT vs. control	No difference	Local recurrence 5% XRT vs. 17% ($P = <.001$)
Emami, 1987 (19)	Stage I-III 69	<50 Gy vs. 50–59 Gy vs. >60 Gy	No difference 3-yr survival radiation vs. surgery alone	3-yr survival 73% if >60 Gy vs. 35% if <60 Gy
Martini, 1992 (16)	Stage II 81	XRT vs. control		XRT most significant predictor of poor outcome ($P = .0005$) (retrospective)
Gebitekin, 1994 (9)	Stage I–III positive margins 40	XRT vs. control	26% no difference	
Lafitte, 1996 (20)	T2N0 163	XRT vs. control	44.2% no difference	
Smolle-Juettner, 1996 (15)	M0 and curative resection 155	50–56 Gy XRT vs. control	24% no difference	Local recurrence 5% XRT vs. 17% ($P = <.001$)

[a]Five-year survival unless otherwise specified.

Table 3 Adjuvant Chemotherapy for Resected NSCLC[a]

Reference	Stage/# treated	Treatment	Overall Survival	Relapse-free survival	Comments
Shields, 1977 (23)	Stage I–III 417	CTX 8 mg/kg/day × 5 d q 5 wk × 18 mo vs. CTX 8 mg/kg/d q 5 wk × >18 mo vs. MTX 10 mg/kg/d × 5 d q 5 wk × 18 mo	24.5% 25.7% 23.5% (NS)		
Shields, 1982 (24)	Stage I–III 865	CCNU 70 mg/m² D1 q 6 wk + hydrea 1 g/m² D1, 4 × 1 yr vs. observation	35% 46%		Includes small cell lung cancer
Girling, 1985 (25)	Stage I–III 123	Busulfan 3–4 mg/d × 2 yr vs. CTX 150–200 mg/d × 2 yr vs. placebo	41% 39% 43%	42% 44% 425	Includes small cell lung cancer
Ayoub, 1987 (26)	Stage I–III 68	VDS 2 mg/m² and CDDP 60 mg/m² × 6 cycles + XRT vs. XRT		61.2% 48.6% at 1 year	*18 mos follow-up
LCSG 791, 1988 (21)	Incomplete resection or N2 172	CTX 400/dox 40/CDDP 40 mg/m² q 4 wk × 6 + XRT 40 Gy split course vs. 40 Gy split-course XRT	43.6% 33.88% (NS)	35.9% 23.3% (p = 0.004)	*Only 51% completed chemo
Klingman, 1990 (33)	T1–2N1 37	CTX 300/dox 20/MTX 15 mg/m² D1,8 + DTIC 100 mg/m² PO D3-13 q 28 d × 1 yr and XRT 30 Gy (CAMP) vs. XRT 30 Gy vs. observation	45.9% 28.6% NR		Median survival: 45.5 mos vs. 19 mos vs. 13.5 mos (p = 0.005)
Ichinose, 1991 (6)	T1–3N0-2 86	PAP or CAP-M or PV vs. observation	58% any chemo 58%		Avg 2.3 cycles of chemo given
Gradishar, 1992 (34)	Stage II 49	CTX 300/dox 20/MTX 15 mg/m² D1,8 + DTIC 100 mg/m² PO D3-13 q 28 d × 1 yr and XRT 30 Gy vs. XRT 30 Gy vs. observation	13% 18% 7%		Median survival: 24 mos vs. 19 mos vs. 6 mos (p = 0.006) *Retrospective

Reference	Stage	No.	Treatment		Comments
Niiranen, 1992 (29)	T1–3N0	110	CTX 400/dox 40/CDDP 40 mg/m² q 4 wk × 6 (CAP) vs. observation	5 year: 67% vs. 56% (P = .05) 10 year: 61% vs. 48% (P = .05)	70% received > 3 cycles
Karp, 1993 (36)	Marginally resectable Stage II–III	34	CDPP/VP-16 and XRT preoperative vs. XRT preoperative		*75% resectable with chemo + XRT **43% resectable with XRT
Holmes, LCSG 772, 1993 (28)	Stage II–III	141	CTX 400/dox 40/CDDP 40 mg/m² q 4 wk × 6 vs. placebo (BCG and levam)	32% 18% Median survival: 23 mo vs. 16 mo (P = .032)	62% 49% (p = 0.047) *24% received no chemo **58% received planned dose chemo
Feld LCSG 801 1994 (30)	T1N1/T2N0	283	CTX 400/dox 40/CDDP 60 mg/m² q 3 wk × 4 vs. observation	56% 53%	53% received 4 cycles chemo
Figlin LCSG 853 1994 (31)	T1–2N1, any N2, any T3	186	Immediate CTX 400/dox 40/CDDP 40 mg/m² q 4 wk × 4 (CAP) vs. delayed CAP	32.7 mo median survival	19.5 mo median relapse-free survival	Immediate CAP decreased RFS by 12% and OS by 18% (NS)
Dautzenberg 1995 (35)	Stage I–III	267	60 Gy XRT + COPAC vs. 60 Gy XRT	18% 19%	16.5 mo 13.3 mo	Median survival 14.9 mo vs. 15.4 mo (NS)
Chuba Study Group 1995 (40)	Stage I–III	309	CDDP 66/dox 26 mg/m² D1 × 1 then UFt 8 mg/kg/d vs. observation	61.8% 57.4% (NS)	61.8% 58.1%	Significantly more node + in chemo arm

Table 3 Continued

Reference	Stage/ # treated	Treatment	Overall survival	Relapse-free survival	Comments
Wada 1996 (37)	Stage I–III 323	CDDP 50 mg/m^2 D1/VDS 2–3 mg/kg D 1, 15, 29 then UFt 400 mg/kg/d × 1 yr vs. UFT 400 mg/kg/d × 1 yr vs. observation	60.6% 64% 49% (P = .053)	39% 39% 42.9% (NS)	
Kimura 1996 (39)	Stage II–III 82	IL-2/LAK cells and MVP vs. observation	58.2% 31.5% (P = .0038)		
Tanaka 1997 (38)	Stage I–IIIa 236	Oral Ft vs. observation	78.1% 69% (P = .046)		No benefit to adjuvant chemo if p53 overexpressed

CAP-M, (CTX, DOX, CDDP, mito-C); CCNU, lomustine; CDDP, cisplatin; COPAC, (cycle 1 and 3: DOX, VCR, CDDP, CCNU cycle 2: VCR, CDDP, CTX); CTX, cyclophosphamide; DOX, doxorubicin; DTIC, procarbazine; FT, tegafur; LAK, lymphocyte activated killer cell; Mito-C, mitomycin C; MVP, (CDDP, VDS, mito-C); MTX, methotrexate; PAP, (CDDP, DOX, pepleomycin); PV, (CDDP, VDS); VCR, Vincristine; VDS, Vindesine; VP-16, etoposide; UFT, uracil and tegafur.

[a]Five-year survival unless otherwise specified

resected NSCLC. Comparison among the trials and to historical controls is difficult, as different definitions of stage were frequently used. In the early studies, stratification for prognostic factors was not performed. Additionally, until the LCSG studies, intraoperative staging was rarely performed. The majority of these trials also included patients with stage III disease, who have an overall worse prognosis (see Table 1). Other potential problems include the use of chemotherapy regimens that are generally thought to be inferior in efficacy to newer combinations such as cisplatin or carboplatin with etoposide, taxanes, or vinca alkaloids. Thus, part of the lack of efficacy may be due to the choice of drug therapy. The toxicity of the chemotherapy given frequently prevented a substantial number of patients from completing the intended treatment. In one study, only 51% of assigned patients completed six planned cycles of chemotherapy (21). Other studies had similar problems, with 50% to 75% of patients completing the intended therapy. The limiting toxicity in the majority of these studies was gastrointestinal symptoms, including nausea and vomiting. The use of newer antiemetics (granisetron or ondansetron with dexamethasone) should make adjuvant therapy more tolerable and allow for more dose-intensive chemotherapy regimens in the future. Finally, the current studies may have lacked the statistical power to identify even a small difference with treatment. In order to detect a 20% to 30% benefit in survival, >2000 patients may be required (22).

Over 30 years ago, the Veterans Administration Surgical Adjuvant Group began a series of adjuvant trials with agents, including single-agent cyclophosphamide, single-agent methotrexate, and a combination of CCNU and hydroxyurea. No benefit with any adjuvant chemotherapy was seen (23,24). Similarly, Girling et al. (25) evaluated oral single-agent busulfan versus oral single-agent cyclophosphamide for 2 years versus placebo, and found no difference in overall or relapse-free survival with either chemotherapy regimen. Ayoub et al. (26), in 1987, presented initial data on the use of adjuvant cisplatin and vindesine with radiation therapy versus radiation therapy alone. A benefit in relapse-free survival was seen in the combination chemoradiotherapy arm (61.2% vs. 48.6% at 1 year of follow-up).

With the advent of more effective therapy for advanced NSCLC in the 1970s, the LCSG designed a series of prospective, randomized trials. In these studies, a careful and uniform surgical staging procedure was mandated for the first time. Protocol LCSG 772 randomized 141 patients with stage II–III disease to cyclophosphamide, doxorubicin (Adriamycin), and cisplatin (CAP) every 4 weeks for six cycles versus intrapleural BCG and levamisole. The BCG and levamisole arm was subsequently considered a control arm when an earlier study, LCSG 771 (27), failed to demonstrate a benefit with immunotherapy. A 7-month delay in time to relapse was seen with chemotherapy, which was identical to the time spent on chemotherapy. Relapse-free survival, at 7.5 years of follow-up, was 62% with chemotherapy versus 49% in the immunotherapy arm ($P = .047$). Overall survival was also improved with CAP chemotherapy. At 7.5 years of follow-up, overall survival was 32% in the chemotherapy arm versus 18% in the immunotherapy arm; this translates into a median survival of 23 months with chemotherapy versus 16 months without (P = .032). In this study, however, only 58% completed the planned chemotherapy (28).

The Lung Cancer Study Group, in LSCG 791, utilized the same chemotherapy (CAP for six cycles) in combination with split-course radiation therapy to 40 Gy versus the split-course radiation therapy alone. This trial was designed to evaluate specifically those patients who either had incomplete resection or N2 disease. There was no benefit in overall survival with the addition of CAP chemotherapy to radiation (43.6% vs. 33.8%; NS), but a benefit in relapse-free survival was seen at 18 months of follow-up with chemoradiotherapy (35.9% vs. 23.3%). Of note, in this study only 51% received six cycles of chemotherapy (21). Other studies using CAP chemotherapy include that by Niiranen et al. (29). This study evaluated CAP for six cycles in 110 patients with T1–3, node-negative disease. A benefit in overall survival was seen at 5 years with chemotherapy (67% vs. 56%; P = .05) and, similarly, at 10 years (61% vs. 48%; P = .05) (29). In this study, at least 70% of patients received three or more of the planned chemotherapy treatments.

Subsequently, two other LCSG studies have evaluated CAP. Protocol LCSG 801 evaluated CAP every 3 weeks for four cycles versus observation in 283 patients with T1N1 or T2N0 disease. This chemotherapy included an escalation in the cisplatin dose from the prior CAP dose of 40 mg/m^2 to 60 mg/m^2 with each cycle. No benefit was seen in survival at 5 years with chemotherapy (56% vs. 53%); however, only 53% of patients were able to complete the intended four cycles of chemotherapy (30). Protocol LCSG 853 evaluated, in 186 patients with any N2 or T3 disease or T1–2N1 disease, the use of CAP every 4 weeks for four cycles, either immediately after surgery or at the time of first relapse. The immediate chemotherapy decreased relapse-free survival by 12% and improved overall survival by 18%, both of which were nonsignificant benefits (31).

The most remarkable aspect of these studies is the poor tolerance of the CAP chemotherapy. This is manifest by the significant number of patients who were unable to complete the chemotherapy. Perhaps, with better-tolerated chemotherapy, or better medication to control symptoms, especially cisplatin-induced nausea and vomiting, a greater benefit might have been possible. Interestingly, while there was a significant dropout rate due to toxicity in the chemotherapy arms of LSCG 801 and 853, a companion study by Ruckdeshel and Piantodosi found no significant impact of a short course of chemotherapy on quality of life (32).

Other chemotherapy regimens have also been evaluated as adjuvant therapy. Klingman and DeMeester (32) evaluated 37 patients with T1–2N1 disease and found a benefit in median survival with the addition of CAMP (cyclophosphamide, doxorubicin, methotrexate, and procarbazine) chemotherapy to 30 Gy of radiation therapy versus 30 Gy radiation therapy alone versus observation (45.5 months vs.

19 months vs. 13.5 months, respectively; $P = .005$). Gradishar et al (34), in a retrospective study of identical design, in 49 stage II patients, again found a survival benefit with chemo-radiotherapy (median survival: 24 months versus 19 months versus 6 months; $P = .006$). Ichinose et al. (6), on the other hand, found no benefit with any of three different chemotherapy regimens in 86 patients with T1–3N0-2 disease (60% stage I). The chemotherapy was left to the discretion of the investigator and included cisplatin, doxorubicin, and pepleomycin (PAP) or cyclophosphamide, doxorubicin, cisplatin, and Mitomycin-C (CAP-M), or cisplatin and vindesine (PV). The 5-year overall survival was identical (58% with all of the chemotherapy treatments combined vs. 58% in the untreated population). Dautzenberg et al. (35), similarly, in 267 patients with stage I–III disease found no benefit in overall survival (OS) or relapse-free survival (RFS) with the addition of COPAC chemotherapy (cycle 1 and 3: doxorubicin, vincristine, cisplatin, lomustine; cycle 2: vincristine, cisplatin, and cyclophosphamide) to 60 Gy radiation versus the 60 Gy radiation therapy alone (OS: 18% vs. 19%, and RFS: 16.5 months vs. 13.3 months).

Karp et al. (36) evaluated 34 marginally resectable clinical stage II or III patients. Patients were randomized to cisplatin and etoposide preoperatively with 60 Gy radiation or preoperative radiation therapy alone. More patients were resectable with the combination of chemotherapy and radiation (75%) than with radiation alone (43%). Median survival was also significantly improved, 44+ months versus 22+ months, respectively ($P = .01$). Unfortunately, this is a small study with few early-stage patients.

More recent studies have utilized newer agents. Wada et al. (37) randomized 323 stage I–III patients to one cycle of cisplatin and vindesine followed by UFT (oral uracil and tegafur) for 1 year versus UFT alone versus observation. No benefit in RFS was seen (39% vs. 39% vs. 43%), but an improvement in overall survival was seen with both chemotherapy arms compared to observation (60.6% vs. 64% vs. 49%; $P = .053$). The Chuba Study Group (40) found no significant benefit in overall or RFS with the combination of one cycle of cisplatin and doxorubicin followed by 1 year of oral UFT when compared with control. Unfortunately, however, there were significantly more node-positive patients in the arm that received the adjuvant chemotherapy. Tanaka et al. (38) evaluated 236 patients with stage I–IIIA disease with oral tegafur (FT) compared to observation. A significant benefit in overall survival was again seen with adjuvant chemotherapy (78.1% vs. 69%; $P = .046$). An interesting subset analysis in this study demonstrated no benefit with chemotherapy when it was given to patients who overexpressed p53. An even greater benefit with chemotherapy was seen in the patients who did not overexpress p53 and who received tegafur (87.1% vs. 75.6%; $P = .036$). Finally, Kimura and Yamaguchi (39) evaluated 82 stage II–III patients with a combination of interleukin-2, LAK (lymphocyte-activated killer) cells and cisplatin, vindesine, and mitomycin-C (MVP) versus observation alone. Initially, a third arm of MVP alone was included, but this was discontinued due to a suboptimal outcome in those patients. A significant benefit in 5-year overall survival was seen in patients receiving the chemoimmunotherapy (58.2% vs. 31.5%; $P = .0038$).

In 1995 the Non-Small Cell Lung Cancer Collaborative Group published a meta-analysis of randomized chemotherapy adjuvant trials in NSCLC (41). The studies were divided into early-stage and stage III disease. In the analysis of surgery versus surgery and chemotherapy in early-stage NSCLC patients, 4357 patients were evaluated in 14 trials. Five studies used long-term alkylating agents, six used cisplatin-based chemotherapy, and three other trials were grouped together. With the long-term alkylating agents, a negative effect was found with chemotherapy and surgery compared to surgery alone (hazard ratio of death 1.15; $P = .005$). On the other hand, chemotherapy with cisplatin-based chemotherapy favored the chemotherapy and surgery arm with a hazard ratio of 0.87 ($P = .08$). This represented a 13% reduction in the risk of death with chemotherapy, or an absolute benefit in survival of 3% at 2 years and 5% at 5 years. The other chemotherapy group (including UFT) also favored the chemotherapy arm with a hazard ratio of 0.89 ($P = .3$). In this analysis a trend toward a benefit was seen with chemotherapy other than alkylating agents, but it did not reach statistical significance. In the analysis of surgery and radiation versus surgery, radiation, and chemotherapy in early-stage NSCLC, there were seven eligible trials with 887 patients. Six of these studies included cisplatin-containing regimens. Overall, there was a slight trend toward benefit with the multimodality arm versus radiation alone with a hazard ratio of 0.98 ($P = .76$). In the cisplatin-based chemotherapy with surgery and radiation evaluation there was a similar nonsignificant trend toward benefit seen with the multimodality approach (hazard ratio 0.94; $P = .46$) (41).

Therefore, based on data to date, no clear recommendation for adjuvant chemotherapy can be made. Several studies have shown that, perhaps with more effective and less toxic regimens, chemotherapy may prove to be a fruitful adjuvant therapy. Agents that have specifically been shown to be radiation sensitizers may also be worthwhile to evaluate. Further studies in this area are warranted.

IV. Adjuvant Immunotherapy

The concept of immunotherapy as adjuvant therapy for NSCLC began after Ruck-deschel et al. (42) noted that patients with a postoperative empyema had a superior 5-year survival. A variety of agents have been evaluated as immunotherapeutic agents: bacillus Calmette-Guerrin (BCG) both intrapleural and intradermal with isoniazide; intrapleural and intravenous *Corynebacterium parvum;* bestatin, *Streptococcus pyogenes* (OK-432); krestin (PSK), *Nocardia rubra* cell wall; and retinol. While the agents vary, the theory remains the same. By stimulating the host immune response with these agents, it is hoped that an enhanced immune antitumor effect will occur and that this will translate into improved disease-free and overall survival. Unfortunately, the studies in Table 4 represent many negative studies and only a few studies where a slight benefit was seen. Bacillus Calmette-Guerrin (BCG) was found to significantly improve survival in one of seven studies. Soresi et al. (43) evaluated 124 patients with stage I–IIIA disease and administered BCG intradermally, with a 15-year overall survival of 8.2% in the BCG arm and 3.3% in the control arm ($P = .005$). In another study, the Ludwig Lung Cancer Study Group did find an improved median disease-free survival with intrapleural BCG when compared to control (3 years vs. 4.6 years; $P = .044$), but no improvement in overall survival was seen (4.5 years vs. 5.1 years; $P = .1$) (44). With a different agent, adjuvant krestin (PSK) combined with radiation therapy versus radiation therapy alone, Hayakawa et al. (45) found a significant 5-year survival advantage (39% vs. 16%; $P = .005$). Pastorino et al. (46) found a borderline survival benefit at 5 years with adjuvant retinol palmitate used for 1 year (64% vs. 51%; $P = .054$). Most recently, Fujisawa and Yamaguchi (47) demonstrated a significant disease-specific survival benefit in the adjuvant use of transfer factor and *Nocardia rubra* cell wall when compared to controls at 5 and 10 years (10-year DSS: 85% vs. 64%; $P = .041$).

At this time, immunotherapy has shown limited benefit in its use as an adjuvant therapeutic agent for resected NSCLC. Perhaps newer agents, or the combination of immunotherapy with either chemotherapy or radiation, may prove more beneficial in the future.

A. Combined Modality Approach

No individual adjuvant therapy has been able to demonstrate a consistent benefit in either disease-free or overall survival. Therefore, it follows that the addition of multiple adjuvant modalities could improve the benefit seen; alternatively, combination therapy could also increase toxicity with little increased benefit.

Radiation therapy and chemotherapy have been the most frequent combination of adjuvant agents after surgery for stage I and II NSCLC. These data are included in Table 3. The study by Ayoub et al. (26) demonstrated an improvement in RFS with the addition of vindesine and cisplatin to radiation therapy. The LCSG (21) in LCSG 791 also demonstrated a benefit in RFS with the addition of CAP chemotherapy to radiation in patients with incomplete resection or N2 disease. This did not, however, translate into an improved survival. Klingman and DeMeester (33) and Gradishar et al. (34) both demonstrated a benefit in median survival with CAMP chemotherapy and radiation therapy. More recently, however, Dautzenberg et al. (35) failed to demonstrate a benefit in either disease-free or overall survival with the addition of COPAC chemotherapy to radiation. These studies show that combinations of radiation, chemotherapy, and surgery, however, do show promise and should be the focus of future studies.

Table 4 Adjuvant Immunotherapy for Resected NSCLC[a]

Reference	Stage/# treated	Treatment	Overall survival	Comments
McNealy 1976 (48)	Stage I–III 101	IP BCG vs. control	33% 66%	3 yr follow-up
Poillart 1979 (49)	Stage I–II 43	ID BCG vs. control	38% (NS) 66%	2 yr follow-up
Hadzieve 1982 (50)	Stage I–II 860	BCG vs. control	13.2% 13.7%	Control was surgery, XRT, chemo
LLCSG 1986 (44)	Stage I–II 407	IP BCG vs. control	4.5 yr 5.1 yr median overall survival ($P = .1$)	22% empyema with BCG vs. 3% DFS: 3 yr vs. 4.6 yr median disease-free survival ($P = .044$)
LLCSG 1986 (51)	T1–2N0-1 128	IP + IV *C. parvum* vs. control	5.4 yr median survival 4.6 yr ($P = .67$)	High% ARDS with *C. parvum*
Little 1986 (52)	T1–2N0 29	BCG vs. control	85.9% 63.9% ($P = .075$)	
Hollingshead 1986 (53)	Any N0-1 232	TAA + FcA vs. control		Improved DFS in N0 immune group ($P < .0002$)
Millar 1988 (54)	Stage II 96	ID BCG × 5 yr vs. control vs. off-study	85.9% 63.9% 69.9% ($P = .075$)	

Mouritzen 1990 (55)	Stage I-II	464	Bestatin 90 mg PO 2 ×/wk × 5 yr vs. control	NS	Started presurgery; median DFS 1531 days bestatin vs
Whyte 1992 (56)	Stage I-III	63	IM transfer factor q 3 mo + XRT vs. XRT (50–60 Gy)	5 yr: 64% vs. 43% 10 yr: 53% vs. 23% ($P = .08$)	
Hayakawa 1993 (45)	Stage I-III	185	PSK + XRT vs. XRT alone	2 yr: 86% vs. 32% 5 yr: 39% vs. 16% ($P = .005$)	
Pastorino 1993 (46)	Stage I	307	Retinol palmitate 300,000 IU PO q d × 1 yr vs. control	64% 51% ($P = .054$)	DFS: 62% vs. 54% ($P = .44$)
Gail LCSG 771 1994 (27)	T1–2N0/T1N1	473	IP BCG vs. IP saline	NS with 10.9 yr follow-up	
Soresi 1994 (43)	Stage I-IIIa	124	ID BCG vs. control	6.7 yr: 52.5% vs. 39.7% 15 yr: 8.2% vs. 3.3% ($P = .005$)	
Lee 1994 (57)	Stage I-IIIa	93	OK-432 IP vs. control	61% 71% (NS)	
Fujisawa 1996 (47)	Stage I	83	TF + *Nocardia rubra* cell wall vs. control	5 yr DSS: 85% vs. 72% 10 yr DSS: 85% vs. 64% ($P = .041$)	

BCG, bacillus Calmette-Guerrin; DFS, disease-free survival; DSS, disease-specific survival; IP, intrapleural; ID, intradermal; TAA + FCA, Freund's adjuvant + allogeneic tumor antigen; PSK, krestin; TF, transfer factor.
[a]Five-year survival unless otherwise specified.

Immunotherapy has similarly been paired with both radiation and chemo-therapy. Table 4 includes the combination of immunotherapy and radiation in several studies. The use of radiation therapy and transfer factor by Whyte et al. (56) did not significantly improve survival. The study by Hayakawa et al. (45), on the other hand, showed a 2- and 5-year benefit with the use of adjuvant krestin and radiation therapy. Finally, Kimura and Yamaguchi (39) combined MVP chemotherapy with IL-2 and LAK cells, resulting in a significant survival benefit.

Thus, the combination of multiple adjuvant agents holds promise and should serve as the basis for future studies.

B. Prognostic Factors

Table 1 demonstrated that 5-year survival for stage I and II disease can range any-where from 25% to 83%. Clearly, this represents a wide biological activity of dis-ease within this subset of non-small-cell lung cancers. It is easy to see how the chance selection of a nonuniform subset of patients could skew the outcome and result in the wide differences of benefit seen in the previous adjuvant trials. Iden-tification of patients most likely to relapse, or, on the other hand, identification of patients unlikely to require adjuvant therapy, would thus be very helpful in the future design of adjuvant studies.

Table 5 presents review data on putative prognostic factors in NSCLC in stage I disease. These data represent univariate analysis of these prognos-tic factors. No one knows at this time how to integrate all of these different factors.

Harpole et al. (59) have also performed a multivariate analysis of prognostic factors that affect outcome in stage I NSCLC. Independent risk factors that affect overall and disease-free survival in descending order of significance include symptomatic disease at time of presentation, vascular invasion, visceral pleura invasion, high mitotic rate, and tumor size >3 cm.

A similar study from the same institution found in 250 consecutive stage I NSCLC patients the following variables to be significant predictors of recurrence on a univariate analysis: lymphatic vessel invasion ($P = .0007$); adenocarcinoma subtype ($P = .013$); and p53 immunostaining ($P = .033$). Stepwise Cox regression analyses confirmed that these were independent predictors of recurrent disease. Atelectasis, RB staining, and differentiation also approached statistical signifi-cance. The remainder of the factors analyzed were not significant: tumor size, blood vessel invasion, plasma cell infiltration, mitotic index, pleural involvement, lymphoid infiltration, presence of tumor giant cells, K-ras mutations, bcl-2 immunostaining, p185neu immunostaining, and flow cytometry (60).

Stratification in future trials based on these or other factors may help to ensure a homogeneous population being evaluated.

Table 5 Prognostic Factors and 5-Year Survival in Stage I NSCLC

Factor	Favorable	Intermediate	Unfavorable
Tumor size (clinical)	T1N0 62%		T2N0 36%
Tumor size (path)	T1N0 73%		T2N0 54%
Histology	Squamous 77%		Adeno/large cell 66% ($P = .014$)
Differentiation	Well-differentiated 78%	Moderately differentiated 54%	Poorly differentiated 28% ($P = .001$)
Lymphatic vessel invasion	Negative 3 yr OS 61%		Positive 42%
Blood vessel invasion	Negative 84%		Positive 49% ($P = .002$)
K-ras mutation	Negative 3 yr OS 68%		Positive 37% ($P = .002$)
Her-2-neu (adenocarcinoma only)	Negative 52%		Positive 30% ($P = <.01$)
p53 (stage I–III)	Negative 3 yr OS 51%		Positive 28% ($P = .01$)
Rb (stage I–III)	Positive 32 mo median survival		Negative 18 mo median survival
Blood group A or AB t	A antigen expressed; 71 mo median survival		A antigen negative; 15 mo median survival
Blood group O or B		39 mo median survival	
Pleural invasion	Negative 67%		Positive 44%
Symptomatic presentation	Negative 74%		Positive 41%
Flow cytometry	Diploid 70%		Aneuploid 33% ($P = .001$)

Source: Ref. 58.

V. Conclusion

Therapy for patients with stage I and II NSCLC remains unsatisfactory. Multiple studies, with many different combinations of agents, have been evaluated as adjuvant therapy for resected stage I and II disease without a clear benefit in survival. These studies are hampered in part by the changing definition of stage and staging

Table 6 Current Adjuvant Studies for Resected NSCLC

PDQ Ref.	Stage	Treatment planned	Comments
NCI-H96-0002	In situ stage I	Dietary intervention with 4 daily fruits and 4 daily vegetables	Squamous cell lung or head and neck Endpoint = reduction in 2nd malignancies
EORTC-08871	Curatively treated	Retinol palmitate vs. N-acetylcysteine vs. both vs. none	Laryngeal, oral cavity, and head and neck cancer Endpoint = reduction in frequency of 2nd malignancies
EU-90042	Limited	Chemotherapy with mito/IFF/CDDP + Radiation vs. radiation alone	Endpoint = compare duration and quality of survival
NCI-P92-0014	Stage I	Isotretinoin (13-CRA) vs. placebo	Endpoint = evaluate toxicity and compare overall survival
NCI-V94-0492	T_2N_0 $T_{1-2}N_1$	Navelbine and cisplatin adjuvant vs. observation	Endpoint = confirm significance of ras mutations. Measure toxicity, QOL, survival
EU-94043	Stage I, II, III	Mito/vindesine/CDDP vs. control ± radiation	Radiation randomized by institution to 50 Gy Endpoint = change in survival.
INT-0115	Stage II, IIIa	Radiation therapy to 50 Gy ± CDDP/etoposide	
NCI-T95-048N	Stage II, III	Vaccine with immune adjuvant Q521	In patients expressing mutant ras protein
C-9333	T_2N_0	Carboplatin and taxol vs. none	Endpoint = evaluate toxicity and compare overall survival

Mito, mitomycin-C; IFF, ifosphamide; CDDP, cisplatin.

procedures over the years. They are also hampered by the wide natural variability of survival within this subset of lung cancer.

Adjuvant radiation therapy has resulted in improved RFS in several studies with no difference in overall survival seen. This local benefit may be particularly useful to build upon in future trials using radiation-sensitizing chemotherapy agents to improve local control, and effective chemotherapy to reduce distant failure. Table 6 presents the study designs of several ongoing adjuvant trials.

Adjuvant immunotherapy has failed to date to demonstrate a benefit in an adjuvant setting. Identification of new agents and tumor vaccines will be areas to explore in future immunotherapy trials.

Adjuvant chemotherapy should not be considered a standard therapeutic treatment in 1999. There is no clear, consistent benefit to chemotherapy in the adjuvant setting for stage I and II NSCLC. Problems with the studies performed to date include: a lack of chemotherapeutic agents with sufficient chemotherapeutic activity in lung cancer; inadequate drug delivery (frequently <70% of patients received the complete intended chemotherapy course); and insufficient patient numbers. A modest 20% to 30% reduction in mortality in the first 5 years after diagnosis would be difficult to detect in trials of <2000 patients.

It is to be hoped that with the advent of newer chemotherapeutic drugs and better medical management of the side effects of chemotherapy, future studies will demonstrate a significant survival benefit with adjuvant therapy. Stage I and II NSCLC encompasses a heterogeneous mixture of tumors, and the selection and randomization based on significant prognostic factors are also important in future trials.

Adjuvant therapy for NSCLC continues to hold the promise of benefit in the future. Ideally, eligible patients with completely resected stage I and II NSCLC will be entered into well-designed randomized clinical trials rather then empirically starting therapy that "looks promising."

References

1. Landis, SH, Murray, T, Bolden, S, Wingo PA. Cancer Statistics, 1998. CA Cancer J Clin 1998; 48:6–29.
2. Jessup JM, McGinnis LS, Winchester DP, et al. Clinical highlights from the National Cancer Data Base: 1996. CA Cancer J Clin 1996; 46:185–192.
3. Ichinose Y, Hara N, Ohta M, Motohiro A, Kuda T, Aso H. Postoperative chemotherapy in non-small cell lung cancer: prognostic value of DNA ploidy and post recurrence survival. J Surg Oncol 1991; 46:15–20.
4. Mountain CF, Lukeman JM, Hammer SP, et al. Lung cancer classification: the relationship of disease extent and cell type to outcome in a clinical trial population. J Surg Oncol 1987; 35:147–156.
4a. Mountain, CF. Revisions in the International System for Staging Lung Cancer. Chest III; 1710–1717, 1997.
5. Naruke T, Goya T, Tsuchiya R, Suemasu K. Prognosis and survival in resected lung

cancer based on the new international staging system. J Thorac Cardiovasc Surg 1988; 96:440–447.

6. Matthews MJ, Kanhouwa S, Pickren J, Robinette D. Frequency of residual and metastatic tumor in patients undergoing curative surgical resection for lung cancer. Cancer Chemother Rep 1973; 4:63–67.

7. Bromley LL, Szur I. Combined radiotherapy and resection for carcinoma of the bronchus, experience with 66 patients. Lancet 1955; 5:937–940.

8. Shields TW. Pre-operative radiation in the treatment of bronchial carcinoma. Cancer 1972; 30:1388–1394.

9. Gebitekin C, Gupta K, Satur CM, et al. Fate of patients with residual tumor at the bronchial resection margin. Eur J Cardio-Thorac Surg 1994; 8:339–342.

10. Kirsh MV, Sloan H. Mediastinal metastasis in bronchogenic carcinoma: influence of post-operative radiation, cell type, and location. Ann Thorac Surg 1981; 5:459–463.

11. Choi NC, Grillo H, Gardiello M, Scannell JG Wilkins EW Jr. Basis for new strategic postoperative radiation of bronchogenic carcinoma. Int J Radiol Oncol Biol Phys 1980; 6:31–35.

12. Green N, Kurohara SS, George FW III, Crews QE Jr. Post-resection irradiation for primary lung cancer. Radiology 1975; 116:405–407.

13. Weisenberger TH, Gail M. Effects of postoperative mediastinal radiation on completely resected stage II and stage III epidermoid cancer of the lung. N Engl J Med 1986; 315:1377–1381.

14. Van Houtte P, Rocmans P, Smets P, Goffin JC. Postoperative radiation therapy in lung cancer: a controlled trial after resection of curative design. Int J Radiat Oncol Biol Phys 1980; 6:983–986.

15. Smolle-Juettner FM, Mayer R, Pinter H. "Adjuvant" external radiation of the mediastinum in radically resected non-small cell lung cancer. Eur J Cardio-Thorac Surg 1996; 10:947–950.

16. Martini N, Burt ME, Bains MS, McCormack PM, Rusch VW, Ginsberg RJ. Survival after resection of stage II NSCLC. Ann Thorac Surg 1992; 54:460–466.

17. Bangma PJ. Postoperative radiotherapy. In: Deeley TJ, ed. Carcinoma of the Bronchus. New York: Appleton Century Crofts, 1971; 163–170.

18. Warram J. Preoperative irradiation of cancer of the lung. Final report of a therapeutic trial. A collaborative study. Cancer 1975; 36:914–925.

19. Emami B, Kim T, Roper C, Simpson JR, Piepich MV, Hederman MA. Postoperative radiation therapy in the management of lung cancer. Radiology 1987; 164:251–253.

20. Lafitte JJ, Ribert ME, Prevost BM, Gosselin BH, Copin MC, Bricket AH. Postresection irradiation for T2N0M0 non-small cell carcinoma: a prospective, randomized study. Ann Thorac Surg 1996; 62:830–834.

21. Anonymous. The benefit of adjuvant treatment for resected locally advanced non-small cell lung cancer. The Lung Cancer Study Group. J Clin Oncol 1988; 6:9–17.

22. Johnson DH. Adjuvant chemotherapy for non-small cell lung cancer. Chest 1994; 106:313S-317S.

23. Shields TW, Humphrey EW, Eastridge CE, Keehn RJ. Adjuvant cancer chemotherapy after resection of carcinoma of the lung. Cancer 1977; 40:2057–2062.

24. Shields TW, Higgins GA Jr, Humphrey EW, Matthews MJ, Keehn RJ. Prolonged

intermittent adjuvant chemotherapy with CCNU and hydroxyurea after resection of carcinoma of the lung. Cancer 1982; 50:1713–1721.

25. Girling DJ, Stott H, Stephens RJ, Fox W. Fifteen-year follow-up of all patients in a study of postoperative chemotherapy for bronchial carcinoma. Br J Cancer 1985; 52:867–873.

26. Ayoub J, Duranceau A, Lorange G. Effectiveness of adjuvant chemotherapy in operable non-small lung cancer. Proceedings of the Fifth International Conference on the Adjuvant Therapy of Cancer. Tuscon, AZ, March 1987:36.

27. Gail MH. Placebo-controlled randomized double blind study of adjuvant intrapleural BCG in patients with resected T1N0, T1N1, T2N0 squamous cell, adenocarcinoma, or large cell carcinoma of the lung. Chest 1994; 106:287S–290S.

28. Holmes EC. Surgical adjuvant therapy for stage II and stage III adenocarcinoma and large cell undifferentiated carcinoma. Chest 1994; 106:293S–296S.

29. Niiranen A, Niitamo-Korhonen S, Kouri M, Assendelft A, Mattson K, Pyrohonen S. Adjuvant chemotherapy after radical surgery for non-small cell lung cancer: a randomized study. J Clin Oncol 1992; 10:1927–1932.

30. Feld R, Rubinstein L, Thomas PA. Adjuvant chemotherapy with cyclophosphamide, doxorubicin, and cisplatin in patients with completely resected stage I non-small cell lung cancer: an LCSG trial. Chest 1994; 106:307S–309S.

31. Figlin RA, Piantodosi S. A phase 3 randomized trial of immediate combination chemotherapy vs delayed combination chemotherapy in patients with completely resected stage II and III non-small cell carcinoma of the lung. Chest 1994; 106:310S-313S.

32. Ruckdeshel JC, Piantodosi S. Quality of life in lung cancer surgical adjuvant trials. Chest 1994; 6:324S–328S.

33. Klingman RR, DeMeester TR. Surgical approach to non-small cell lung cancer stage I and II. Heme Oncol Clin North Am 1990; 4:1079–1091.

34. Gradishar WJ, Mick R, Hoffman PC, et al. The impact on survival by adjuvant chemotherapy and radiation therapy in stage II non-small cell lung cancer. Am J Clin Oncol 1992; 15:405–411.

35. Dautzenberg B, Chastong C, Arriagada A, et al. Adjuvant radiotherapy versus combined sequential chemotherapy followed by radiation in the treatment of resected NSCLC. A randomized trial of 267 patients. GETCB. Cancer 1995; 76:779–786.

36. Karp DD, Daly BD, Robert NJ. Long term safety of cisplatin and etoposide (CE) plus concentrated XRT (Rad) as adjuvant therapy in non-small cell lung cancer. Proc Am Soc Clin Oncol 1993; 12:A1202.

37. Wada H, Hitomi S, Teramatsu T. Adjuvant chemotherapy after complete resection in non-small cell lung cancer. West Japan Study Group for Lung Cancer Surgery. J Clin Oncol 1996; 14:1048–1054.

38. Tanaka F, Yamaguchi K, Ohtabe Y, Fukuse T, Hitomi S, Wada H. p53 status predicts the efficacy of post-operative oral administration of tegafur (FT) for completely resected non-small cell lung cancer (NSCLC). Proc Am Soc Clin Oncol 1997; A1746.

39. Kimura N, Yamaguchi Y. Adjuvant chemo-immunotherapy after curative resection of stage II and IIIa primary lung cancer. Lung Cancer 1996; 14:301–314.

40. Study Group of Adjuvant Chemotherapy for Lung Cancer (Chuba, Japan). A ran-

domized trial of postoperative adjuvant chemotherapy in non-small cell lung cancer (the second cooperative study). Eur J Surg Oncol 1995; 21:69–76.

41. Non-Small Cell Lung Cancer Collaborative Group. Chemotherapy in non-small cell lung cancer: a meta analysis using updated data on individual patients from 52 randomized clinical trials. BMJ 1995; 311:900–909.

42. Ruckdeschel JC, Codish SD, Stranaham A, McKneally MF. Post-operative empyema improves survival in lung cancer: documentation and analysis of a natural experiment. N Engl J Med 1972; 287:1013–1017.

43. Soresi E, Borghini U, Schialdi GF, Boffi R, Invernizzi G, Ravini M. Long-term results of adjuvant immunotherapy with intradermal bacillus calmette guerrin (BCG) in resected NSCLC. Cuneo Lung Cancer Study Group. First international lung cancer conference: non-small cell lung cancer management—open questions and controversies, Oct. 7–8, 1994, Alba, Cuneo, Italy.

44. Ludwig Lung Cancer Study Group. Immuno-stimulation with intrapleural BCG as adjuvant therapy in resected non-small cell lung cancer. Cancer 1986; 58:2411–2416.

45. Hayakawa K, Mitsuhashi N, Saito Y, et al. Effect of krestin (PSK) as adjuvant therapy on the prognosis after radical radiotherapy in patients with non-small cell lung cancer. Anticancer Res 1993; 13:1815–1820.

46. Pastorino V, Infante M, Maioloi M, et al. Adjuvant therapy of stage I lung cancer with high dose vitamin A. J Clin Oncol 1993; 11:1216–1222.

47. Fujisawa T, Yamaguchi Y. Postoperative immunostimulation after complete resection improves survival of patients with stage I non-small cell lung cancer. Cancer 1996; 78:1892–1898.

48. McKneally MF, Mayer C, Kausel HW. Regional immunotherapy with intrapleural BCG in lung cancer. Lancet 1976; 1:377–379.

49. Pouillart P, Palangie T, Huguenin P. Adjuvant non-intrapleural BCG In: Muggia F, Rosencweig M, eds. Cancer: Progress in Therapeutic Research. New York: Raven Press, 1979:477.

50. Hadziev S, Mandulova P, Kavaklieva-Dimitrova J, Penev K, Spassova M, Madzarova S. BCG immunotherapy of lung cancer in a district oncology dispensary. I. Study of 860 patients with histologic diagnosis. Neoplasma 1982; 29:93–110.

51. Anonymous. Intrapleural and intravenous *Corynebacterium parvum* in patients with resected stage I and II non-small cell carcinoma of the lung. The Ludwig Lung Cancer Study Group. Cancer Immunol Immunother 1986; 23:1–4.

52. Little AG, DeMeester TR, Ferguson MK, et al. Modified stage I (T1N0M0, T2N0M0), non-small cell lung cancer: treatment results, recurrence patterns, and adjuvant immunotherapy. Surgery 1986; 100:621–628.

53. Hollingshead AC. Immunotherapy: a report of an adjuvant phase III lung cancer immunotherapy trial. Adv Oncol 1986; 2:1–5.

54. Millar JW, Roscoe P, Pearce SJ, Ludgate S, Horne NW. Five-year results of a controlled study of BCG immunotherapy after surgical resection in bronchial carcinoma. Thorax 1982; 37:57–60.

55. Mouritzen C. Bestatin as adjuvant treatment in operated stage I and stage II non-small cell lung cancer. Acta Oncol 1990; 29:817–820.

56. Whyte RI, Schork A, Sloan H, Orringer MB, Kirsh MM. Adjuvant treatment using

transfer factor for bronchogenic carcinoma: long term follow-up. Ann Thorac Surg 1992; 53:391–396.

57. Lee YC, Luh SP, Wu RM, Lee CJ. Adjuvant immunotherapy with intrapleural strep pyogenes (OK-432) in lung cancer patients after resection. Cancer Immunol Immunother 1994; 39:269–274.

58. Strauss GM, Kwaitkowsi DJ, Harpole DH, Lynch TJ, Skarin AT, Sugarbaker DJ. Molecular and pathologic markers in stage I non-small-cell carcinoma of the lung. J Clin Oncol 1995; 13:1265–1279.

59. Harpole DH, Herndon JE, Young GW. Stage I non-small cell lung cancer in multi-variate analysis of treatments methods and patterns of recurrence. Cancer 1995; 76:87–96.

60. Kwiatkowski DJ, Harpole DH, Godleski J, et al. Prognostic factor analysis of 250 stage I NSCLC patients: pathologic features are more important than molecular analyses. Proc Am Soc Clin Oncol 1997; 16:1644A.

8

Superior Pulmonary Sulcus Tumors

HAROLD C. URSCHEL, JR.

University of Texas Southwestern Medical School and
Baylor University Medical Center
Dallas, Texas

I. Introduction

Superior pulmonary sulcus tumors include a wide variety of pathological entities
that are encompassed by the term "Pancoast's syndrome." The classic syndrome
includes pain in the shoulder, arm, and hand in the distribution of C8 and T1 nerve
roots; weakness and atrophy of the hand muscles; Horner's syndrome; and first-rib
erosion secondary to Pancoast's tumor in the superior thoracic inlet.

Anatomically, the superior pulmonary sulcus is the area on the superior surface of the lung traversed by the subclavian vessels and encircled by the first rib
and spine. It may also be described as the thoracic outlet or thoracic inlet.

The treatment of choice is preoperative irradiation (3000r over 2 to 3 weeks)
followed by surgical en bloc resection of the lung, chest wall, lower brachial
plexus, and vertebrae at 1-month intervals. This affects approximately 35% 5-year
survival with N0–1 stage.

II. History

Edward Hare in 1838 described a patient with pain and numbness in the area of his
left ulnar nerve with Horner's syndrome and associated with a tumor in the left

159

side of his neck (1). Henry K. Pancoast, a radiologist, in 1924 described the clinical-radiographic findings of four patients with pain in the upper extremity, Horner's syndrome, and erosion of the first rib and vertebra secondary to cancer in the superior pulmonary sulcus (2). He presented seven patients in 1932 from which resulted the eponym Pancoast's tumor and Pancoast's syndrome (3). He localized the lesions to tumors in the thoracic outlet or inlet. He coined the term "superior pulmonary sulcus tumor" rather than apical chest tumor but mistakenly felt that these tumors came from embryonic cell rest of the fifth branchial cleft. Tobias recognized that these tumors produced a "painful apical costovertebral syndrome" and were secondary to cancers of pulmonary origin (4). Pancoast's syndrome may be produced by both benign and malignant lesions but most frequently are secondary to carcinomas of bronchogenic origin.

In the early 1950s these tumors were considered unresectable and were treated primarily by irradiation therapy only. Few patients survived. Midway through the irradiation therapy of one patient in 1951, the patient became extremely ill, irradiation was stopped, and, because the pain was still severe, Dr. Robert Shaw (my senior partner), elected to resect the lesion. This was done empirically approximately 4 weeks after the 3000r had been delivered in 2-week period. The patient subsequently became pain-free and lived 15 years thereafter without evidence of disease, expiring from another cause. Because of this, in our group several other cases were treated in similar fashion with 3,000r to the tumor and mediastinal lymph nodes over a period of 2 to 3 weeks followed by a waiting period of 2 to 4 weeks. This allows time for the benefits of irradiation, which theoretically include shrinking of the tumor, blocking of the lymphatics, and weakening cells that might be left after surgery since the margins are extremely close in such tumor resections. In 1961, 14 cases were reported with approximately 40% 5-year survival shown (5). Chardack and MacCallum presented a case in 1953 and 1956 that had been resected and treated successfully with *post*operative irradiation therapy (6,7). This, however, has not been as reproducible in other centers as a successful technique.

III. Diagnosis

A. Clinical Presentation

The vast majority of patients present with shoulder and elbow pain because of the involvement of the lower trunk of the brachial plexus. The discomfort often follows the distribution of the ulnar nerve because of malignant invasion of T1 and C8 nerve roots and extension into the parietal pleura and first rib (8–17). Weakness and atrophy of the intrinsic muscles in the hand along with pain and paresthesias in the medial aspect of the arm and fourth and fifth digits (distribution of the ulnar nerve), sometimes associated with a loss of the triceps reflex, is also caused by C8 and T1 nerve root involvement. Pain may radiate into the neck, head, and posteriorly into the scapular area or anteriorly into the chest (Fig. 1).

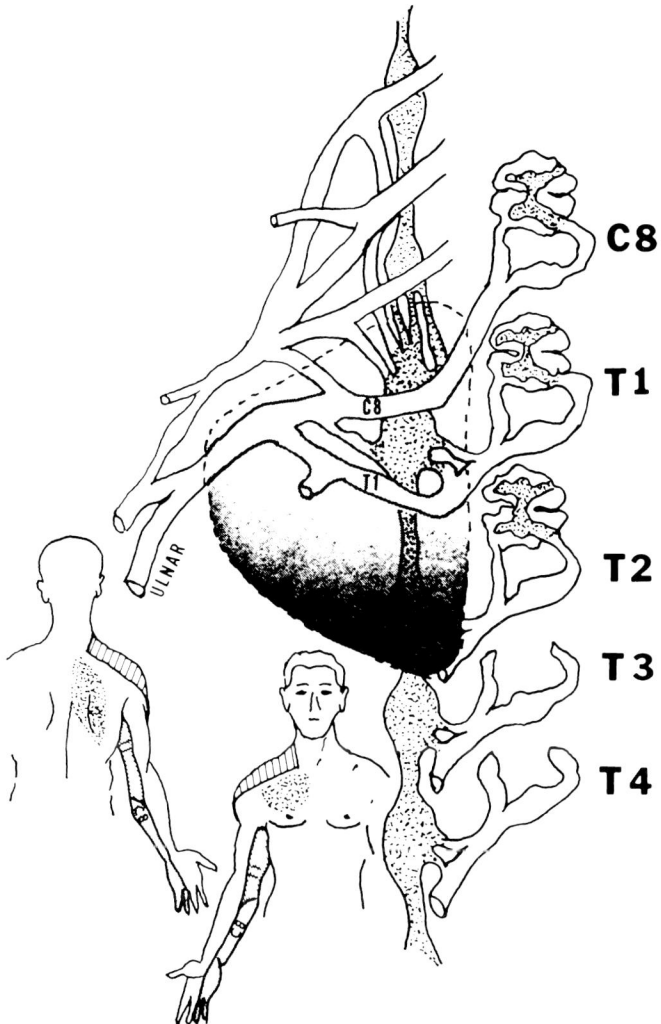

Figure 1 Neural involvement of the typical superior pulmonary sulcus carcinoma: peripheral nerves C8, T1, T2 distribution and sympathetic nerves C8, T1, T2 ganglion.

Classically, the patient presents holding the elbow with the other arm to support the shoulder and take the pressure off the brachial plexus for symptomatic relief (3,10,16–18) (Fig. 2). Frequently, the diagnosis is missed because of concentration on cervical osteoarthritis, disks, or other differential diagnoses, often delaying recognition of the true etiology. Horner's syndrome is classically present as an ipsi-

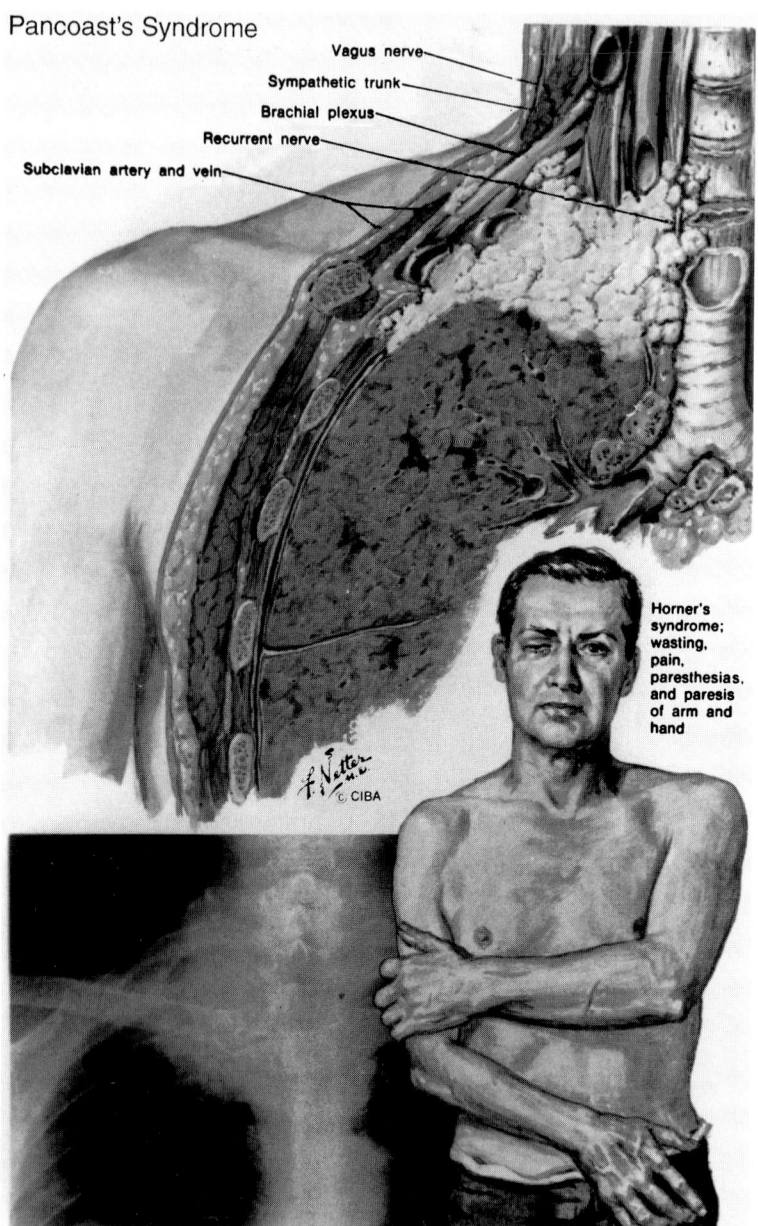

Pancoast's Syndrome

Vagus nerve
Sympathetic trunk
Brachial plexus
Recurrent nerve
Subclavian artery and vein

Horner's syndrome; wasting, pain, paresthesias, and paresis of arm and hand

Figure 2 Composite illustration (by Frank Netter) of a patient with clinical manifestations, chest radiograph of tumor with superior sulcus location, and gross pathologic diagnostic demonstration of the lung carcinoma invading the chest wall, brachial plexus, and sympathetic nerves. (Copyright 1979. CIBA-GEIGY Corporation. Reproduced with permission from The CIBA Collection of Medical Illustrations by Frank H. Netter, M.D. All rights reserved.)

lateral ptosis, narrowing of the palpebral fissure, myosis, and anhydrosis. It is produced by involvement of the sympathetic chain in the area of C7 and C8, the upper
two-thirds of the stellate ganglion (8,9,10–13,16,19–22). Vertebral involvement
and spinal cord compression with paralysis (paraplegia) are occasionally observed.
Phrenic or recurrent laryngeal nerve invasion is infrequently present, producing
diaphragmatic paralysis or hoarseness. Superior vena cava syndrome may result if
anterior tumors are present. This leads to swelling of the face and distension of the
neck and upper chest wall veins. Primary pulmonary tumors may also produce the
usual symptoms of cough, hemoptysis, dypsnea, wheeze, or weight loss.

B. Radiographic Observations

Chest roentgenographs (PA and lateral) are the simplest methods of discerning an
apical mass (Fig. 3). Apical lordotic chest views are valuable following the screening procedure. Computerized tomography (CT) of the chest provides additional
information, particularly about bone invasion (including the first rib) and vertebral
involvement. It also may be used to delineate lung and liver metastases. Magnetic
resonance imaging (MRI) is particularly helpful in soft tissue areas such as invasion of the brachial plexus and chest wall as well as lymph node metastases in the
mediastinum (23) (Figs. 4, 5).

C. Diagnostic Tests

The definitive diagnosis is established by a transthoracic needle biopsy, usually
through the supraclavicular space or the posterior superior chest between the

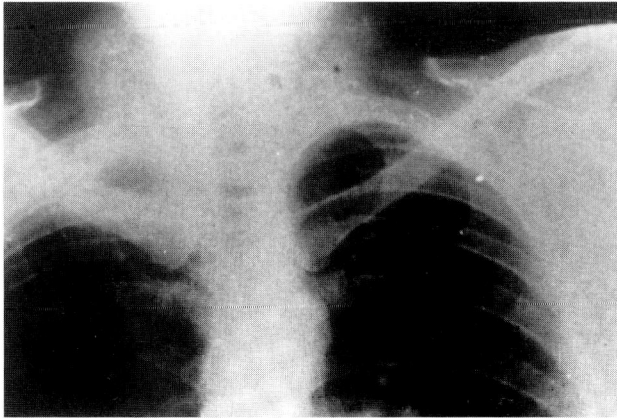

Figure 3 Chest radiograph of right superior pulmonary sulcus carcinoma invading the
first rib.

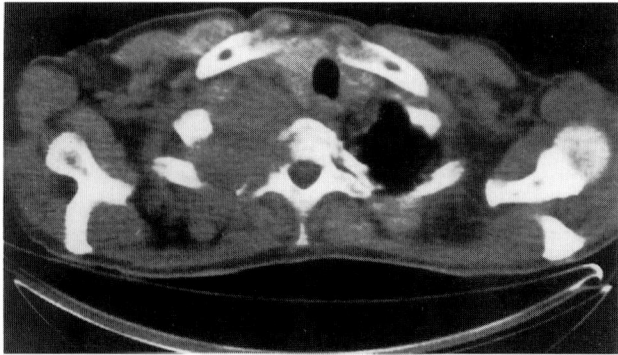

Figure 4   CT scan of right superior pulmonary sulcus carcinoma invading the first rib and vertebra.

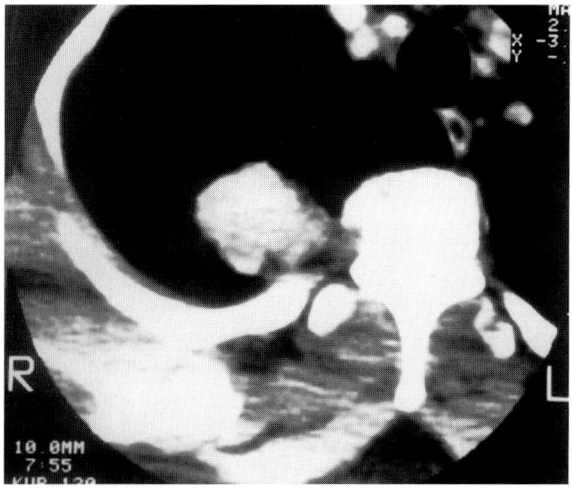

Figure 5   MRI scan of right superior pulmonary sulcus carcinoma invading the first rib and vertebra.

scapula and spine. These small needles are guided by fluoroscopy, ultrasound, or CT in most cases. The first description of transcervical biopsy via the supraclavicular approach was reported by McGoon in 1964 (24). Biopsy may be performed under local or general anesthesia. The diagnostic yield for needle biopsy is >90%. Video-assisted thoracoscopy (VATS) may be used for diagnosis, but patients may also be treated without a diagnosis if the symptoms are classical and the needle biopsies are negative (10).

Diagnostic yield from sputum cytology is <20% and for bronchoscopy (fiberoptic or rigid) <30% (25,26). This is because most of these tumors are peripheral.

D. Staging and Perioperative Assessment

Cervical mediastinal lymph node exploration is necessary before treatment in these patients to establish whether the lymph nodes are positive. The suggestion of enlarged nodes on either the CT or MRI may be helpful, but the staging of actual metastases is critical (27). False positives are present in both directions. If the mediastinal nodes are positive for a right upper lobe lesion, it is still treated as an operable case because they are assumed to be "regional" lymph nodes. Contrarily, for a left upper lobe metastasis to the mediastinal lymph node, surgical therapy is less likely to be successful. Perinodal lymph node metastasis portends a worse prognosis than intranodal metastases (10).

Invasion of the vertebral body (T4) demonstrated by CT usually renders a patient inoperable because "no reported cures" have resulted with vertebral involvement in our experience (23). Distant metastases are suspected by history and physical examination, and by blood tests including liver chemistries as well as CT and MRI of the mediastinum, retroperitoneum, liver, and adrenal glands.

Cell types encountered are predominantly squamous cell carcinoma, with large cell the second and adenocarcinoma the third most commonly observed (28–35). Many may begin as "scar" carcinomas or be secondary to other malignancies (36–49). Metastatic carcinoma from other organs may produce similar symptoms in this area. Various other etiologies include benign tumors and infections such as actinomycosis, tuberculosis, escharhea infection, cryptococcosis, or hydatid cyst (50–61). Vascular aneurysms (62) or amylordosis (63) may also produce the syndrome.

E. Differential Diagnosis

Differential diagnosis includes thoracic outlet syndrome (TOS), which may mimic the symptoms of ulnar paresthesias and pain. First-rib resection has been carried out for TOS mistakenly in patients with superior sulcus tumor of the lung (10). Esophageal and cardiac disease can also mimic symptoms of superior pulmonary sulcus tumors, and these areas should be ruled out in the differential diagnosis (10).

IV. Indications for Surgery

If the patient has a tumor in the area of the superior pulmonary sulcus with or without rib involvement, with or without lower brachial plexus involvement, and staged as a T3 N0 or N1, he or she is operable. N2 disease is operable if it is in the right upper lobe and the mediastinal nodes are considered to be intranodal metastases. Involvement of the vena cava, subclavian artery, or vein are not contraindications for surgery.

Contraindications include vertebral involvement because there have been no "reported" cures, extensive involvement of the brachial plexus, mediastinal perinodal involvement, significant invasion of soft tissues of the neck, and distant metastasis. Palliative resection is occasionally performed for intractable pain (23).

V. Treatment

A. Preoperative Radiotherapy Followed by Surgery

After the 3000r in 2 to 3 weeks followed by a 4-week waiting period, surgical extirpation with an "en bloc" resection of the pulmonary tumor, chest wall, lower brachial plexus, and vertebrae through the posterior thoracoplasty approach is performed (64,65) (Figs. 6–14). The en bloc resection of the pulmonary tumor and chest wall is accompanied by resection of the sympathetic chain, the lower trunk of the brachial plexus in most cases (T1 nerve root in most cases; C8 nerve root less frequently), and, rarely, the subclavian artery with an interposed graft. A margin of vertebral body is removed with all tumors. A segmentectomy, subsegmental resection, lobectomy, or pneumonectomy is performed to complete the en bloc

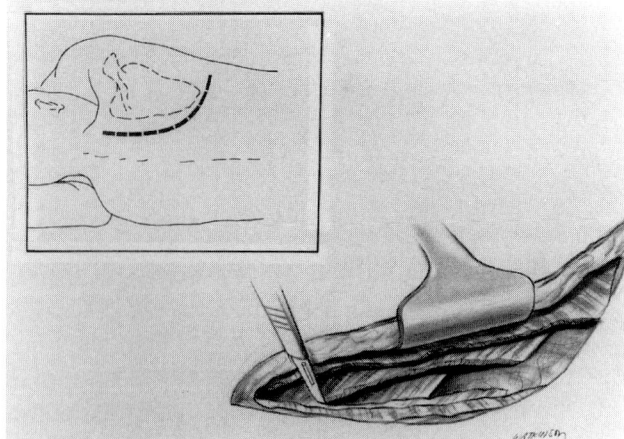

Figure 6 The patient is placed in the lateral position with an axillary roll under the "down" side. The incision is made from above the angle of the scapula, halfway between it and the spinous processes (thoracoplasty technique), inferiorly angling anteriorly around the tip of the scapula. The subcutaneous tissue and the trapezius and rhomboid muscles are divided. The posterior superior serratus muscle is divided.

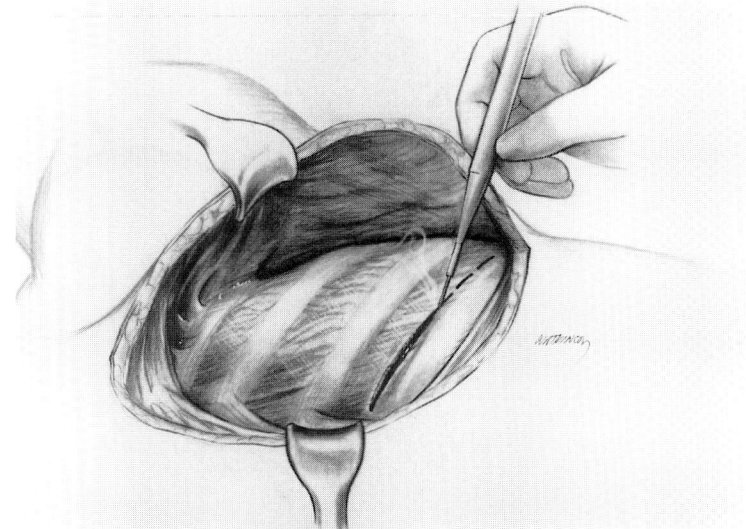

Figure 7 After incising the intercostal muscle on top of the fourth rib, a Finochietto retractor is placed between the top of the fourth rib and the scapula. A double-lumen tube is employed so that the lung is collapsed.

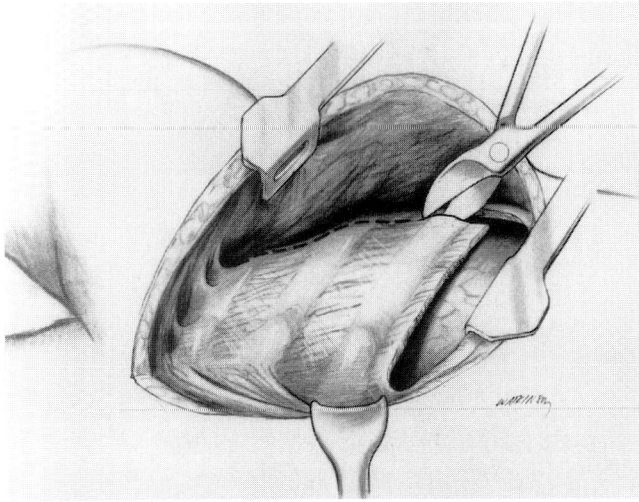

Figure 8 The fourth interspace is opened. With a hand in the chest, the tumor is palpated to ascertain its extent and the number of ribs, as well as the length of each rib to be resected. If the tumor is larger, a lower interspace may be used.

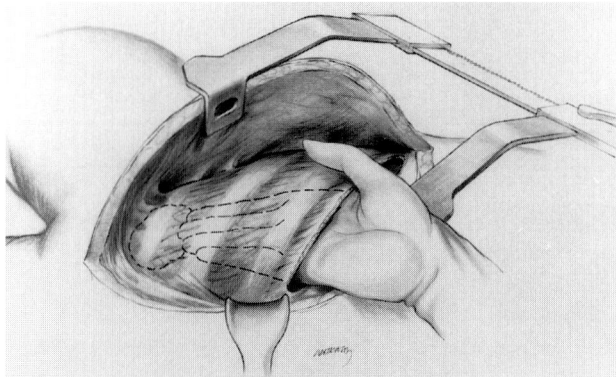

Figure 9 Anteriorly, the ribs are divided with the rib shears after ligating, dividing, or clipping the neurovascular bundle under each rib. The dissection is carried up to and through the first rib.

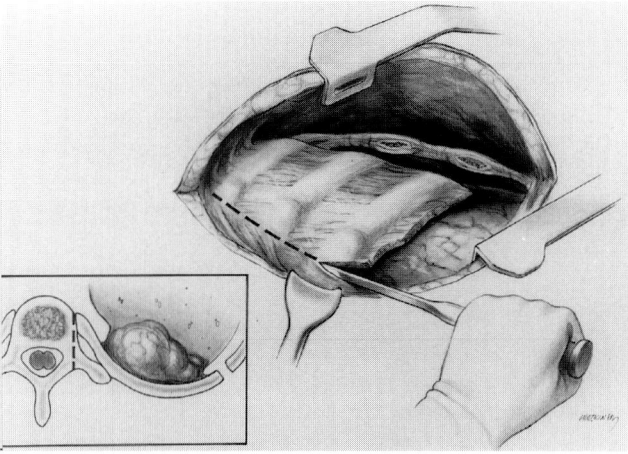

Figure 10 Posteriorly, the ribs are sheared off with an osteotome, taking the rib at the level of the transverse processes or small segment of vertebrae if necessary. The intercostal bundles may be cauterized or clipped. This is carried through the third, second, and first ribs. (Preoperatively, if the tumor is invading the vertebrae by CT scan, the patient is considered "inoperable.") If the tumor is adjacent to the vertebrae, a margin of vertebrae is taken with the osteotome.

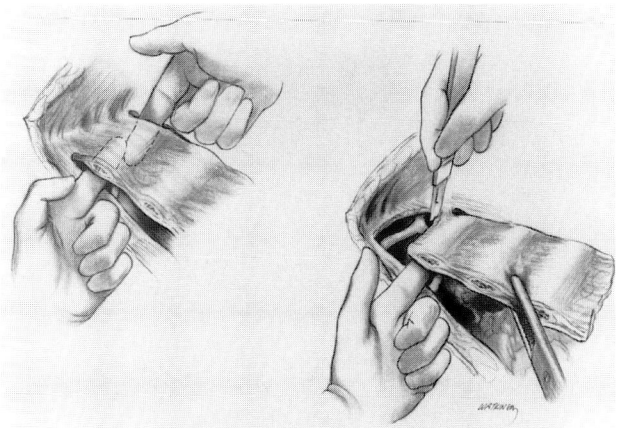

Figure 11   After cutting the first rib anteriorly and posteriorly, one index finger is inserted from the front and one from the back to palpate the tumor and ascertain its relationship to the T1 and C8 nerve roots, the lower trunk of the brachial plexus, and the axillary subclavian artery and vein. The scalenus anticus and medius muscles are divided with the finger holding the en bloc section anteriorly and inferiorly. Care is taken not to injure the artery or vein.

dissection. Chest wall replacement is required occasionally for anterior tumors, but usually not for those lying under the scapula. If six or more ribs are taken, posterior reconstruction with Marlex or other synthetic material is important to keep the scapula from sticking inside the chest (64).

The anterior cervical approach championed by Dartevelle involves a median sternotomy and cervical resection of the clavicle, and en bloc resection of the artery, often the vein, and the tumor (65,66) (Figs. 15–19). The long-term results have not been gratifying.

B.   Chemotherapy

Since the interest in induction neoadjuvant chemotherapy in the treatment of locally advanced bronchogenic carcinoma, the efficacy in the treatment of superior sulcus tumors has not been demonstrated. Only small groups have been studied, one involving 18 patients with stage 3A and 3B superior sulcus tumors which were treated with neoadjuvant chemotherapy and preoperative irradiation therapy followed by surgery (67). Another group of 16 patients had cysplatinum, etoposide, and cyclophosphamide followed by surgery and subsequently irradiation therapy (68). There was no improvement of survival rates or local control in either

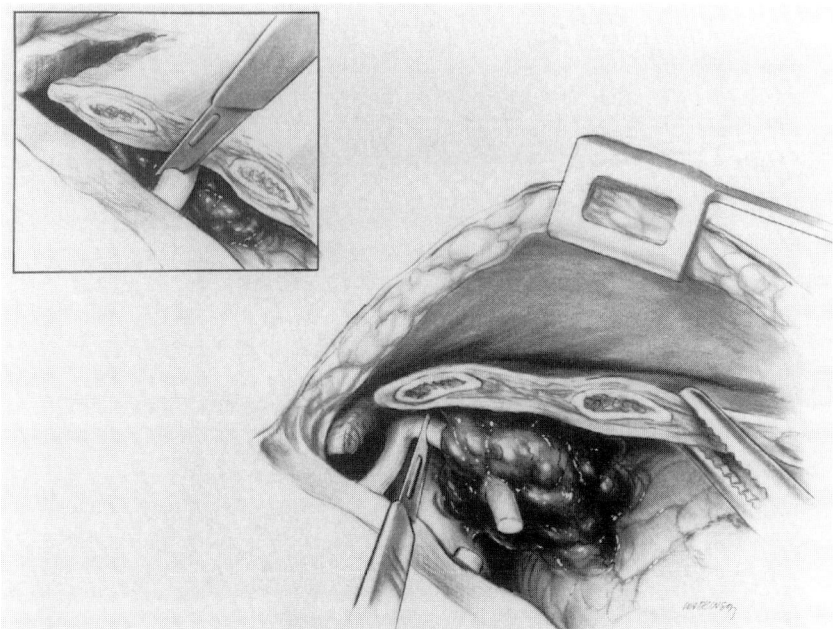

Figure 12 The T1 nerve root is divided posteriorly, and the segment is lifted up with the tumor. The C8 nerve root is visualized and may be divided if necessary. The anterior part of T1 nerve root is divided.

group. A study of 124 patients with superior sulcus tumor who received preoperative platinum-based chemotherapy showed no long-term, disease-free survivors (69). A Phase II trial of induction chemotherapy and radiotherapy followed by surgical resection of superior sulcus tumors of N0 to N1 disease conducted by the Eastern Cooperative Oncology Group has been initiated. No chemotherapy has been established as standard therapy although more lung carcinomas are treated with a platinum-based regimen for a total of four to six cycles. The best therapeutic option for patients with superior sulcus tumors at the present time does *not* include chemotherapy.

C. Complications of Therapy

1. Surgery

Surgical morbidity includes bleeding, atelectasis, infection, thromboembolism, persistent air leak, empyema, spinal fluid leak with pneumocephagram and/or meningitis, chylothorax, ulnar nerve paresis or paralysis, and Horner's syndrome not present preoperatively (70–74).

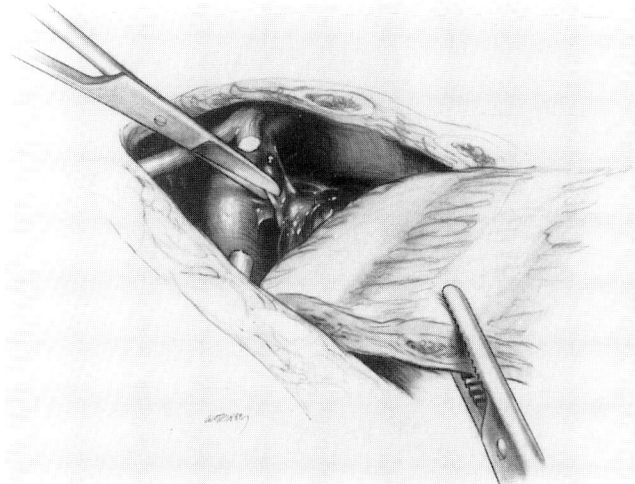

Figure 13   The subclavian artery is dissected from the tumor. If the artery is involved, an interposition graft may be employed (usually autogenous saphenous vein). This is usually not the case because the adventitia protects the artery from tumor invasion.

Interestingly enough, taking T1 or even T2 does not seem to produce much clinical problem, and even C8 does not give the usual severe problems of ulnar plexus injuries. Possibly this is because the slow growth of the tumor allows other nerve roots to assume function. Surgical morbidity is 38% and mortality between 5% and 10% (12,75–79).

2. Irradiation Therapy

Adverse effects of irradiation therapy include skin fibrosis, fatigue, esophagitis, radiation pneumonitis, pulmonary fibrosis, myelitis, and brachial neuritis, all of which may be extremely devastating to the patient (80–91).

3. Chemotherapy

Complications of chemotherapy include myelosuppression, increased risk of bleeding and infection, peripheral or central neuropathy, renal insufficiency, mucositis, nausea, vomiting, diarrhea, and hypersensitive reaction to secondary malignancies (92–95).

4. Recurrence

There is a significant risk of local or regional recurrence and distant metastases following treatment of superior sulcus tumors just as there is on any bronchogenic

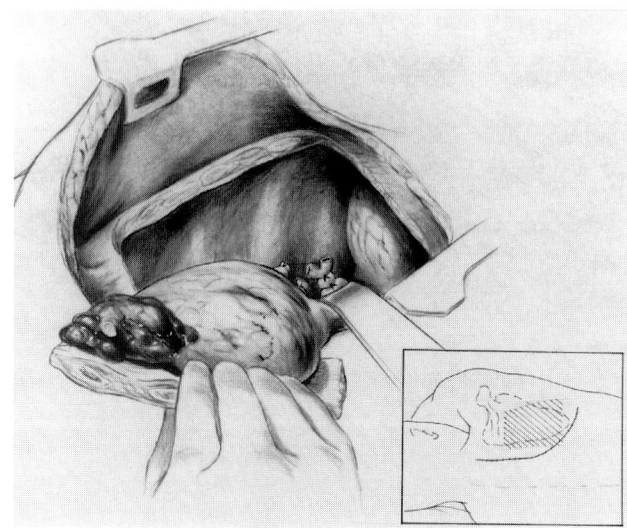

Figure 14 Following completion of the en bloc chest wall resection, a lobectomy or segmental resection of the lung is performed. The chest wall is closed with Marlex if anterior.
However, the scapula covers the posterior area so that usually no chest wall reconstruction
is necessary. If the fifth rib is removed, the scapula tip may get hooked under the sixth rib.
If this appears to be a possibility, the tip of the scapula is excised. The wound is closed in
layers with interrupted 0 Neurlon sutures in a figure-of-eight fashion (Tom Jones stitch),
running 2-0 Vicryl in the subcutaneous tissue, and skin clips in the skin.

carcinomas. Brain metastasis is one of the most common in younger patients with
large-cell and adenocarcinoma (96–102).

D. Survival and Prognostic Factors

Overall 5-year survival rate following combined preoperative radiotherapy and
extended surgical resection is generally around 20% to 35%, but varies from 10%
to 64% with a median survival of 7 to 31 months in different series (3,23,73,
94,103–106). It is directly related to N-stage disease, being 35% for N0–1 disease
(10). Preoperative radiotherapy in the treatment of superior sulcus tumors
improves resectability and survival (10). Several earlier studies comparing preoperative radiotherapy in doses of 3000 to 6000 cGy and surgery alone in the treatment of non-Pancoast's bronchogenic carcinoma have not reported significant differences in survival between these groups (105,106). However, our data reveal a
survival of 35% in 372 patients followed over 5 years and treated with preoperative irradiation and en bloc resection.

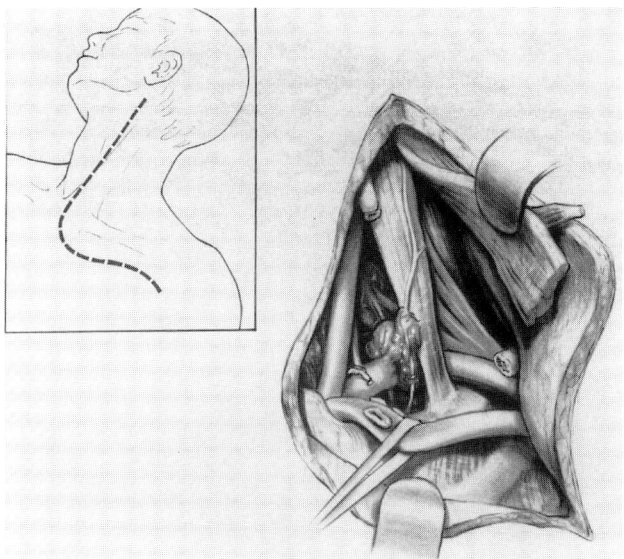

Figure 15 The patient is placed in the supine position, prepared, and draped with the head turned to the right. A pad is placed under the back between the scapulae. The incision is made below the ear anterior to the sternocleidomastoid muscle down to the sternal notch and out laterally in the supraclavicular space in an L-shaped incision. The flap is dissected. The sternocleidomastoid muscle is divided from the sternum. The clavicle is resected, and the subclavian vein is dissected free and retracted. The external jugular vein is divided. The tumor is growing into the lower T1 nerve root, the axillary-subclavian artery, and the scalenus anticus muscle above its attachment to the first rib.

With primary radiotherapy, overall 5-year survival rates reported in the literature vary between 0% and 29% (11,17,35,37,76,86). In these series, a better 5-year survival rate of 40% was generally associated with the absence of mediastinal lymph node and bone involvement, and achievement of local control of the tumor (9,15); the latter was related to higher radiotherapy dose in some studies (16,80). However, many studies of radiotherapy alone have reported 5-year survival rates of 0% to 10%, most likely because of the inclusion of patients with unfavorable prognostic factors and unresectable tumors, making comparisons of primary radiotherapy to combined radiosurgical treatment unreliable (8,21,104). A few studies have not found significant differences in survival between patients treated with irradiation only and irradiation combined with surgery (15,33). Five-year survival rates in these studies have ranged from 18% to 23% for both treatment modalities.

Several clinical features of patients with superior sulcus tumors are impor-

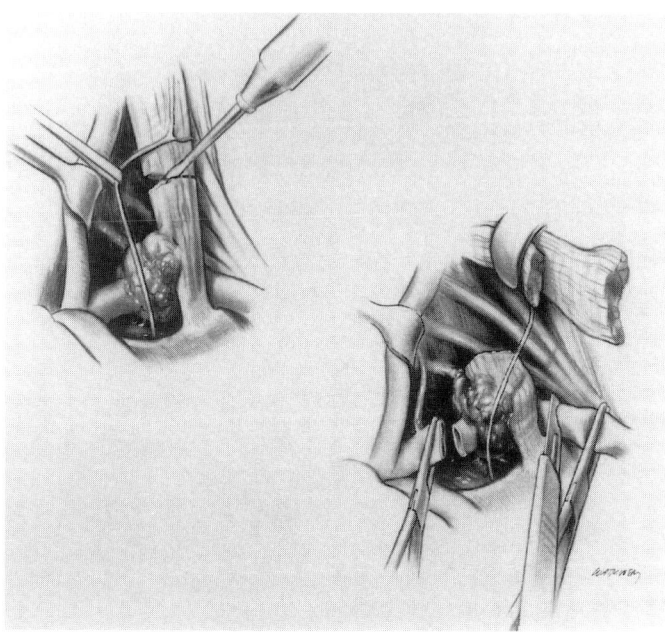

Figure 16 The scalenus anticus muscle is divided high above the tumor, retracting the phrenic nerve away from the area. The subclavian artery is clamped and divided on each side of the tumor, leaving a margin. Heparin is used as a local flush but not systemically.

tant prognostic indicators. The factors associated with a poor prognosis include extension of the tumor into the base of the neck; involvement of the mediastinal lymph nodes (107,108), vertebral bodies, or the great vessels; and the presence of Horner's syndrome (10,18,70). In our series of 372 patients with preoperative irradiation (3000r), 44% of those who had no nodal involvement survived 5 years or more, whereas those with mediastinal lymph node involvement had a reduced survival (18). Komaki et al. noted that patients with clinical and radiographic stage 3A disease had significantly better survival than those who had stage 3B disease (80,109). In contrast, N2 lymph nodal status was not associated with a worse prognosis compared with N0 status in the series reported by Maggi et al. (70) and others (10).

Longer duration of symptoms, most likely as an indicator of advanced disease, has also been found to adversely affect the prognosis (20). In contrast, good performance status and <5% weight loss are associated with better survival (16,80). Finally, local control of the tumor by irradiation and/or surgery and the achievement of pain relief after treatment have been established as important factors for improved survival (9,10,18,32,65,69).

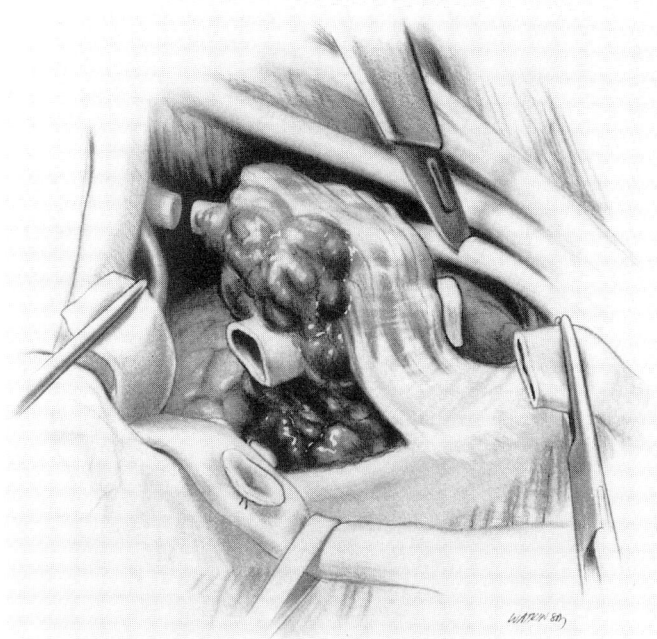

Figure 17 The T1 nerve root is excised on each side of the tumor, leaving a margin.

E. Pathology

The superior sulcus tumor is usually an extension of a pulmonary carcinoma, most of it being outside the lung and involving chest wall, nerve roots, and lower trunk of the brachial plexus, sympathetic chain, ganglion, ribs, and bone. Squamous cell carcinoma occurs most frequently, although large-cell undifferentiated types are also common. Adenocarcinoma is found in this location rarely and can even be metastatic. Involvement of the phrenic or recurrent laryngeal nerve or superior vena caval obstruction is not characteristic of a Pancoast tumor.

In the resected specimen that has received preoperative irradiation, favorable histologic signs include no residual tumor in the specimen, no residual tumor in the chest wall, tumor in the chest wall replaced by fibrosis, or minimal tumor in the chest wall with a strong radiation effect (10,18) (Figs. 20–24).

In contrast, unfavorable pathologic observations in the irradiated resected specimen include a large amount of tumor in the chest wall or in the nerve without significant irradiation effect. In the latter group, all patients have subsequently succumbed, whereas in the former group >95% have survived with negative mediastinal nodes (10,18).

In addition to the three classical bronchogenic carcinomas cell types, Pan-

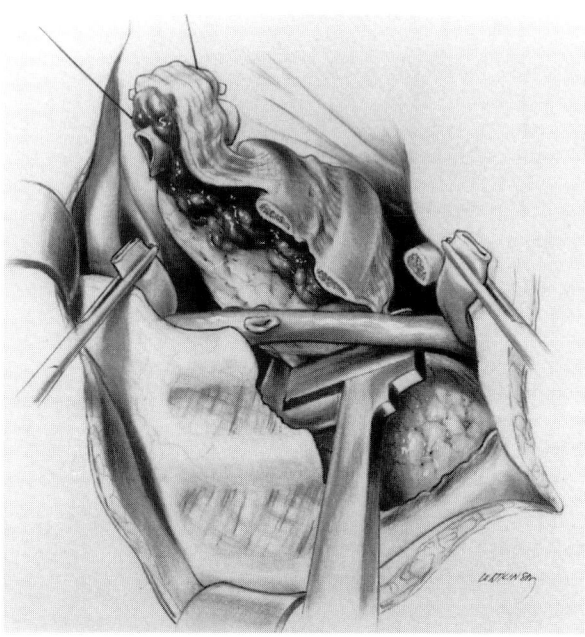

Figure 18   After dividing the ribs with an adequate margin from the tumor secondary to the posterior resection (usually the first three ribs), a saphenous vein or Dacron graft is interposed between the ends of the subclavian artery, using 5-0 Prolene sutures for the anastomoses.

coast's syndrome may be caused by a variety of other neoplasms or benign diseases. Primary pulmonary neoplasms include adenoid carcinoma (36), hemangiopericytoma (37), and metastatic malignancies from various primary sites such as the cervix (38,39), larynx (40), liver (41), thyroid gland (42), and mesotheliomas (40). Hematologic neoplasms such as plasmacytomas (43–45), lymphomatoid granulomatosis (46), and lymphomas (40,47–49), and various infections may also produce in Pancoast's syndrome (50–59). These infections include pseudomonal and staphylococcal (51,52) pneumonia, tuberculosis, actinomycosis (54), aspergillosis (55,56), allescheria infection (57), cryptococcosis (58,59), and hydatid cysts (60,61). Vascular aneurysms and amyloid nodules may also result in Pancoast's syndrome (62,63).

VI.   Conclusion

Pancoast's syndrome is a collection of characteristic symptoms and signs, which include shoulder and arm pain in a specific dermatomal distribution, Horner's syn-

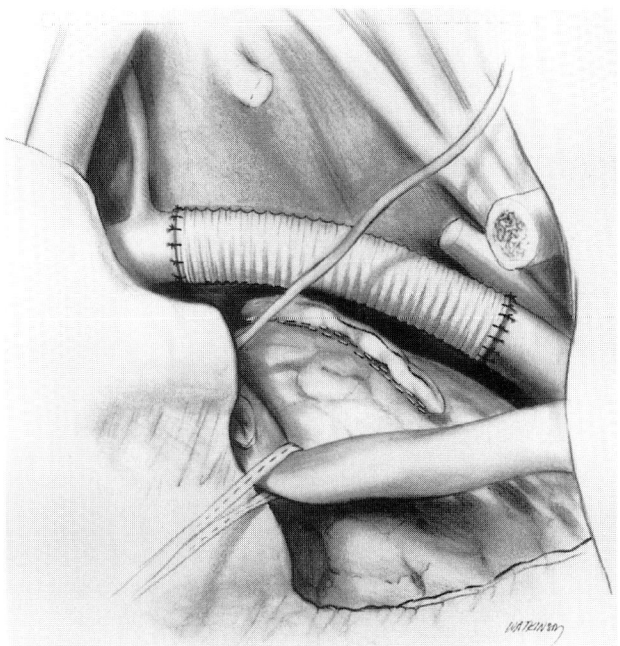

Figure 19 The mass is pulled up out of the chest, and, using a stapler, a wedge resection is carried out. This is a low-grade tumor usually originating in a scar. Usually the first, second, and third ribs had been divided anteriorly and posteriorly to allow the retraction of the tumor up and out of the chest. The stapler is placed across the lung for a subsegmental resection. The clavicle may be completely resected to allow easy exposure. If only the medial one-third is removed, a rod may be placed in the clavicle to provide stability. The vein is allowed to retract back into the field. Hemostasis is secured. Two large round Jackson-Pratt drains and chest tubes are placed.

drome, and weakness and atrophy of the muscles of the hand, most commonly caused by extension of an apical lung tumor located at the superior thoracic inlet. Although the majority of cases are the result of bronchogenic carcinoma, other neoplastic and nonneoplastic causes exist, and a definitive histologic diagnosis should be sought before the consideration of treatment options. Treatment should be attempted after careful evaluation of the extent of the disease and the underlying medical status.

The most effective treatment of Pancoast's syndrome due to bronchogenic carcinoma is clearly preoperative irradiation (3000r) combined with extended en bloc surgical resection (Table 1). Five-year survival for N0–1 disease is 35%. The exact role of adjuvant and neoadjuvant systemic chemotherapy is not established

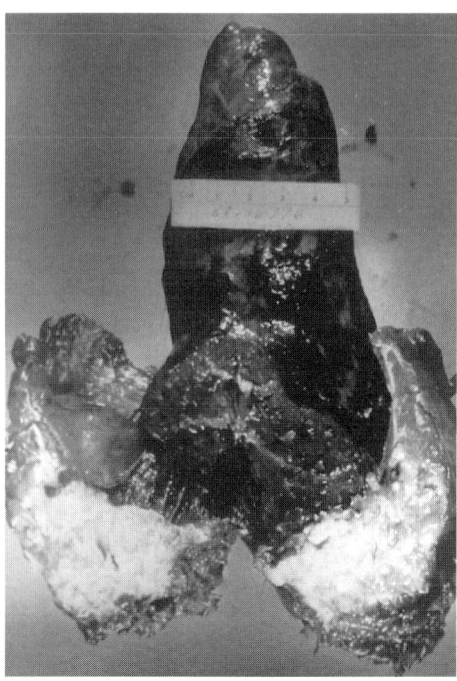

Figure 20 Gross pathologic specimen of superior pulmonary sulcus carcinoma resected en bloc after preoperative irradiation therapy, demonstrating extension of the mass outside of chest wall.

at this time. Preliminary reports with preoperative chemoradiotherapy followed by surgical resection show that this approach is feasible and may be associated with similar survival. Whenever possible, patients with Pancoast's tumors should be enrolled in prospective clinical trials so that we can add to our knowledge about this disease and determine the most effective and optimal therapy.

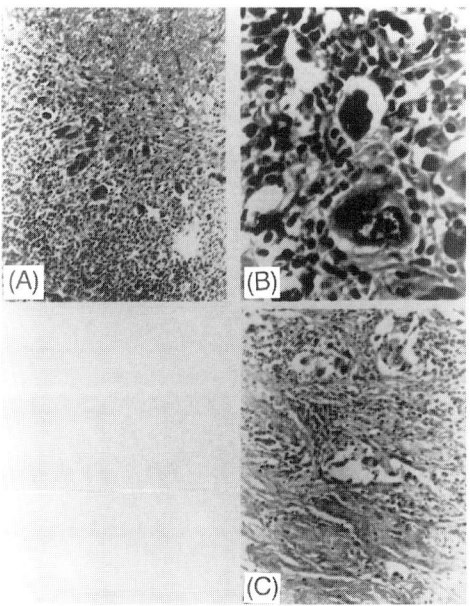

Figure 21 Photomicrograph of a resected superior pulmonary sulcus carcinoma demonstrating postirradiation change of fibrosis-inflammation (A), dark hyperchromic nuclei (B), and giant cells (C).

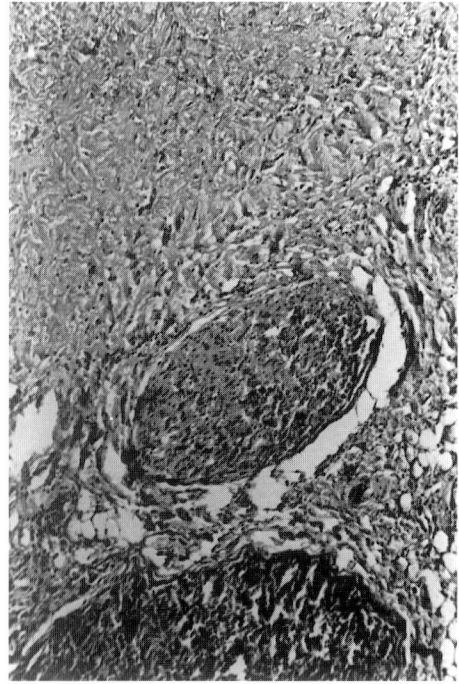

Figure 22   An excellent postirradiation effect of severe fibrosis around a nerve, portending an excellent clinical prognosis.

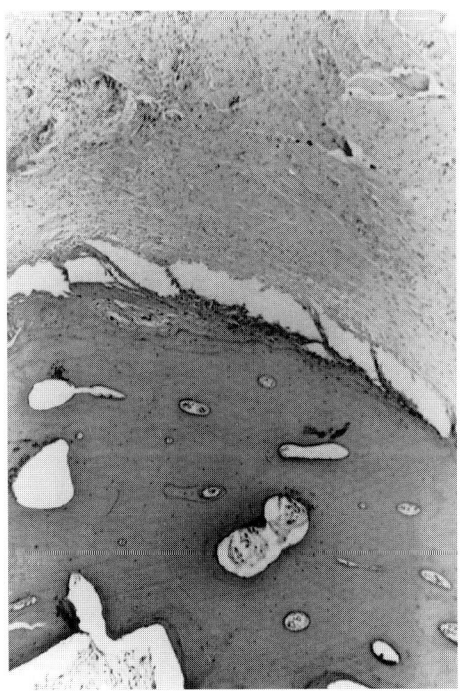

Figure 23 A good postirradiation effect of fibrosis up to the rib that contains no tumor, with a good clinical prognosis.

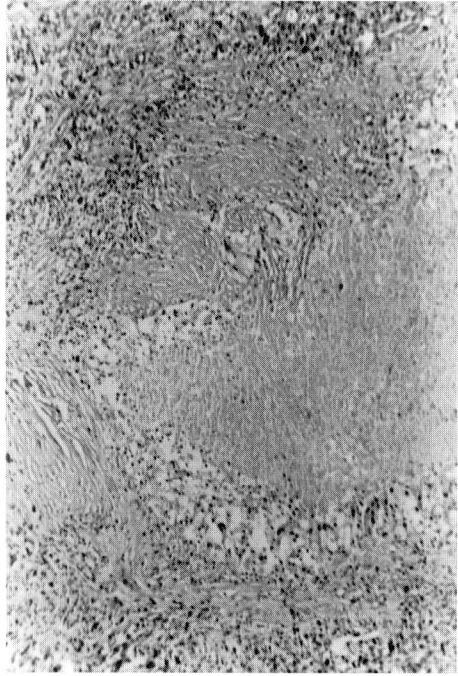

Figure 24   Only a slight postirradiation effect with recognizable carcinoma cell present, portending a poor clinical prognosis.

Table 1 Superior Pulmonary Sulcus Diagnosis and Treatment Algorithym

	Diagnosis and Staging	Treatment
History	Bronchoscopy	*Preop Irradiation*
Pain	Mediastinoscopy—cervical (right)	(3000 rads in 2–3 weeks)
Localized shoulder	—second interspace (left)	
Vertebral border scapula	Biopsy—supraclavicular or posterior cervical	
Ulnar distribution in arm and hand		Delay 2–4 weeks
Smoking		
Physical Examination	*Pathology (Carcinoma)*	*Resection*
Horner's syndrome	Squamous	Chest wall en bloc
Laboratory Studies	Large-cell undifferentiated	Lower trunk of brachial plexus
CBC	Adeno	Lung—segmental
Urinalysis		—lobectomy
SMA 20		
Sputum cytology		PROGNOSIS *5-year survival*
Roentgenographic Evaluation		1. *Lymph nodes*
Chest x-rays	T3	N0-1 35%
CT and magnetic resonance scans (neck, chest, upper abdomen)	N0-1	
Vertebral polytomes	M0	N2 (right) 15%
Arteriogram where specifically indicated		2. *Radiation effect*
Venogram		EXCELLENT >50%
Scans		
Liver		
Bone		
Brain		
Gallium		

References

1. Hare ES. Tumor involving certain nerves. London Med Gazette 1838; 23:16–18.
2. Pancoast HK. Importance of careful roentgen-ray investigations of apical chest tumors. JAMA 1924; 83:1407–1411.
3. Pancoast HK. Superior pulmonary sulcus tumor. JAMA 1932; 99:1391–1396.
4. Tobias JW. Sindrome apico-costo-vertebral dolorosa por tumor apexiano: su valor diagnostico en el cancer primitivo pulmonar. Rev Med Lat Am 1932; 17:1522–1556.
5. Shaw RR, Paulson DL, Kee JL. Treatment of the superior sulcus tumor by irradiation followed by resection. Ann Surg 1961; 154:29–40.
6. Chardack WM, MacCallum JD. Pancoast syndrome due to bronchogenic carcinoma: successful surgical removal and postoperative irradiation. J Thorac Surg 1953; 25:402–412.
7. Chardack WM, MacCallum JD. Pancoast tumor. Five-year survival without recurrence or metastases following radical resection and postoperative irradiation. J Thorac Surg 1956; 31:535–542.
8. Attar S, Miller JE, Satterfield J, et al. Pancoast tumor: irradiation or surgery? Ann Thorac Surg 1979; 28:578–586.
9. Van Houtte P, MacLennan I, Pouter C, Rubin P. External radiation in the management of superior sulcus tumor. Cancer 1984; 54:223–227.
10. Urschel HC Jr. Superior pulmonary sulcus carcinoma. Surg Clin North Am 1988; 68:497–509.
11. Shahian DM, Neptune WB, Ellis FH Jr. Pancoast tumors: improved survival with preoperative and postoperative radiotherapy. Ann Thorac Surg 1987; 43:32–38.
12. Kanner RM, Martini N, Foley KM. Incidence of pain and other clinical manifestations of superior pulmonary sulcus (Pancoast) tumors. In: Bonica J, ed. Advances in Pain Research and Therapy. Vol. 4. New York: Raven Press, 1982:27–39.
13. Walls WJ, Thornbury JR, Naylor B. Pulmonary needle aspiration biopsy in the diagnosis of Pancoast tumors. Radiology 1974; 111:99–102.
14. Miller JI, Mansour KA, Hatcher CR Jr. Carcinoma of the superior pulmonary sulcus. Ann Thorac Surg 1979; 28:44–47.
15. Komaki R, Roh J, Cox JD, Da Conceicao AL. Superior sulcus tumors: results of irradiation of 36 patients. Cancer 1981; 48:1563–1568.
16. Komaki R. Preoperative radiation therapy for superior sulcus lesions. Chest Surg Clin North Am 1991; 1:13–35.
17. Grover FL, Komaki R. Superior sulcus tumors. In: Roth JA, Ruckdeschel JC, Weisenburger TH, eds. Thoracic Oncology. 2nd ed. Philadelphia: W.B. Saunders, 1995:225–238.
18. Paulson DL. Carcinomas in the superior pulmonary sulcus. J Thorac Cardiovasc Surg 1975; 70:1095–1104.
19. Hepper NGG, Herskovic T, Witten DM, Mulder DW, Woolner LB. Thoracic inlet tumors. Ann Intern Med 1966; 64:979–989.
20. Anderson TM, Moy PM, Holmes EC. Factors affecting survival in superior sulcus tumors. J Clin Oncol 1986; 4:1598–1603.
21. Stanford W, Barnes RP, Tucker AR. Influence of staging in superior sulcus (Pancoast) tumors of the lung. Ann Thorac Surg 1980; 29:406–409.

22. Sundaresan N, Hilaris BS, Martini N. The combined neurosurgical-thoracic management of superior sulcus tumors. J Clin Oncol 1987; 5:1739–1745.
23. Urschel HC Jr. New approaches to Pancoast and chest wall tumors. Chest 1993; 103: 360S–361S.
24. McGoon DC. Transcervical technique for removal of specimen from superior sulcus tumor for pathologic study. Ann Surg 1964; 159:407–410.
25. Maxfield RA, Aranda CP. The role of fiberoptic bronchoscopy and transbronchial biopsy in the diagnosis of Pancoast's tumor. NY State J Med 1987; 87:326–329.
26. Pratt DS. Diagnosis of a thoracic inlet tumour by transbronchial biopsy. Thorax 1978; 33:803–805.
27. O'Connell RS, McLoud TC, Wilkins EW. Superior sulcus tumor: radiographic diagnosis and work up. AJR 1983; 140:25–30.
28. Ginsberg RJ, Payne DG, Shamji F. Superior sulcus tumors. In: Aisner J, ed. Comprehensive Textbook of Thoracic Oncology. Baltimore: Williams & Wilkins, 1996:375–387.
29. Remmen HJ, Lacquet LK, Van Son JA, Morshuis WJ, Cox AL. Surgical treatment of Pancoast tumor. J Cardiovasc Surg 1993; 34:157–161.
30. Fuller DB, Chambers JS. Superior sulcus tumors: combined modality. Ann Thorac Surg 1994; 57:1133–1139.
31. Hilaris BS, Martini N, Wong GY, Nori D. Treatment of superior sulcus tumor (Pancoast tumor). Surg Clin North Am 1987; 67:965–977.
32. Komaki R, Barber-Derus S, Perez-Tamayo C, Byhardt RW, Hartz A, Cox JD. Brain metastasis in patients with superior sulcus tumors. Cancer 1987; 59:1649–1653.
33. Devine JW, Mendenhall WM, Million RR, Carmichael MJ. Carcinoma of the superior pulmonary sulcus treated with surgery and/or radiation therapy. Cancer 1986; 57:941–943.
34. Lands RH, Patel N, Maran S, Karnad A. Small cell lung cancer presenting as a Pancoast tumor. J Tenn Med Assoc 1991; 84:113–114.
35. Johnson DH, Hainsworth JD, Greco FA. Pancoast's syndrome and small cell lung cancer. Chest 1982; 82:602–606.
36. Hatton MQ, Allen MB, Cooke NJ. Pancoast syndrome: an unusual presentation of adenoid cystic carcinoma. Eur Respir J 1993; 6:271–272.
37. Chong KM, Hennox SC, Sheppard MN. Primary hemangiopericytoma presenting as a Pancoast's tumor. Ann Thorac Surg 1993; 55:9.
38. Amin R. Bilateral Pancoast's syndrome in a patient with carcinoma of the cervix. Gynecol Oncol 1986; 24:126–128.
39. Omenn GS. Pancoast syndrome due to metastatic carcinoma from the uterine cervix. Chest 1971; 60:268–270.
40. Herbut PA, Watson JS. Tumor of the thoracic inlet producing the Pancoast syndrome: a report of seventeen cases and a review of the literature. Arch Pathol 1946; 42:88–103.
41. Chocarro A, Labanda F, Martinez E, Pereda JM. Pancoast syndrome as the initial manifestation of a hepatocarcinoma. Med Clin 1986; 86:822.
42. Rabano A, La Sala M, Hernandez P, Barros JL. Thyroid carcinoma presenting as Pancoast's syndrome. Thorax 1991; 46:270–271.

43. Brenner B, Carter A, Freidin N, Malberger E, Tatarsky I. Pancoast's syndrome in multiple myeloma. Acta Haematol 1984; 71:353–355.

44. Chen KT, Padmanbhan A. Pancoast syndrome caused by extramedullary plasmacytoma. J Surg Oncol 1983; 24:117–118.

45. Wilson KS, Cunningham TA, Alexander S. Myeloma presenting with Pancoast's syndrome. Br Med J 1979; 1:20.

46. Dolan G, Smith J, Reilly JT. Extrapulmonary lymphomatoid granulomatosis presenting as Pancoast's syndrome. Postgrad Med J 1991; 67:914–915.

47. Wang JC, Finn NG, Nimmagadda N, Reddy D. Pancoast syndrome in a patient with malignant lymphoma. Cancer 1989; 64:2588–2590.

48. Mills PR, Han LY, Dick R, Clarke SW. Pancoast syndrome caused by a high grade lymphoma. Thorax 1994; 49:92–93.

49. Arcasoy SM, Bajwa MK, Jett JR. Non-Hodgkin's lymphoma presenting as Pancoast's syndrome. Resp Med. In press.

50. Vandenplas O, Mercenier C, Trigaux JP, Delaunois L. Pancoast's syndrome due to *Pseudenomas aeruginosa* infection of the lung apex. Thorax 1991; 46:683–684.

51. Silverman MS, MacLeod JP. Pancoast's syndrome due to staphylococcal pneumonia. Can Med Assoc J 1990; 141:343–345.

52. Gallagher KJ, Jeffrey RR, Kerr SM, Steven MM. Pancoast syndrome: an unusual complication of pulmonary infection by *Staphylococcus aureus*. Ann Thorac Surg 1992; 53:903–904.

53. Vamos G, Papp A. Pancoast's syndrome and pulmonary tuberculosis. Schweiz Z Tuberk 1960; 17:423–430.

54. Stanley SL Jr, Lusk RH. Thoracic actinomycosis presenting as a brachial plexus syndrome. Thorax 1985; 40:74–75.

55. Collins PW, de Lord C, Newland AC. Pancoast's tumour due to aspergilloma. Lancet 1990; 336:1595.

56. Simpson FG, Morgan M, Cooke NJ. Pancoast's syndrome associated with invasive aspergillosis. Thorax 1986; 41:156–157.

57. Winston DJ, Jordan MC, Rhodes J. *Allescheria boydii* infections in the immunosuppressed host. Am J Med 1977; 63:830–835.

58. Mitchell DH, Sorrell TC. Pancoast's syndrome due to pulmonary infection with *Cryptococcus neoformans* variety *gattii*. Clin Infect Dis 1992; 14:1142–1144.

59. Ziomek S, Weinstein W, Margulies M, Braun RA. Primary pulmonary crytococcosis presenting as a superior sulcus tumor. Ann Thorac Surg 1992; 53:892–893.

60. Gotterer N, Lossos I, Breuer R. Pancoast's syndrome caused by primary pulmonary hydatid cyst. Respir Med 1990; 84:169–170.

61. Aletras H, Papaconstantinou C. Pancoast syndrome following an intrapleural rupture of a hepatic ecchinococcus cyst. Scand J Thorac Cardiovasc Surg 1982; 16:283–287.

62. Rong SH. Carotid pseudoaneurysm simulating Pancoast tumor. AJR 1984; 142:495–496.

63. Gibney RT, Connoly TP. Pulmonary amyloid nodule simulating pancoast tumor. J Can Assoc Radiol 1984; 35:90–91.

64. Urschel HC Jr, Cooper JD, eds. Atlas of Thoracic Surgery. New York: Churchill Livingstone, 1995:180–193.

65. Shaw RR. Pancoast's tumor. Ann Thorac Surg 1984; 37:343–345.

66. Dartevelle PG, Chapelier AR, Macchiarini P, et al. Anterior transcervical-thoracic approach for radical resection of lung tumours invading the thoracic inlet. J Thorac Cardiovasc Surg 1993; 105:1025–1034.
67. Martinez-Monge R, Herreros J, Aristu JJ, Aramendia JM, Azinovic I. Combined treatment in superior sulcus tumors. Am J Clin Oncol 1994; 17:317–322.
68. Temeck BK, Okunieff PG, Pass HI. Chest wall disease including superior sulcus tumors. In: Pass HI, Mitchell JB, Johnson DH, Turrisi AT, eds. Lung Cancer: Principles and Practice. Philadelphia: Lippincott-Raven, 1996:585–601.
69. Ginsberg RJ, Martini N, Zaman M, et al. Influence of surgical resection and brachytherapy in the management of superior sulcus tumor. Ann Thorac Surg 1994; 57:1440–1445.
70. Maggi G, Casadio C, Pischedda F, et al. Combined radiosurgical treatment of Pancoast tumor. Ann Thorac Surg 1994; 57:198–202.
71. Derbekyan V, Novales-Diaz J, Lisbona R. Pancoast tumor as a cause of reflex sympathetic dystrophy. J Nucl Med 1993; 34:1992–1994.
72. Delreux V, Kevers L, Callewaert A. Paroxysmal hemicrania preceding Pancoast's syndrome. Rev Neurol 1990; 145:151–152.
73. Sartori F, Rea F, Calabro F, Mazzucco C, Bortolotti L, Tomio L. Carcinoma of the superior pulmonary sulcus: results of irradiation and radical resection. J Thorac Cardiovasc Surg 1992; 104:679–683.
74. Ginsberg RJ. Resection of a superior sulcus tumor. Chest Surg Clin North Am 1995; 5:15–31.
75. McLaughlin JS. Superior sulcus tumors. In: Baue AE, ed. Glenn's Thoracic and Cardiovascular Surgery. 6th ed. Connecticut: Appleton & Lange, 1996; 445–458.
76. Neal CR, Amdur RJ, Mendenhall WM, Knauf DG, Block AJ, Million RR. Pancoast tumor: radiation therapy alone versus preoperative radiation therapy and surgery. Int J Radiol Oncol Biol Phys 1991; 21:651–660.
77. Hilaris BS, Luomanen RK, Beattie EJ Jr. Integrated irradiation and surgery in the treatment of apical lung cancer. Cancer 1971; 27:1369–1373.
78. Martini N. Surgical treatment of non-small cell lung cancer by stage. Semin Surg Oncol 1990; 6:248–254.
79. Ahmad K, Fayos JV, Kirsch MM. Apical lung carcinoma. Cancer 1984; 54:913–917.
80. Komaki R, Mountain CF, Holbert JM, et al. Superior sulcus tumors: treatment selection and results for 85 patients without metastasis (M0) at presentation. Int J Radiat Oncol Biol Phys 1990; 19:31–36.
81. Kirsch MM, Dickerman R, Fayos J, et al. The value of chest wall resection in the treatment of superior sulcus tumors of the lung. Ann Thorac Surg 1973; 15:339–346.
82. Holmes EC, Livingston R, Turrisis A. Neoplasms of the thorax. In: Holddan JF, Frei E, Bast RC, Kufe DW, Morton DL, Weischselbaum RR, eds. Cancer Medicine. 3rd ed. Philadelphia: Lea & Febiger, 1993:1285–1337.
83. Wright CD, Moncure AC, Shephard J-AO, Wilkins EW Jr, Mathisen DJ, Grillo HC. Superior sulcus lung tumors. Results of combined treatment (irradiation and radical resection). J Thorac Cardiovasc Surg 1987; 94:69–74.
84. Haas LL, Harvey RA, Langer SS. Radiation management of otherwise hopeless thoracic neoplasms. JAMA 1954; 154:323–326.

85. Mantell BS. Superior sulcus (Pancoast) tumours: results of radiotherapy. Br J Dis Chest 1973; 67:315–318.

86. Morris RW, Abadir R. Pancoast tumor: the value of high dose radiation therapy. Radiology 1979; 132:717–719.

87. Hilaris BS, Luomanen RK, Mahan GD, Henschke UK. Interstitial irradiation of apical lung cancer. Radiology 1971; 99:655–660.

88. Green N, Kurohara SS, George FW III, Crews QE Jr. Postresection irradiation for primary lung cancer. Radiology 1975; 116:405–407.

89. Chung CK, Stryker JA, O'Neill M Jr, DeMuth WE Jr. Evaluation of adjuvant postoperative radiotherapy for lung cancer. Int J Radiat Oncol Biol Phys 1982; 8:1877–1880.

90. Van Houtte P, Rocmans P, Smets P, et al. Postoperative radiation therapy in lung cancer: a controlled trial after resection of curative design. Int J Radiat Oncol Biol Phys 1980; 16:983–986.

91. Weisenburger TH, Gail M, Lung Cancer Study Group. Effects of postoperative mediastinal radiation on completely resected stage II and stage III epidermoid cancer of the lung. N Engl J Med 1986; 315:1377–1381.

92. Westgate SJ, Perry MC. Toxicity of combined modality therapy. In: Aisner J, ed. Comprehensive Textbook of Thoracic Oncology. Baltimore: Williams & Wilkins, 1996:1002–1018.

93. Jett JR. Current treatment of unresectable lung cancer. Mayo Clin Proc 1993; 68:603–611.

94. Beyer DC, Weisenburger T. Superior sulcus tumors. Am J Clin Oncol 1986; 9:156–161.

95. Hilaris BS, Nori D, Beattie EJ Jr, Martini N. Value of perioperative brachytherapy in the management of non-oat cell carcinoma of the lung. Int J Radiat Oncol Biol Phys 1983; 9:1161–1166.

96. Takasugi JE, Rapoport S, Shaw C. Superior sulcus tumors: the role of imaging. J Thorac Imag 1989; 4:41–48.

97. McLoud TC, Isler RJ, Novelline RA, Putnam CE, Simeone J, Stark P. The apical gap. AJR 1981; 137:299–306.

98. Hamlin JD, Burgener FA. CT, including sagittal and coronal reconstruction, in the evaluation of Pancoast tumors. J Comput Tomogr 1982; 6:43–50.

99. Takasugi JE, Godwin JD, Halvorsen RL, Williford ME, Silverman PM, Putnam CE. Computerized tomographic evaluation of lesions in the thoracic apex. Invest Radiol 1985; 20:260–266.

100. Glazer HS, Duncan-Meyer J, Aronberg DJ, Moran JF, Levitt RG, Sagel SS. Pleural and chest wall invasion in bronchogenic carcinoma: CT evaluation. Radiology 1985; 157:191–194.

101. Pennes DR, Glazer GM, Wimbish KJ, Gross BH, Long RW, Orringer MB. Chest wall invasion by lung cancer: limitations of CT evaluation. AJR 1985; 144:507–511.

102. Heelan RT, Demas BE, Caravelli JF, et al. Superior sulcus tumors: CT and MR imaging. Radiology 1989; 170:637–641.

103. Mansour KA. Extended resection of bronchial carcinoma in the superior pulmonary sulcus. In: Shields TW, ed. General Thoracic Surgery 4th ed. Baltimore: Williams & Wilkins, 1994:572–578.

104. Hilaris BS, Martini N, Luomanen RKJ, Batata M, Beattie EJ Jr. The value of preoperative radiation therapy in apical cancer of the lung. Surg Clin North Am 1974; 54:831–840.
105. Shields TW. Preoperative radiation therapy in the treatment of bronchial carcinoma. Cancer 1972; 30:1388–1393.
106. Warram J. Preoperative irradiation of cancer of the lung: final report of a therapeutic trial. A collaborative study. Cancer 1975; 36:914–925.
107. Martini N, Heelan R, Westcott J, et al. Comparative merits of conventional, computed tomographic, and magnetic resonance imaging in assessing mediastinal involvement in surgically confirmed lung carcinoma. J Thorac Cardiovasc Surg 1985; 90:639–648.
108. Heelan RT, Martini N, Westcott JW, et al. Carcinomatous involvement of the hilum and mediastinum: computed tomographic and magnetic resonance evaluation. Radiology 1985; 156:111–115.
109. Padovani B, Mouroux J, Seksik L, et al. Chest wall invasion by bronchogenic carcinoma: evaluation with MR imaging. Radiology 1993; 187:33–38.

9

Surgery for Advanced Lung Cancer

RAPHAEL BUENO

Brigham and Women's Hospital
Boston, Massachusetts

I.   Introduction

Complete surgical resection is currently the best treatment modality for lung cancer. While technically possible in patients with early-stage lung cancer and helpful in patients without evidence of nodal and distant metastases, surgical resection has proven challenging in patients with locally advanced disease. This chapter provides a brief background look at stage classifications for advanced lung cancer and then presents methods and results of surgical management and multimodality treatment (combinations of surgery with chemotherapy and radiation therapy) strategies for patients with advanced lung cancer. The three advanced stages of lung cancer to be discussed in this chapter are described in the tumor (T), node (N), and metastasis (M) system as: T4 N0–2 M0, any T N3 M0, and T1–3 N0–2 M1 (1,2).

II.   T4 Tumors

T4 tumors are defined as lesions which invade one or more of the following structures: the mediastinum (other than just the parietal pleura), the heart, great vessels, trachea, esophagus, vertebral body, carina, or any tumor accompanied by a malignant pleural effusion (see Chapter 5). In the absence of nodal involvement or distant metastatic disease, these T4 tumors represent, essentially, very locally aggressive lesions that involve vital structures through proximity. It is not known if these cancers invade nonlung tissues because they are biologically more aggressive than earlier lesions (such as T1 and T2) or because they arise near to and then invade into adjacent mediastinal structures, very much like T3 lesions that involve the chest wall. The clinical perception is that these tumors are incurable both because they involve vital, hard-to-resect structures and because the invasion of the structure may be a marker for distant disease. Thus, many clinicians shy away from attempting curative resections of these tumors. Fortunately, some surgeons have utilized advanced techniques to resect these cancers in the hope of achieving long-term survival. Consequently data are available on the outcome of aggressive surgical treatment modalities for advanced lung cancer.

T4 tumors can be divided into two categories. Category 1 includes lesions involving the three structures that connect the lung to the mediastinum, i.e., pulmonary artery (PA), pulmonary vein, and bronchus/trachea. Invasion of these structures can be viewed as more direct extension of the hilar lung cancer into the root of the lung past the pleural and pericardial linings. The remaining structures whose invasion is classified as T4 disease are invaded by direct extension of anatomically adjacent cancer or involved lymph nodes across the pleural planes separately from the hilar structures.

A. Treatment of Tracheal Involved T4 Disease

The oldest and the most commonly accepted form of resection of T4 lung cancer is resection for tumor involving the distal trachea or the carina. A carinal pneumonectomy (or a sleeve pneumonectomy) is the removal of a lung and a distal portion of the trachea followed by the anastomosis of the remaining distal trachea to the main stem bronchus of the contralateral lung (Figure 1). A carinal resection without pneumonectomy refers to such a resection of the trachea and main bronchus with an anastomotic reconstruction of the carina.

These resections were described over 30 years ago (3); consequently data are available from a number of series as to the appropriate indications, techniques, and results. Carinal pneumonectomy is indicated in patients with lung cancer localized to the area of the carina and without evidence of metastatic disease or nodal spread. Patients who have N2 nodes infiltrated by cancer, even when treated with neoadjuvant chemotherapy, have worse survival than patients with negative lymph nodes. At this time, patients with such positive mediastinal lymph nodes on mediastinoscopy are best treated within randomized protocols. Most commonly, the candidate for sleeve pneumonectomy has a hilar mass, usually squamous carcinoma involving the proximal main stem bronchus or the distal trachea. Patient

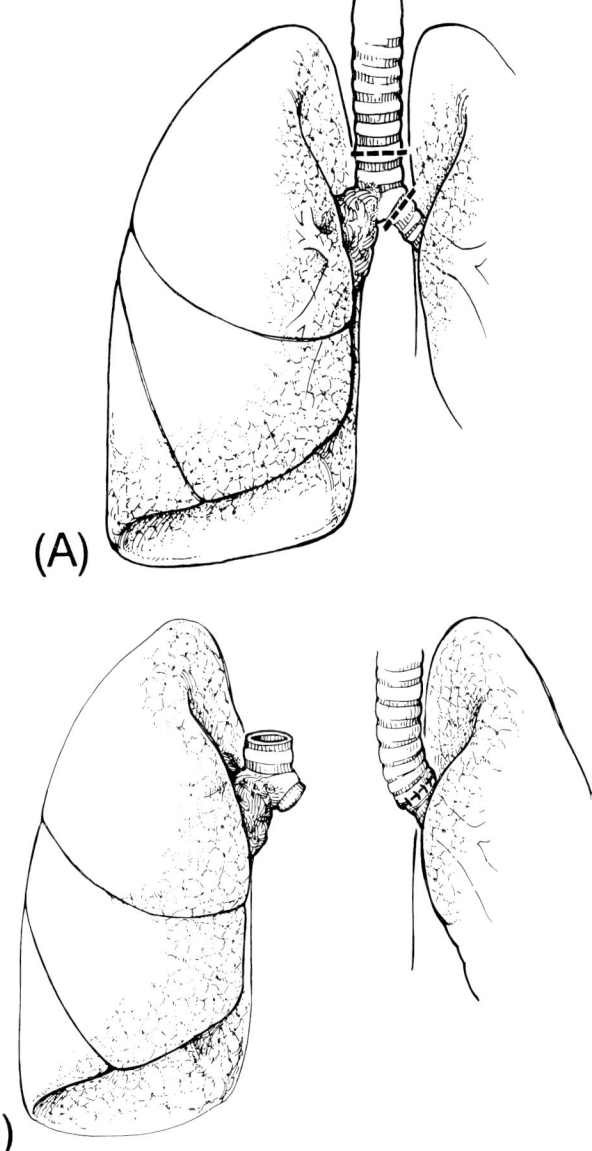

Figure 1 Right sleeve pneumonectomy and reconstruction.

eligibility for resection includes adequate pulmonary reserve and cardiac function to tolerate a pneumonectomy as well as emotional, physical, and nutritional stamina to sustain a meaningful recovery.

The operative procedure is formidable and should be performed only in centers with specialized experience. Intraoperative ventilation is performed utilizing sterile tubing over the field. The resection is performed through the ipsilateral chest, via a median sternotomy or by utilizing a clam shell incision. The length of tracheal and bronchial resection should be <4 cm in order to avoid undue tension and a high likelihood of dehiscence. Complete resection is done with emphasis on preserving the bronchial and tracheal blood supply and nondisruption of the lymphatic drainage if possible. The anastomosis is constructed without tension and, if possible, covered with a viable muscle or pericardial flap. Several maneuvers such as anterior tracheal release and a hilar release are performed to reduce tension. If necessary, other involved structures, most commonly the superior vena cava (SVC) or azygous vein, can be resected en bloc with the specimen. The reported mortality from carinal pneumonectomy varies from 4% to 29%, and the reported 5-year survival ranges from 13% to 43%. The most common causes of death include postpneumonectomy pulmonary edema and septic complications from pneumonia or anastomotic dehiscence. Though challenging, carinal resection in the 1990s can carry 20% to 40% 5-year survival and should certainly be offered to appropriate candidates (3–13).

B. Cardiac Involvement

At the current time, resection of a locally invasive lung cancer into the heart is usually attempted only in cases of left atrial involvement. This is clearly because the left atrium is the closest cardiac structure in communication with the lung and the most likely to be involved with cancer in the absence of metastatic disease. The great majority of patients undergoing a concomitant left atrial resection with the lung resection have a hilar mass extending near or into the atrium and are resected in order to provide a histologically negative margin.

In major series, these patients represent only a small percentage (<5%) of all patients undergoing pulmonary resection for carcinoma of the lung. The major technical concerns in this disease setting include intraoperative hemodynamic instability, injury to the mitral valve, and the obstruction of pulmonary venous flow. Tsuchiya et al. reviewed the outcome of 101 patients who underwent radical pulmonary surgery for advanced lung cancer (14). They reported an impressive series of 44 patients who underwent left atrial resection with 22% 5-year survival. The 30-day and in-hospital mortality were 8% and 13%, respectively. The perioperative morbidity was 42%. Seven patients (18.9%) of a 37-patient subset who underwent resection of the lung and left atrium for pulmonary carcinoma survived >4 years. Four of them had true invasion of the left atrium, and the other three had disease considered T3. Their nodal status was: N0, one patient; N1, four patients; and N2, two patients. Seven patients who had concomitant resections of the lung, left atrium, and another "T4" structure died within 2 years of surgery. The most important factors for long-term survival in their series were the completeness of the resection and the final pathological stage.

These patients were evaluated preoperatively with a chest computed tomogram (CT), a bone scan, a cardiac ECHO, and angiography. In all cases, the left atrial resection was accomplished off cardiopulmonary bypass by utilizing a vascular clamp placed across the atrium which was then sutured directly. (Figure 2)

In a 1994 review from Memorial Sloan-Kettering Cancer Institute, Martini et al. describe 102 patients with T3 and T4 lung cancer and N0–1 nodal status who were explored for resection (15). Forty-four patients had T4 tumors, and of these tumors eight involved the left atrium. Only eight patients with T4 cancers were resected, including three who had a partial left atrial resection. Only one patient of eight (a patient with left atrial resection) was a long-term survivor. Other series reviewing experience with left atrial resection concomitant with pulmonary surgery for lung cancer have reported 5-year survival as high as 22%. It appears that there is a subgroup of patients with locally advanced lung cancer without metastatic disease or lymphatic spread whose tumor developed quite close to the heart as it extended along the pulmonary veins. In these circumstances, it is reasonable to

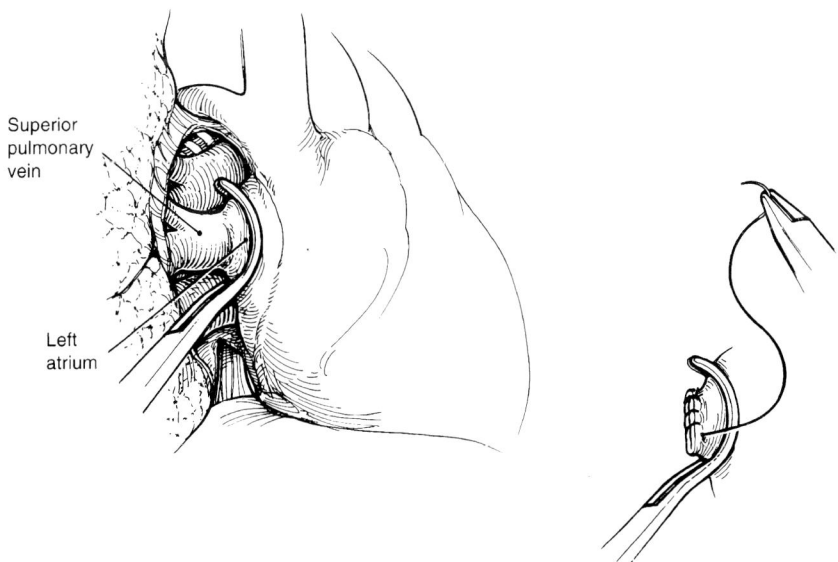

Figure 2 Resection of a tumor invading into the left atrium with clamp control and suturing of the atrial stump.

place a clamp on the left atrium and resect the tumor as long as the resection does not compromise the mitral valve or result in other hemodynamic disturbances (9–11,14,15). I favor using a transesophageal ECHO intraoperatively to help in that assessment. In some of these cases, the resected tumor turns out not to involve the heart, and the resection merely allows for a good margin. In other cases, some left atrial involvement will be documented histologically. Nevertheless, such a resection should be done in patients without metastatic or nodal disease in whom a complete resection can be achieved because such surgery may confer a survival rate of 20% at 5 years, quite better than the 0% to 5% 5-year survival seen in the unresected group of patients with T4 disease.

Finally, patients with involved N2 lymph nodes or involvement of an additional mediastinal structure in the presence of suspected left atrial involvement should be treated with neoadjuvant therapy preferably in the setting of a clinical protocol with demonstration of response prior to resection. Though there are no clear data to demonstrate the success of this therapy, extrapolation of data from treatment of IIIA disease and our experience support this view (16–27).

C. Involvement of the Main Pulmonary Artery (PA)

The data regarding resection of the main pulmonary artery are less readily available probably because such resections are required less frequently. Ricci et al. (28) and Tsuchiya et al. (14) describe subgroups of patients who underwent en bloc resection of their main PA during a pulmonary resection for lung cancer. All the resections were performed with the aid of cardiopulmonary bypass and commonly through a median sternotomy. The defects were repaired with direct suture or with the aid of GORTEX (W.L. Gore, Flagstaff, AZ) or pericardial patches. However, despite a successful technical outcome, there were no long-term survivors. These limited data suggest that invasion of the main PA is a marker of advanced and perhaps unresectable disease.

Macchiarini et al. (21) recently described a cohort of patients with stage IIIB (T4 non-N3) lung cancer who underwent induction chemotherapy with or without radiation therapy prior to resection of the T4 tumors. In a subgroup of patients with intrapericardial vascular invasion, the 3-year survival was 62% with an operative mortality of 18%. Radiation therapy did not impact on survival; only preoperative chemotherapy did. These studies suggest that proximal and main PA involvement are markers for the systemic nature of the disease. Long-term survival is far more likely in patients treated with systemic chemotherapy in whom distant disease has been controlled prior to complete resection.

Surgical resection and reconstruction of the main PA for lung cancer (Figure 3) usually requires the use of cardiopulmonary bypass (29). The approach (i.e., median sternotomy or thoracotomy) is determined by the constraints imposed by the location and extent of the tumor. The surgical candidate must have no evidence

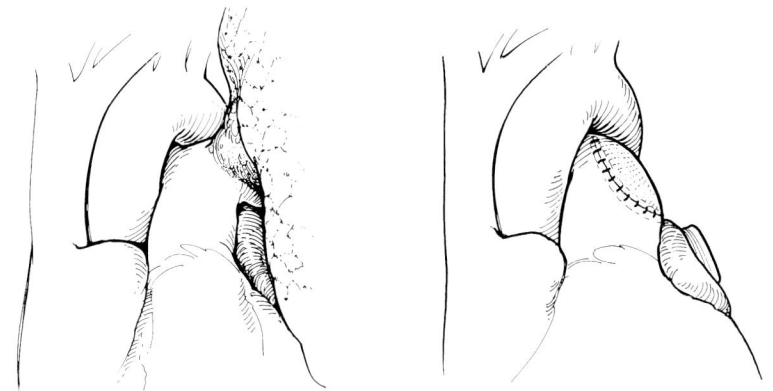

Figure 3 Resection and patch repair of the main pulmonary artery.

of distant disease or lymphatic spread, and should have adequate cardiopulmonary reserve to tolerate the operation. Care must be exercised in avoiding the kinking or narrowing of the main and contralateral pulmonary arteries. Various patching techniques may be tailored to the particular reconstruction if needed. As in the other instances of T4 disease, these operations are best performed by experienced surgeons and under protocol settings. In selected patients, long-term survival may be achieved.

D. Vena Caval Involvement

On occasion, the Superior Vena Cava (SVC) is invaded by hilar and tracheal tumors or by a malignant hilar lymph node (Figure 4). The challenges to en bloc resection of the tumor and a portion of the SVC include the need for adequate replacement of the vein with a conduit of long-term patency, the technical exposure and vascular control of the SVC, and the physiological consideration of clamping of this vessel. Over the past two decades, there has been an increase in technical experience in managing SVC resection for both benign and malignant diseases. Small, noncircumferential segments of vein wall may be resected and repaired primarily or with patches (pericardial or GORTEX). Spiral vein grafts and externally reinforced polytetrafluoroethylene (PTFE) grafts have both been used successfully for SVC replacement with good long-term patency rates (30).

Vascular control of the SVC can be achieved proximally via an intrapericardial approach at its junction with the right atrium and distally just before the confluence of the innominate vessels. A right thoracotomy incision or a sternotomy incision can be used depending on the technical constraints imposed by the anatomical location of the tumor. The physiological concerns associated with clamping of

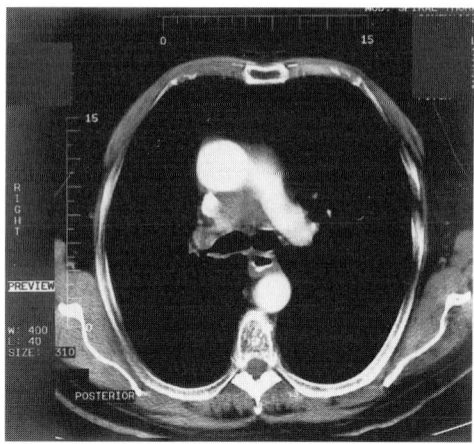

Figure 4   Computed tomography scan depicting vena caval involvement by a hilar mass.

the SVC include acute disruption of venous drainage from the head with adverse neurological sequelae, decreased preload resulting in hypotension, and thrombosis both early and late in the postoperative period. Adequate fluid loading with crystalloid or plasma infusions, as well as intravenous anticoagulation with heparin, will usually allow safe SVC clamping for >60 min. Monitoring of the pressure in the subclavian vein with a standard pressure transducer permits early response to central venous hypertension (>40 mm Hg). In rare circumstances, a temporary venoatrial shunt may be used for decompression of the clamped veins. (Figure 5)

Long-term patency rates for SVC replacement in benign and malignant conditions have been shown to be excellent. Dartevelle and his colleagues reported a 7.1% operative mortality in their series of patients, most of whom underwent a concomitant right pneumonectomy (9,11,31). They also report a 5-year survival rate of 31% and note that none of the long-term survivors had N2 disease. Extrapolating the aforementioned data to patients with positive N2 disease, it may be reasonable to include such patients who respond favorably to neoadjuvant chemoradiation as candidates for aggressive resections. En bloc resection of the SVC can be performed with acceptable morbidity and mortality rates with relatively good outcome for patients who in the recent past would have been deemed inoperable (5,7,9,11,14,30–36).

E.   Resection of the Aorta

There are a number of articles detailing the methods and results of surgical resection of lung cancer en bloc with the involved aorta or other major arteries (5,9,11,14,33,37). Tumors invading the full thickness of the aortic wall require resection with the patient supported by complete or partial cardiopulmonary

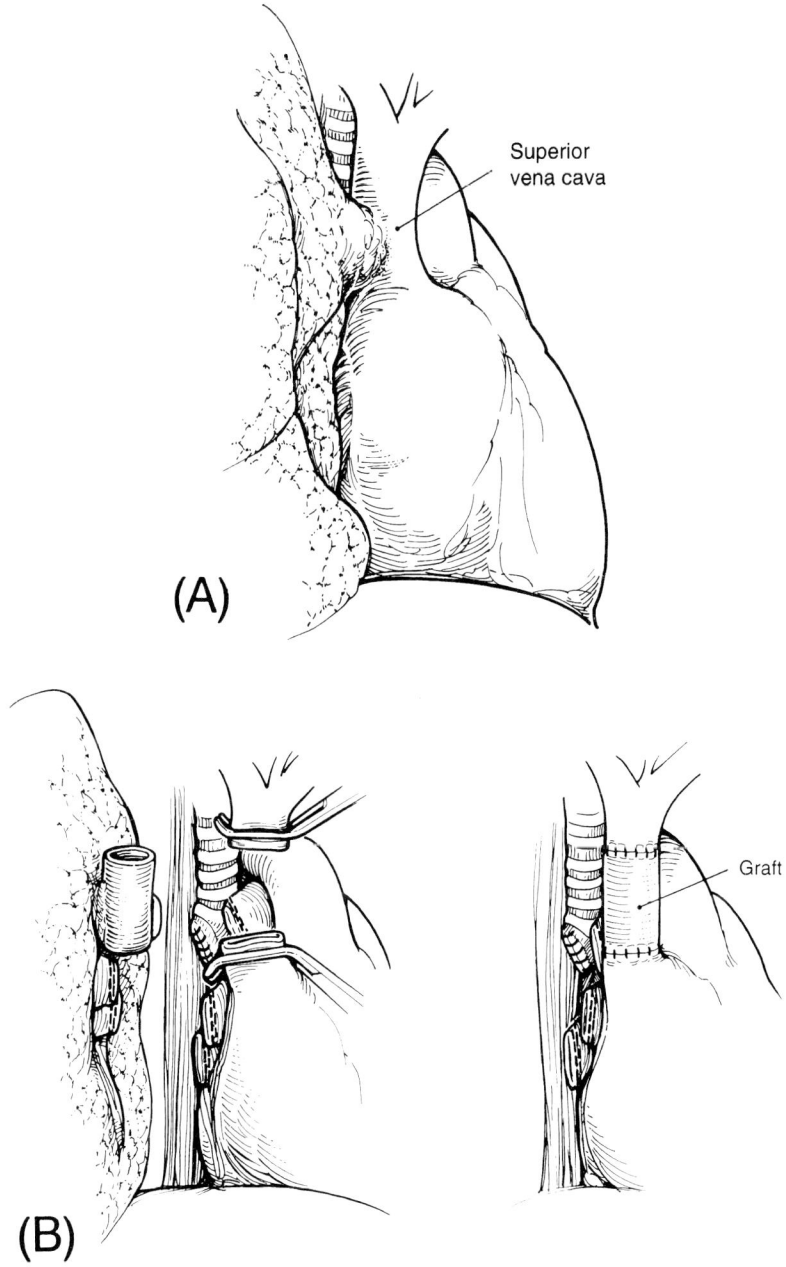

Figure 5 Resection and graft replacement of the superior vena cava.

bypass and the use of a synthetic vascular graft. On occasion, direct suture repair over a clamp or a patch graft may be attempted. In the case where only adventitial resection is required to separate the tumor off the aorta and achieve negative histological margins, it is recommended to wrap the stripped aorta with a prosthetic patch for support. Though the majority of patients who undergo such resection succumb to their disease, there are a few long-term survivors. Aortic involvement indicates advanced, unresectable disease. Resection should only be contemplated in healthy, young patients with no evidence of distant or lymphatic spread and with only minimal aortic involvement. Such resection is best performed by experienced thoracic surgeons and within the confines of clinical protocols. Patients found at thoracotomy to have unexpected aortic involvement probably do well left unresected at exploration, subsequently given neoadjuvant therapy and then resected, if shown to be good responders to neoadjuvant therapy.

F.   Resection of the Esophagus

There are few reports of surgical resection of lung tumors invading into the esophagus. It is more common for esophageal tumors to erode into the lung. Published and personal experience with resection of lung cancer penetrating the esophagus is anecdotal at best (38,39). In the absence of other disease, it may be reasonable in some cases to resect the muscular wall of the esophagus with the lung tumor. However, there is no evidence at present to support concomitant esophagectomy and lobectomy for lung cancer in this setting.

G.   Resection of the Vertebral Body

True vertebral body invasion by adjacent lung cancer is considered a T4 lesion classification of disease. This type of involvement is most commonly seen in patients with Pancoast tumors, a topic discussed more thoroughly in another chapter. DeMeester and his colleagues have published a detailed series of patients with vertebral body involvement (40). The patients in their series presented with pain and were noted to have lung cancer invading into the vertebral body without any evidence for distant or lymphatic disease. The authors point out that it is usually difficult to ascertain the extent of tumor invasion using current radiological imaging modalities and describe their techniques and results with partial resection of the vertebral body. They recommend preoperative radiation therapy (they used 3000 cGy; other investigators up to 4500 cGy) (41) followed by a complete tumor resection. They found that the long-term survival benefit depended on the degree of bony invasion. All patients with vertebral cortex invasion died within a few months of surgery, whereas patients with invasion of the periosteum or parietal pleura enjoyed 5-year survival at a rate up to 42%. These data suggest that it is reasonable to treat patients with isolated vertebral body involvement with neoadjuvant radiation therapy with or without chemotherapy and then proceed with a partial resection of the vertebral body. Unfortunately, an intraoperative frozen section analysis of the margin is impossible due to the need for decalcification. Resection is not indicated in patients who have clear involvement of the cortex of the bone seen on imaging analysis. Patients who are found to have such invasion are unresectable.

III. Stage IIIB: Surgical Treatment for N3 Disease

In general, patients with positive contralateral paratracheal or supraclavicular lymph nodes are at the very least included in stage IIIB disease classification and are considered surgically unresectable. Usually these patients are offered palliative radiation therapy and/or chemotherapy; they have median survival of about 8 months, and 5-year survival of <5% (1,2,18,26).

There are preliminary data from a Phase II study of the Southwest Oncology Group to support surgery in a subgroup of these patients. This study, published in 1995 (25), was designed for patients with stage IIIA and IIIB lung cancer who were treated with neoadjuvant chemotherapy plus radiotherapy followed by surgery. One subset of patients included those with positive N3 disease with both supraclavicular and/or contralateral paratracheal nodes involved. A subgroup of these patients had a complete response to the therapy, and at surgical resection the members of this group of patients were found to have cancer-free (negative) lymph nodes. Those patients in this study whose cancer was downstaged by chemoradiation had improved survival compared with historical controls (for IIIB disease) and with patients in the study with N2 or N3 disease who did not achieve sterilization of the lymph nodes. Certainly, the number of patients in this subgroup is rather small, and the study was not a prospective randomized one. Furthermore, the only N3 downstaged patients who achieved long-term survival were those who initially had positive supraclavicular nodes rather than contralateral paratracheal nodes. Therefore, it is premature to conclude that N3 positive tumors should generally be treated by adjuvant chemoradiation followed by resection. However, it is reasonable to consider, both in a protocol setting and on an individualized basis, that some patients who respond particularly well to up-front chemoradiation and who are otherwise healthy, young, and vigorous, may be candidates for aggressive resection which would include complete resection of the tumor and clearance of their mediastinum. For the great majority of patients with N3 disease, surgery is not currently recommended; chemotherapy with radiotherapy is the current standard of care.

IV. Resection of Lung Cancer in the Presence of Metastatic Disease

A large number of patients with lung cancer present with stage IV disease. These patients are usually offered only palliative chemotherapy and radiation therapy. As a group, their median survival is 6 to 9 months. The most common sites of metastatic disease are the brain, bones, adrenals, and liver. A large majority of patients with stage IV lung cancer have multiple metastases (2,42–44).

There are subsets of patients with single metastatic focus who have been treated aggressively with resection of all disease. The only group of patients among them who benefit from such therapy are those with isolated brain metastasis. In the 1920s (45), Harvey Cushing reported that lung cancer was the most common site from which metastatic disease of the brain arose, and that aggressive resection could result in significantly improved survival. Over the past 20 years, more data have been accumulated to confirm his observations. Patients who have a single metastatic lesion to their brain which can be controlled with neurosurgery and concomitant radiotherapy, are candidates for pulmonary resection as well. Those who do best have T1–2 N0–1 tumors. In several series, these patients have shown a median survival of 11 to 18 months and 5-year survival rates of 21%. These numbers are certainly better than the 1- to 6-month median survival rates of unresected patients in this disease setting.

Our current practice is to stage such patients at the time of craniotomy with a mediastinoscopy. Those who have no distant disease elsewhere, no lymphatic spread, and brain mets (three or less) which can be completely controlled by neurosurgery with radiation therapy, are offered pulmonary resection. There are currently no data to support the addition of chemotherapy for treatment in these patients, but a randomized protocol for this group of patients is certainly warranted (42–44,46–49).

V. Conclusion

Lung cancer is a common malignancy that is not readily curable with chemotherapy or radiation therapy. Unfortunately, a large percentage of patients with lung cancer present with late-stage disease that is not usually amenable to standard surgical therapy. Aggressive downstaging with neoadjuvant therapy and radical resectional surgery allow for improved survival in certain subsets of patients who previously had no hope for cure. New surgical and anesthetic techniques afford thoracic surgeons the ability to push the previously accepted limits of resectability.

References

1. Naruke T, Goya T, Tsuchiya R, Suemasu K. Prognosis and survival in resected lung carcinoma based on the new international staging system. J Thorac Cardiovasc Surg 1988; 96:440–447.
2. Mountain CF. Revisions in the international system for staging lung cancer. Chest 1997; 111:1710–1717.

3. Mathisen DJ, Grillo HC. Carinal resection for bronchogenic carcinoma. J Thorac Cardiovasc Surg 1991; 102:16–23.
4. Maeda M, Nakamoto K, Tsubota N, Okada T, Hiroshi K. Operative approaches for left-sided carinoplasty. Ann Thorac Surg 1993; 56:441–446.
5. Naruke T. Bronchoplastic and bronchovascular procedures of the tracheobronchial tree in the management of primary lung cancer. Chest 1989; 96(suppl):53S–56S.
6. Tsuchiya R, Goya T, Naruke T, Suemasu K. Resection of tracheal carina for lung cancer. Procedure, complications, and mortality. J Thorac Cardiovasc Surg 1990; 99:779–787.
7. Dartevelle PG, Khalife J, Chapelier A, et al. Tracheal sleeve pneumonectomy for bronchogenic carcinoma: report of 55 cases. Ann Thorac Surg 1988; 46:68–72.
8. Roviaro GC, Varoli F, Rebuffat C, et al. Tracheal sleeve pneumonectomy for bronchogenic carcinoma. J Thorac Cardiovasc Surg 1994; 107:13–18.
9. Dartevelle PG. Extended operations for the treatment of lung cancer. Ann Thorac Surg 1997; 63:12–19.
10. Pitz CCM, de la Riviere AB, Elbers HRJ, Westermann CJJ, van den Bosch JM. Results of resection of T3 non-small cell lung cancer invading the mediastinum or main bronchus. Ann Thorac Surg 1996; 62:1016–1020.
11. Dartevelle P, Marzelle J, Chapelier A, Loc'h F. Extended operations for T3-T4 primary lung cancers. Indications and results. Chest 1989; 1 (Suppl):51S–53S.
12. Ayabe H, Tagawa Y, Tsuji H, et al. Results of carinal resection for bronchogenic carcinoma. Tohoku J Exp Med 1995; 175:91–99.
13. Grillo HC, Tsuchiya R. Invited letter concerning: Resection of tracheal carina for lung cancer. J Thorac Cardiovasc Surg 1990; 99(letters):940–941.
14. Tsuchiya R, Asamura H, Kondo H, Goya T, Naruke T. Extended resection of the left atrium, great vessels, or both for lung cancer. Ann Thorac Surg 1994; 57:960–965.
15. Martini N, Yellin A, Ginsberg RJ, et al. Management of non-small cell lung cancer with direct mediastinal involvement. Ann Thorac Surg 1994; 58:1447–1451.
16. Naruke T, Suemasu K, Ishikawa S. Lymph node mapping and curability at various levels of metastasis in resected lung cancer. J Thorac Cardiovasc Surg 1978; 76:832–839.
17. Faber LP. Current status of neoadjuvant therapy for non-small cell lung cancer. Chest 1994; 106(suppl):355S–358S.
18. Green MR. New adjuvant strategies for the management of resectable non-small-cell lung cancer. Chest 1993; 103(suppl):352S–355S.
19. Eagan RT. Management of regionally advanced (stage III) non-small cell lung cancer. Chest 1994; 106(suppl):340S–343S.
20. Weiden L, Piantadosi S. Preoperative chemotherapy (cisplastin and fluorouracil) and radiation therapy in stage III non-small cell lung cancer. Chest 1994; 106(suppl):344S–347S.
21. Macchiarini P, Chapelier AR, Monnet I, et al. Extended operations after induction therapy for stage IIIb (T4) non-small cell lung cancer. Ann Thorac Surg 1994; 57:966–973.
22. Martini N, Flehinger BJ. The role of surgery in N2 lung cancer. Surg Clin North Am 1987; 67:1037–1049.
23. Rosell R, Gomez-Codina J, Camps C, et al. A randomized trial comparing preopera-

tive chemotherapy plus surgery with surgery alone in patients with non-small-cell lung cancer. New Engl J Med 1994; 330:153–158.

24. Dillman RO, Seagren SL, Propert KJ, et al. A randomized trial of induction chemotherapy plus high-dose radiation versus radiation alone in stage III non-small-cell lung cancer. New Engl J Med 1990; 323:940–945.

25. Albain KS, Rusch VW, Crowley JJ, et al. Concurrent cisplastin/etoposide plus chest radiotherapy followed by surgery for stages IIIA (N2) and IIIB non-small-cell lung cancer: mature results of Southwest Oncology Group Phase II study 8805. J Clin Oncol 1995; 13:1880–1892.

26. Wagner H, Lad T, Piantadosi S, Ruckdeschel JC. Randomized phase 2 evaluation of preoperative radiation therapy and preoperative chemotherapy with mitomycin, vinblastine, and cisplastin in patients with technically unresectable stage IIIA and IIIB non-small cell cancer of the lung. Chest 1994; 106(suppl):347S–354S.

27. Roth JA, Fossella F, Komaki R, et al. A randomized trial comparing perioperative chemotherapy and surgery with surgery alone in resectable stage IIIA non-small-cell lung cancer. J Natl Cancer Inst 1994; 86:673–680.

28. Ricci C, Rendina EA, Venuta F, Ciriaco PP, De Giacomo T, Fadda GF. Reconstruction of the pulmonary artery in patients with lung cancer. Ann Thorac Surg 1994; 57:627–633.

29. Warren WH. Surgical techniques in the dissection and reconstruction of the pulmonary artery. Chest Surg Clin North Am 1995; 5:333–344.

30. Dartevelle P, Chapelier A, Navajas M, et al. Replacement of the superior vena cava with polytetrafluoroethylene grafts combined with resection of mediastinal-pulmonary malignant tumors. Report of thirteen cases. J Thorac Cardiovasc Surg 1987; 94:361–366.

31. Dartevelle PG, Chapelier AR, Pastorino U, et al. Long-term follow-up after prosthetic replacement of the superior vena cava combined with resection of mediastinal-pulmonary malignant tumors. J Thorac Cardiovasc Surg 1991; 102:259–265.

32. Inoue H, Shohtsu A, Koide S, Ogawa J, Inoue HI. Resection of the superior vena cava for primary lung cancer: 5 years' survival. Ann Thorac Surg 1990; 50:661–662.

33. Nakahara K, Ohno K, Mastumura A, et al. Extended operation for lung cancer invading the aortic arch and superior vena cava. J Thorac Cardiovasc Surg 1989; 97:428–433.

34. Abner A. Approach to the patient who presents with superior vena cava obstruction. Chest 1993; 103(suppl):394S–397S.

35. Thomas P, Magnan PE, Moulin G, Giudicelli R, Fuentes P. Extended operation for lung cancer invading the superior vena cava. Eur J Cardiothorac Surg 1994; 8:177–182.

36. Dartevelle P, Macchiarini P, Chapelier A. Technique of superior vena cava resection and reconstruction. Chest Surg Clin North Am 1995; 5:345–358.

37. Horita K, Itho T, Ueno T. Radical operation using cardiopulmonary bypass for lung cancer invading the aortic wall. J Thorac Cardiovasc Surg 1993; 41:130–132.

38. Burt ME, Pomerantz AH, Bains MS, et al. Results of surgical treatment of stage III lung cancer invading the mediastinum. Surg Clin North Am 1987; 67:987–1000.

39. VanRaemdonck DE, Schneider A, Ginsberg RJ. Surgical treatment for higher stage non-small cell lung cancer. Ann Thorac Surg 1992; 54:999–1013.

40. DeMeester TR, Albertucci M, Dawson PJ, Montner SM. Management of tumor adherent to the vertebral column. J Thorac Cardiovasc Surg 1989; 97:373–378.

41. Wright CD, Moncure AC, Shepard JO, Wilkins EW Jr, Mathisen DJ, Grillo HC. Superior sulcus lung tumors. Results of combined treatment (irradiation and radical resection). J Thorac Cardiovasc Surg 1987; 94:69–74.

42. Read RC, Boop WC, Yoder G, Schaefer R. Management of nonsmall cell lung carcinoma with solitary brain metastasis. J Thorac Cardiovasc Surg 1989; 98:884–891.

43. Mandell L, Hilaris B, Sullivan M, et al. The treatment of single brain metastasis from non-oat cell lung carcinoma. Surgery and radiation versus radiation therapy alone. Cancer 1986; 58:641–649.

44. Burt ME. Role of surgery in the treatment of patients with solitary metastasis from non-small cell lung cancer. In: Aisner J, Arriagada R, Green MR, Martini N, Perry MC, eds. Comprehensive Textbook of Thoracic Oncology. Baltimore: Williams & Wilkins, 1996:416–425.

45. Fried BM, Buckley RC. Primary carcinoma of the lungs IV. Intracranial metastasis. Arch Pathol 1930; 9:483–527.

46. Sarma DP, Weilbaecher TG. Long-term survival after brain metastasis from lung cancer. Cancer 1986; 58:1366–1370.

47. Yokoi K, Miyazawa N, Arai T. Brain metastasis in resected lung cancer: value of intensive follow-up with computed tomography. Ann Thorac Surg 1996; 61:546–551.

48. Noordijk EM, Vecht CJ, Haaxma-Reiche H. The choice of treatment of single brain metastasis should be based on extracranial tumor activity and age. Int J Radiat Oncol Biol Phys 1994; 29:711–717.

49. Harpole D, Amos A, Alexander E, et al. Stage of the primary is important when treating isolated brain metastases from lung cancer. Prog Proc Am Soc Clin Oncol 1996; A1143 (Abstr.)

10

Multimodality Therapy for Stage IIIA and IIIB Non-Small-Cell Lung Cancer

GARY M. STRAUSS

Dana-Farber Cancer Institute
Harvard Medical School, Boston, and
Memorial Hospital
Worcester, Massachusetts

ELIZABETH H. BALDINI

Brigham and Women's Hospital
Dana-Farber Cancer Institute
Boston, Massachusetts

I. Introduction

The treatment of regionally advanced non-small-cell lung cancer (NSCLC) has evolved significantly over the last decade. Until 1986, the American Joint Committee on Cancer (AJCC) staging system (1), which grouped regionally advanced NSCLC along with distant metastatic disease in a single stage III category, was utilized. At that time, however, the AJCC system was replaced by the International Staging System (ISS). The ISS subdivided regionally advanced stage III disease into stage IIIA and IIIB subcategories (2).

The intent of the ISS was to subdivide regionally advanced disease into groups that were potentially resectable (stage IIIA) and those that were categorically unresectable (stage IIIB). Based on the 1986 classification, stage IIIA was composed of T3N0, T3N1, T1N2, T2N2, and T3N2 disease. Stage IIIB consisted of tumors without distant metastases, that were associated with either a T4 primary lesion or N3 disease.

However, in 1997, the ISS was revised in several respects (Table 1) (3). The revision in the ISS relevant to stage IIIA is that T3N0 lesions are no longer classified as stage IIIA, but have been downstaged into a new stage IIB category. Accordingly, at present, stage IIIA NSCLC comprises T3N1 and T1–T3N2 lesions. The definition of stage IIIB NSCLC has not changed with the new revision. However, in the era of multimodality therapy, certain subsets of patients with stage IIIB disease can be considered potentially resectable.

In addition to changes in the staging classification, new guidelines for grouping regional lymph node stations in the mediastinum have also been published (4,5). The objective is to provide for greater consistency and reproducibility of lymph node mapping within the mediastinum.

Despite the revisions in the ISS, regionally advanced NSCLC continues to include a heterogeneous group of diseases. Moreover, there has historically been no "standard therapy" for such patients, because the vast majority have been destined to die of their disease. However, an increasing number of therapeutic options are becoming available for patients with both stage IIIA and stage IIIB NSCLC.

In addition to anatomic factors, heterogeneity remains substantial with respect to such patient characteristics as performance status, degree of weight loss, pulmonary function, and comorbid disease. These various tumor and patient factors have repeatedly been shown to significantly influence prognosis (6–11). Consequently, in the development and evaluation of treatment strategies it is important to focus on subgroups of patients with regionally advanced NSCLC that are as homogeneous as possible.

II. Single-Modality Treatment

A. Radiation Therapy

Historically, radiotherapy (RT) had been considered to represent "standard treatment" for stage III NSCLC. Conventional RT for NSCLC consists of once-daily treatments of 1.8 to 2 Gy to a total dose of about 60 Gy. This convention was defined by the RTOG 73-01 randomized study, which showed that 60 Gy delivered in a continuous course was superior to a split-course technique and lower-dose continuous courses (12). Conventional RT first-course treatment volumes include the primary tumor with a 2 cm margin, the ipsilateral hilum, mediastinum, subcarinal region, and, for middle and upper lobe tumors, the supraclavicular regions. Boost or second-course volumes typically include the primary tumor and involved nodes only (13).

It has been clearly shown that the efficacy of RT alone is quite limited. Median survival is generally <12 months, and 5-year survival rates range between 5% and 8% (12,14). Local control is also a major problem. With radiotherapy alone, local failure ranges between 75% and 83% (15–21).

One new strategy for the delivery of RT is hyperfractionation (HFX). In this technique, multiple fractions of RT (usually two) are delivered daily. Late toxicity is minimized because normal "late-responding" tissues (spinal cord, lung) are able to repair sublethal damage in the 4 to 6 hours between daily fractions. Acute toxicity and tumor control, however, are theoretically increased since "early-respond-

Table 1 International Staging System for Lung Cancer—Revised 1997

Primary tumor (T)	
T1	Tumor <3 cm diameter without invasion more proximal than lobar bronchus
T2	Tumor >3 cm diameter, or tumor of any size with any of the following:
	Invades visceral pleura
	Atelectasis of less than entire lung
	Proximal extent at least 2 cm from carina
T3	Tumor of any size with any of following:
	Invasion of chest wall
	Involvement of diaphragm, mediastinal pleural, or pericardium
	Atelectasis involving entire lung
	Proximal extent within 2 cm of carina
T4	Tumor of any size with any of following:
	Invasion of mediastinum
	Invasion of heart or great vessels
	Invasion of trachea or esophagus
	Invasion of vertebral body or carina
	Presence of malignant pleural effusion

Nodal involvement (N)	
N0	No regional node involvement
N1	Metastasis to ipsilateral hilar nodes
N2	Metastasis to ipsilateral mediastinal or subcarinal nodes
N3	Metastasis to contralateral mediastinal or hilar nodes, or ipsilateral or contralateral supraclavicular nodes

Metastases (M)	
M0	Distant metastases absent
M1	Distant metastases present

Stage groupings of TNM subsets	
Stage IA	T1 N0 M0
Stage IB	T2 N0 M0
Stage IIA	T1 N1 M0
Stage IIB	T2 N1 M0
	T3 N0 M0
Stage IIIA	T3 N1 M0
	T1–3 N2 M0
Stage IIIB	Any T N3 M0
	T4 any N M0
Stage IV	Any T any N M1

Source: Ref. 3.

ing" tissues (esophageal mucosa, tumor) are generally not capable of repair during these interfraction intervals. Hyperfractionated RT was evaluated in the RTOG 83-11 trial which randomized patients to five different arms of 1.2 Gy b.i.d. treatment to total doses of 60 Gy, 64.8 Gy, 69.6 Gy, 74.4 Gy, and 79.2 Gy (22). No significant differences were seen for the groups as a whole, but subset analysis showed a survival advantage for "favorable" patients (good performance status and minimal weight loss) who received 69.6 Gy (23).

Another nonconventional RT approach is accelerated hyperfractionation. This technique incorporates the features of hyperfractionation with reduced overall treatment time. The rationale for the approach is to prevent accelerated repopulation of tumor cells during treatment. Two British trials have piloted the use of continuous hyperfractionated accelerated radiotherapy (CHART). The first trial was a Phase I study which defined the tolerability of the following regimen: 1.5 Gy delivered three times daily with 6 hours between treatments for 12 consecutive days to a total dose of 54 Gy (24). The second trial randomized patients between conventional RT of 60 Gy (given in 2 Gy once-daily fractions) and the CHART t.i.d. regimen. Preliminary results show a significant 2-year survival advantage for the CHART arm (25).

Yet another approach consists of the "concomitant boost" technique. RTOG 83-12 is a Phase I/II trial which delivered 1.8 Gy daily to a traditional first-course RT volume (described above) immediately followed by an additional 0.88 Gy to a boost volume consisting of the primary tumor and involved nodes. Over 5.5 weeks (28 fractions) the large field received 50.4 Gy and the gross tumor volume received 75 Gy (26). Results were comparable to other reports in the literature.

Other innovative ways to deliver RT include the use of three-dimensional treatment planning with dose escalation. However, as doses are escalated, the treatment volumes must be reduced. A lot is still unknown about the relative trade-offs of volume and dose in terms of both toxicity and efficacy. The use of radiosensitizers during the delivery of RT is another avenue of research. Radiosensitizers act to increase the sensitivity of tumors to radiation, and they include standard chemotherapeutic agents as well as novel agents.

B. Surgery

Since the majority of patients with NSCLC who achieve long-term survival undergo resection, surgery is believed to represent the most effective modality in the treatment of NSCLC. As previously stated, patients with stage IIIA disease compose a heterogeneous group with varying prognoses. Prior to the revisions in the ISS, T3N0 tumors were classified as stage IIIA disease. However, patients with T3N0 lesions have a superior prognosis to those with nodal involvement. Such differences in prognosis represent the basis of downstaging such patients into a new stage IIB category (3).

Patients with T3 primaries, based on chest wall involvement, probably have the most favorable outlook with surgical resection(27). Reports from the Mayo Clinic and from the Brigham and Women's Hospital indicate 5-year survivals in excess of 50% for resected T3N0 chest wall lesions (28,29). Similarly, superior sulcus tumors without regional node involvement enjoy respectable long-term survival rates following resection (30).

With respect to N2 disease, the results are less favorable. Several series demonstrate 5-year survival rates ranging from 15% to 29% among highly selected groups of patients undergoing resection of N2 disease (27,28,31). The largest experience pertaining to the role of surgery in N2 disease comes from Memorial Sloan-Kettering Cancer Center (MSKCC) (6). Of 706 patients judged to have N2 disease by either clinical or pathologic criteria (mediastinoscopy was not routinely performed), 404 underwent thoracotomy and 151 were completely resected. Approximately 90% of all resected patients also received postoperative radiation to the ipsilateral hilum and mediastinum (40 to 45 Gy). The bulk of mediastinal node involvement significantly affected the likelihood of complete resection and outcome. The overall 5-year survival for the entire group of resected N2 patients was 30%. For those who were clinically N0 or N1, the 5-year survival was 34%. For those with clinically overt N2 disease, the 5-year survival was 9%; this 9% figure is not very different from that achievable with radiation alone.

A series from Toronto General Hospital on the surgical treatment of 141 patients with stage IIIA disease demonstrated that cervical mediastinoscopy is extremely useful in selecting patients for surgical resection (7). All patients underwent preoperative cervical mediastinoscopy in order to surgically stage the mediastinum. In 62 patients, mediastinoscopy was negative, but mediastinal node involvement was found at the time of resection. The actuarial 5-year survival in this group was 24%. In contrast, for patients with a positive mediastinoscopy, the 5-year survival was only 9%.

Accordingly, the data support the conclusion that surgical resection rate is high in certain N2 subsets. Moreover, long-term survival is achieved in some of these patients. On the other hand, the results with resection are not sufficiently compelling for surgery to automatically be considered "standard" treatment, particularly in patients with clinically overt N2 disease.

III. Combined Modality Treatments

A. Surgery and Radiation

The rationale for combining radiation and surgery is to improve local-regional control. An improvement in local control in theory could lead to an improvement in overall survival, although such has not been the case in most adult solid tumors. Radiation has been combined with surgery both preoperatively and postoperatively. Two large randomized trials comparing preoperative radiation therapy followed by surgery to surgery alone were conducted in the 1960s and 1970s (32,33). Both trials failed to demonstrate any benefit for preoperative radiation; however, modern radiographic and surgical staging was not employed in either study, and patients with small-cell lung cancer were included in these trials. Sherman et al. reported the results of a Phase II trial of preoperative radiation followed by surgical resection in stage III NSCLC (34). Fifty-three patients received 30 to 40 Gy preoperative radiation followed by resection and postoperative radiation. Five-year survival was 18% for the entire cohort of 53 patients, and 27% for 38 patients who underwent successful resection. The role of postoperative radiation was most definitively evaluated by the Lung Cancer Study Group, in LCSG protocol 773 (35). Patients with completely resected stage II or III squamous cell carcinoma were randomized to receive 50 Gy postoperative radiation or no further therapy. Postoperative radiation therapy significantly reduced the incidence of isolated local-regional recurrences to the ipsilateral lung and mediastinum from 41% to 3%. However, this did not translate into a survival advantage.

B. Chemotherapy and Radiation

The role of chemotherapy combined with thoracic radiation for stage IIIA NSCLC has been extensively studied, and many Phase II and Phase III studies have been reported. Some of the positive studies are detailed below.

Perhaps the most influential Phase III trial in stage III NSCLC is the trial conducted by Cancer and Leukemia Group B (CALGB 84-33) (16,17). Eligibility for this trial was limited to patients with favorable pretreatment characteristics including good performance status (ECOG PS of 0 or 1) and minimal weight loss (<5% of body weight in the preceding 3 months). Patients were randomized to receive 60 Gy of radiation in 6 weeks or two cycles of induction chemotherapy with cisplatin and vinblastine followed by the identical radiation treatment. A recent update of this trial showed that the group randomized to induction chemotherapy achieved a significant improvement in median survival (13.7 vs. 9.6 months) as well as in the proportion of patients surviving out to 7 years (13% vs. 6%).

Le Chevalier et al. reported the results of a multicenter French study involving 353 patients who were randomized to 65 Gy radiation or three cycles of induction chemotherapy using cisplatin, vindesine, cyclophosphamide, and CCNU given prior to radiation followed by three additional cycles of chemotherapy (18,19). Three-year survival for the combined chemotherapy/radiation arm was 11%, while for the radiation-alone arm it was 5% ($P = .08$).

The Radiation Therapy Oncology Group (RTOG) and Eastern Cooperative Oncology Group (ECOG) have conducted a confirmatory three-arm trial involving 452 eligible patients who were randomized to the same two treatment arms employed in CALGB 84-33 as well as a third arm which included hyperfractionation radiation to a total dose of 69.6 Gy (36). Preliminary results of this trial indicate that 1-year and median survival is superior in the group randomized to receive induction chemotherapy compared to the other two groups ($P = .03$). The 1-year survivals for the three groups are as follows: induction chemotherapy and RT, 60%; hyperfractionation, RT 51%; and standard RT, 46%.

The European Organization for Research and Treatment of Cancer (EORTC) conducted a three-arm study in 331 patients comparing 50 Gy thoracic radiation in one arm, to two other arms which utilized concurrent cisplatin and radiation on one of two schedules (20). In one arm, cisplatin was administered daily (6 mg/m^2/day) along with radiation, while in the other it was administered weekly (30 mg/m^2/week). There was a significant improvement ($P = .009$) in survival for daily cisplatin/radiation compared to radiation alone (3-year survivals, 16% vs. 2%, respectively). For weekly cisplatin/radiation, survival was intermediate (3-year survival, 13%) but was not significantly different from either of the other arms. Interestingly, the survival benefit observed with daily cisplatin/radiation appeared to be secondary to improved local control ($P = .003$).

Jeremic reported a randomized trial consisting of the following three treatment arms: hyperfractionated RT alone (1.2 Gy bid to 64.8 Gy); the same hyperfractionated RT and weekly carboplatin and etoposide; the same RT and alternate-week carboplatin and etoposide (37). The middle arm of RT and continuous chemotherapy was superior in terms of local control and survival (but not distant recurrence rate). For the three arms, the local recurrence rates were 88%, 66%, and 76%, respectively; the 3-year overall survival rates were 6.6%, 23%, and 16%, respectively. Thus, this is the second trial demonstrating that improved local control rates correlate with improved survival.

In addition to the above-cited positive trials which show a benefit for chemoradiation compared to radiation alone, there are several trials which fail to demonstrate a significant difference (38–40). A meta-analysis has been published which includes data from 2589 patients enrolled in 14 randomized trials that compared chemotherapy and radiation to radiation alone in regionally advanced stage III NSCLC (41). Overall, the meta-analysis demonstrated that the use of combination chemotherapy and radiation reduced the risk of death by 17% at 3 years. This corresponds to a mean gain of life expectancy of about 2 months. The magnitude of benefit was similar independent of whether chemoradiation was delivered sequentially or concurrently. Kubota et al. performed a phase III trial asking a different question—what is the role of RT for patients receiving chemotherapy? Patients with stage III disease were initially randomized to one of three cisplatin-based chemotherapy regimens. Then they underwent a second randomization to receive RT (50 to 60 Gy) or not. The 3-year overall survival rate was significantly improved for patients who received RT (29% vs. 3%) (42).

Despite encouraging data for combined chemoradiation, many important questions remain. These unanswered questions include the choice of the chemotherapy regimen, the optimal sequencing of chemotherapy and radiation, the role of hyperfractionated radiation, and the choice of radiation treatment volumes and total doses.

C. Phase II Trials of Induction Chemotherapy, Radiation, and Surgery

Numerous phase II trials of induction chemotherapy and surgical resection in regionally advanced stage III NSCLC have been conducted. However, these trials vary considerably with respect to many factors. The variability relates to the use of surgical staging of the mediastinum, the delivery of radiation sequentially with chemotherapy vs. concurrently, the choice and dose of chemotherapeutic agents, radiation dose schedules, and definitions of resectable disease. Such inconsistencies have led to considerable difficulties in interpretation of these trials.

Table 2 lists 11 phase II trials of induction chemotherapy and surgery with or without radiation in stage IIIA NSCLC (43–53). (Two trials also included patients with stage IIIB disease [43; Albain, 1995 #981].) Each of the trials listed utilized a cisplatin-based combination chemotherapy regimen. Seven of the trials used preoperative radiation (six given concurrently with chemotherapy and one sequentially), two trials used only postoperative radiation, and two did not employ radiation at all.

Overall, response rates to induction therapy were quite impressive, varying from 39% to 77%. Resectability rates exceeded 50% in each of these trials. The highest resectability rate (93%) was noted in a trial that utilized hyperfractionated radiation concurrently with induction chemotherapy (48). Many trials report pathologic complete response rates in the range of 10% to 20% following induction therapy. Median survival and long-term survival rates varied significantly among the trials, but it is clear that a minority of patients enjoyed long-term survival and possible cure. Moreover, two multi-institutional trials showed that patients who were found to have negative N2 nodes at the time of resection had a significantly better survival rate than those with persistent N2 positive disease at resection (47, Albain, 1995 #981).

None of these trials were designed to evaluate the therapeutic role of surgery in the context of regionally advanced disease, but the addition of surgery to the locoregional treatment regimen almost certainly accomplishes an improvement in local control. Local recurrence has generally been observed in <50% of patients who undergo trimodality therapy. This contrasts with an 80% to 90% rate of persistent or recurrent local-regional disease among those who are not resected (12,17,18,20). Thus, these Phase II trials employing chemotherapy, radiation, and surgery demonstrate a shift in recurrence patterns from both local and distant to predominantly distant. Furthermore, improved local control rates may result in significant overall survival gains, as has been demonstrated by the reports of Schaake-Koning (20) and Jeremic (37).

D. Phase III Trials of Induction Chemotherapy

Reports of small randomized trials comparing induction chemotherapy followed by surgical resection to resection without systemic treatment have been influential in modifying the perception of the role of chemotherapy in the management of regionally advanced NSCLC.

A study from Barcelona, Spain, randomized patients to an induction chemotherapy regimen of cisplatin, mitomycin C, and ifosfamide followed by resection and postoperative radiation therapy (50 Gy) compared to resection and the same postoperative radiation therapy. There was a dramatic, threefold survival advantage for those randomized to receive induction chemotherapy (54). In the group randomized to chemotherapy, median survival was 26 months; in the surgery plus RT group, it was (a lower than expected) 8 months ($P < .001$).

In a similar trial conducted at M.D. Anderson, patients were randomized to receive induction chemotherapy consisting of three cycles of cyclophosphamide, etoposide, and cisplatin followed by resection, or surgical resection alone (55). Of note, radiation therapy was given to >50% of patients in both arms. The group that received chemotherapy achieved an estimated median survival that was almost sixfold greater than that of patients randomized to surgery alone (64 months compared to 11 months; $P < .008$). Similarly, 3-year survival was 56% for the induction chemotherapy group compared to 15% for the surgery-alone group.

While receiving much less attention than the other two trials, a third randomized trial from NCI had preceded the other two (56). In this trial, the experimental group was treated with induction cisplatin and etoposide chemotherapy followed by resection and postoperative chemotherapy. The control group underwent immediate surgical resection and postoperative radiation therapy (54 to 60 Gy). Patients treated with induction chemotherapy had a superior survival, but the difference was not statistically significant (28.7 vs. 15.6 months, respectively).

A fourth randomized trial, which was conducted by the CALGB, is not yet fully mature (57). The experimental arm of this study consisted of induction chemotherapy with cisplatin and etoposide for two cycles followed by resection, two additional cycles of chemotherapy, and subsequent radiation therapy (54 or 60 Gy). The control arm consisted of preoperative radiation therapy (40 Gy), resection, and postoperative radiation therapy (to a total dose of 54 or 60 Gy). Preliminary results show that the median overall survival was 19 months for the group undergoing induction chemotherapy, compared to 23 months for the group receiving preoperative radiation. While the trend toward reduced survival in the group receiving induction chemotherapy was not statistically significant, the results of CALGB 9134 conflict with the results of the other three randomized trials that suggest a dramatic benefit with the use of induction chemotherapy.

Although three of the four randomized trials did show a survival benefit with the use of induction chemotherapy (including two in which the differences were

Table 2 Phase II Trials on Induction Chemotherapy and Surgery in Stage IIIA Disease

Group or institution	Reference	Number of patients	Induction chemotherapy regimen	Radiation	Response to induction therapy	Resectability	Median survival	Percent long-term survival
CAP I trial (DFCI)	(43)	41	Cisplatin, cytoxan, adriamycin	After induction chemotherapy but prior to resection (and postoperatively)	53%	83%	32 mo	31% (5 yr)
CAP II trial (DFCI)	(44)	54	Cisplatin, cytoxan, adriamycin	given postoperatively	39%	54%	17.9 mo	22% (5 yr)
PFL (DFCI)	(45)	34	Cisplatin, 5-fluorouracil, leukovorin	given postoperatively	65%	52%	18 mo	18% (4 yr)
CALGB 8634	(46,59)	41	Cisplatin, vinblastine, 5-FU	concurrent with induction chemotherapy (and postoperatively)	51%	61%	15.5 mo	22% (9 yr)
CALGB 8935	(47,60)	74	Cisplatin, vinblastine	given postoperatively	88% (PR or stable disease)	62%	15 mo	23% (3 yr)
MGH	(48)	42	Cisplatin, vinblastine, 5-FU	twice daily radiation given concurrently with induction chemotherapy (and postoperatively)	73%	93%	25 mo	37% (5 yr)
MSKCI	(49)	136	Mitomycin, vindesine, cisplatin	Not routinely utilized	77%	65%	19 mo	17% (5 yr)
Toronto	(50)	39	Mitomycin, vindesine, cisplatin	Not routinely utilized	64%	56%	18.6 mo	26% (3 yr)

Rush	(51)	129 83 stage IIIA 46 stage IIIB	Cisplatin, 5-FU, ± VP-16	Concurrent with induction chemotherapy	Not reported	72%a	17.6 mo	32% (3 yr)
LCSG	(52)	85	Cisplatin, 5-FU	Concurrent with induction chemotherapy	56%	52%	13 mo	20% (3 yr)
SWOG 8805	(53)	126 75 stage IIIA 51 stage IIIB	Cisplatin, VP-16	Concurrent with induction chemotherapy (and postop)	59%	71% 76% stage IIIA 63% stage IIIB	13 mo stage IIIA 17 mo stage IIIB	27% (3 yr) stage IIIA 24% (3 yr) stage IIIB

a72% resectability achieved among 86 patients deemed ''eligible for surgery'' at outset. Resectability was 47% among all 129 patients.

statistically significant), these studies have significant limitations which raise important questions as to whether induction chemotherapy has been proven to be beneficial. One major problem relates to the fact that each of the trials enrolled small numbers of patients (Barcelona, 60 patients; M.D. Anderson, 60; NCI, 27; CALGB, 57). The Barcelona and M.D. Anderson trials were discontinued before the projected accrual goal was reached because of early stopping rules. The highly publicized beneficial effects observed in the Barcelona and M.D. Anderson trials were most likely responsible for difficulty in accruing to CALGB 9134, leading to its premature closure. Furthermore, the absolute magnitude of the survival differences seen in the M.D. Anderson and Barcelona trials was far greater than could be reasonably expected from the modestly effective chemotherapy regimens employed. These extreme results should raise caution. A plausible explanation for the magnitude of the differences seen in these studies is that despite the process of randomization, there may have been an imbalance of prognostic factors between the arms. In the Barcelona study, it was demonstrated that the group of patients randomized to surgery alone included a higher fraction of tumors with the more virulent characteristics of K-ras mutations (42% vs. 15%) and DNA aneuploidy (70% vs. 29%) (54,58). Hence, it is possible that an excess of biologically virulent tumors in the group randomized to surgery alone in the Barcelona study is responsible for the observed outcome differences rather than a beneficial effect of the induction chemotherapy per se. While there is no direct evidence for a similar imbalance in the M.D. Anderson trial, prognostically important molecular markers were not considered in this study. An imbalance of some unmeasured prognostic variable might have contributed to the magnitude of the differences seen in this trial.

Cumulatively, these four Phase III studies evaluating the role of induction chemotherapy followed by surgery have included a total of only 204 patients. The results are surprising and conflicting. Accordingly, the benefit of induction chemotherapy, although suggested, has not been definitively demonstrated. The 11 Phase II studies listed in Table 2 include 781 patients. While the results of these trials vary, there is greater consistency in the results of the phase II trials than of the randomized trials.

IV. Conclusions

Despite the limitations of the randomized induction chemotherapy and surgery trials in stage IIIA NSCLC, they do lend some support to the conclusion that for favorable patients with stage IIIA NSCLC, induction chemotherapy followed by resection (±RT) may enhance disease outcome compared to that achieved with resection (±RT). While the magnitude of the survival advantages added by chemotherapy are very likely to have been exaggerated, particularly in the M.D. Anderson trial, numerous Phase II trimodality studies support a similar conclusion, though with a modest degree of effectiveness. In addition, these results for induction chemotherapy with surgery are consistent with numerous Phase III studies that have demonstrated that induction chemotherapy with definitive radiation improves outcome when compared to thoracic radiation therapy alone.

Whether induction chemotherapy is now standard therapy is debatable, but there is a clear suggestion of benefit, and additional clinical trials evaluating this approach will be difficult to accomplish. The role of resection in stage IIIA disease remains unproved, but local control appears improved in multimodality programs that include resection, and patients found to have negative N2 nodes at resection do quite well. A Phase III trial designed to evaluate the efficacy of surgical resection in the context of induction chemoradiation in stage IIIA NSCLC is ongoing by several cooperative groups under the leadership of the SWOG. Conventional radiation treatment approaches are probably not optimal. Hyperfractionated radiation and concurrent chemoradiation schemes may prove to be superior, but the toxicities, logistical difficulties, and costs of these aggressive approaches must not be minimized. Further investigation of these RT techniques and the use of three-dimensional treatment planning with dose escalation should be supported.

The recent results of both phase III and phase II trials have provided a basis for optimism that real therapeutic progress is finally being achieved in regionally advanced NSCLC. Further study of therapeutic strategies which incorporate aggressive systemic treatment and maximal local-regional therapy in stage IIIA NSCLC is clearly warranted. Patients most likely to benefit from these aggressive strategies are those in the favorable prognosis subgroups—patients with good performance status and minimal weight loss. Given the heterogeneities of patient and tumor characteristics in stage IIIA NSCLC, future trials investigating aggressive treatment strategies should clearly stratify patients to define homogeneous groups for study.

References

1. American Joint Committee on Cancer, Task Force on Lung Staging of Lung Cancer. Chicago: American Joint Committee on Cancer, 1979.
2. Mountain CF. A new international staging system for lung cancer. Chest 1986; 89:225S–233S.
3. Mountain CE. Revisions in the international system for staging lung cancer. Chest 1997; 111:1710–1717.
4. Mountain CF, Dresler CM. Regional lymph node classification for lung cancer staging. Chest 1997; 111:1718–1723.
5. Jette JR. What's new in staging of lung cancer? Chest 1997; 111:1486–1487.
6. Martini N, Flehinger BJ. The role of surgery in N2 lung cancer. Surg Clin North Am 1987; 67:1037–1049.

7. Pearson F, Delarue N, Ives R, et al. Significance of positive superior mediastinal nodes identified at mediastinoscopy in patients with resectable cancer of the lung. Thorac Cardiovasc Surg 1982; 83:1–11.

8. Albain KS, Crowley JJ, Leblanc M, et al. Survival determinants in extensive stage non-small cell lung cancer: the Southwest Oncology Group experience. J Clin Oncol 1991; 9:1618–1626.

9. Stanley KE. Prognostic factors for survival in patients with inoperable lung cancer. J Natl Cancer Inst 1980; 65:25–32.

10. Paesmans M, Sculier JP, Lilbert P, et al. Prognostic factors for survival in advanced non-small cell lung cancer; univariate and multivariate analyses including recursive partitioning and amalgamation algorithm: the European Lung Cancer Working Party. J Clin Oncol 1995; 13:1221–1230.

11. Sorensen JB, Olsen BJHJ, Srensen JB. Prognostic factors in inoperable adenocarcinoma of the lung: a multivariate regression analysis of 259 patients. Cancer Res 1989; 49:5748–5754.

12. Perez CA, Bauer M, Edelstein S, et al. Impact of tumor control on survival in carcinoma of the lung treated with irradiation. Int J Radiat Oncol Biol Physics 1986; 12:539–547.

13. Perez CA, Brady LW, eds. Principles and Practice of Radiation Oncology. 2nd ed. Philadelphia: J.B. Lippincott, 1992.

14. Perez CA, Stanley K, Grundy G. Impact of irradiation technique and tumor extent in tumor control and survival of patients with unresectable non-oat cell carcinoma of the lung: report by the Radiation Oncology Group. Cancer 1982; 50:1091–1099.

15. Schaake-Koning C, Schuster-Uitterhoeve L, Hart G, et al. Prognostic factors of inoperable localized lung cancer treated by high dose radiotherapy. Int J Radiat Oncol Biol Physics 1983; 9:1023–1028.

16. Dillman RO, Herndon J, Seagren SL, Eaton WL, Green MR, Improved survival in stage III non-small cell lung cancer: seven-year followup of Cancer and leukemia Group B (CALGB) 8433 trial. J Natl Cancer Inst 1996; 88:1210–1215.

17. Dillman RO, Seagren S, Propert K, et al. A randomized trial of induction chemotherapy plus high-dose radiation versus radiation alone in stage III non-small cell lung cancer. N Engl J Med 1990; 323:940–945.

18. Le Chevalier T, Arriagada R, Quoix E, et al. Radiotherapy alone versus combined chemotherapy and radiotherapy in nonresectable non-small-cell lung cancer: first analysis of a randomized trial in 353 patients. J Natl Cancer Inst 1991; 83:417–423.

19. Le Chevalier T, Arriagada R, Tarayre M, et al. Correspondence-significant effect of adjuvant chemotherapy on survival in locally advanced non-small cell lung carcinoma. J Natl Cancer Inst 1992; 84:58.

20. Schaake-Koning C, Van den Bogaert W, Dalesio O, et al. Effects of concomitant cisplatin and radiotherapy on inoperable non-small cell lung cancer. N Engl J Med 1992; 326:524–530.

21. Arriagada R, LeChevalier T, Quoix E, et al. Astro plenary: effect of chemotherapy on locally advanced non-small cell lung carcinoma: a randomized study of 353 patients. Int J Radiat Oncol Biol Physics 1991; 20:1183–1190.

22. Cox JD, Azarnia N, Byhardt RW, et al. N2 (clinical) non-small cell carcinoma of the

lung: prospective trials of radiation therapy with total doses 60 Gy by the radiation therapy oncology group. Int J Radiat Oncol Biol Physics 1991; 20:7–12.

23. Cox JD, Azarnia N, Byhardt RW, et al. A randomized phase I–II trial of hyperfractionated radiation therapy with total doses of 60.0 Gy to 79.2 Gy: possible survival benefit with >69.6 Gy in favorable patients with radiation therapy oncology group stage III non-small cell lung carcinoma: report of radiation therapy oncology group 83-11. J Clin Oncol 1990; 8:1543–1555.

24. Saunders MI, Dische S. Continuous hyperfractionated, accelerated radiotherapy (CHART) in non-small cell carcinoma of the bronchus. Int J Radiat Oncol Biol Physics 1990; 19:1211–1215.

25. Saunders MI, Dische S, Barrett A, et al. Randomised multicentre trials of CHART versus radiotherapy in head and neck and non-small cell lung cancer: an interim report. Br J Cancer 1996; 73:1455–1462.

26. Graham MV, Pajak TE, Herskovic AM, Emami B, Perez CA. Phase I/II study of treatment of locally advanced (T3/T4) non-oat cell lung cancer with concomitant boost radiotherapy by the Radiation Oncology Group (RTOG-83-12): long term results. Int J Radiat Oncol Biol Physics 1995; 13:1221–1230.

27. Pairolero P, Trastek V, Payne W. Treatment of bronchogenic carcinoma with chest wall invasion. Surg Clin North Am 1987; 67:959–964.

28. Piehler J, Pairoler P, Weiland L, et al. Bronchogenic carcinoma with chest wall invasion. Factors affecting survival following en bloc resection. Ann Thorac Surg 1982; 34:684–691.

29. Sleckman B, Harpole D, Strauss G, Sugarbaker D. Multimodality therapy for chest wall invasive lung cancer. In: Proceedings of 47th Annual Cancer Symposium, Society of Surgical Oncology, 1994.

30. Grover F, Komaki R. Superior sulcus tumors. In: Roth J, Ruckdeschel J, Weisenburger, eds. Thoracic Oncology. Philadelphia: W.B. Saunders, 1989:263–279.

31. Ginsberg RJ, Goldberg M, Waters PF. Surgery for non-small cell lung cancer. In: Roth J, Ruckdeschel J, Weisenburger, eds. Thoracic Oncology Philadelphia: W B Saunders, 1989:177–199.

32. Shields TW. Preoperative radiation therapy in the treatment of bronchial carcinoma. Cancer 1972; 30:1388–1393.

33. Collaborative study. Properative irradiation of cancer of the lung: final report of a therapeutic trial. Cancer 1975; 3:914–925.

34. Sherman DM, Neptune W, Weishselbaum R, et al. An aggressive approach to marginally resectable lung cancer. Cancer 1978; 41:2040–2045.

35. Lung Cancer Study Group. Effects of postoperative mediastinal radiation on completely resected stage II and stage III epidermoid cancer of the lung. N Engl J Med 1986; 315:1377–1381.

36. Sause W, Scott C, Taylor S, et al. Radiation Therapy Oncology Group (RTOG) 88-08 and Eastern Cooperative Oncology Group (ECOG) 4588: preliminary results of a phase III trial in regionally advanced, unresectable non-small cell lung cancer. J Natl Cancer Inst 1995; 87(3):198–205.

37. Jeremic B, Shibamoto Y, Acimovic L, Djuric L. Randomized trial of hyperfractionated radiation therapy with or without concurrent chemotherapy for stage III non-small cell lung cancer. J Clin Oncol 1995; 13:452–458.

38. Soresi E, Clerci M, Grilli R, et al. A randomized clinical trial comparing radiation therapy versus radiation therapy plus cis-dichorodiammine platinum (II) in the treatment of locally advanced non-small cell lung cancer. Semin Oncol 1988; 15(suppl 7):20–25.

39. Morton RF, Jett JR, Maher L, et al. Randomized trial of thoracic radiation therapy with or without chemotherapy for treatment of locally unresectable non-small cell lung cancer (NSCLC). ASCO Proc 1988; 7:200.

40. Mattson K, Holsti LR, Holsti P, et al. Inoperable non-small cell lung cancer: radiation with or without chemotherapy. Eur J Cancer Clin Oncol 1988; 24:477–482.

41. Pritchard RS, Anthony SP. Chemotherapy plus radiotherapy compared with radiotherapy alone in the treatment of locally advanced, unresectable, non-small cell lung cancer. Ann Intern Med 1996; 125:723–729.

42. Kubota K, Furuse K, Kawahara M, et al. Role of radiotherapy in combined modality treatment of locally advanced non-small cell lung cancer. J Clin Oncol 1994; 12:1547–1552.

43. Skarin A, Jochelson M, Sheldon T, et al. Neoadjuvant chemotherapy in marginally resectable stage III M0 non-small cell lung cancer: long-term follow-up in 41 patients. J Surg Oncol 1989; 40:266–274.

44. Elias AD, Skarin AT, Gonin P, et al. Neoadjuvant treatment of stage IIIA non-small cell lung cancer: long-term results. Am J Clin Oncol 1994; 17:26–36.

45. Elias AD, Skarin AT, Leong T, et al. Neoadjuvant therapy for surgically staged IIIA N2 non-small cell lung cancer (NSCLC). Lung Cancer 1997; 17:147–161.

46. Strauss GM, Herndon JE, Sherman DD, et al. Neoadjuvant chemotherapy and radiotherapy followed by surgery in stage IIIA non-small cell carcinoma of the lung: report of a Cancer and Leukemia Group B phase II study. J Clin Oncol 1992; 10:1237–1244.

47. Sugarbaker DJ, Herndon J, Kohman LJ, Krasna MJ, Green MR. Results of Cancer and Leukemia Group B Protocol 8935: a multiinstitutional phase II trimodality trial for stage IIIA (N2) non-small cell lung cancer. J Thorac Cardiovasc Surg 1995; 109: 473–485.

48. Choi NC, Carey RW, Daly W, et al. Potential impact on survival of improved tumor downstaging and resection rate by preoperative twice-daily radiation and concurrent chemotherapy in stage IIIA non-small cell lung cancer. J Clin Oncol 1997; 15:712–722.

49. Martini N, Kris M, Flehinger B, et al. Preoperative chemotherapy for stage IIIa (N2) lung cancer: the Sloan-Kettering experience with 136 patients. Ann Thorac Surg 1993; 55:1365–1374.

50. Burkes RL, Ginsberg RJ, Sheperd FA, et al. Induction chemotherapy with mitomycin, vindesin, and cisplatin for stage III unresectable non-small cell lung cancer: results of a Toronto phase II trial. J Clin Oncol 1992; 10:580–586.

51. Reddy S, Lee MS, Bonomi P, et al. Combined modality therapy for stage III non-small cell lung cancer: results of treatment sand patterns of failure. Int J Radiat Oncol Biol Phys 1992; 24:17–32.

52. Weiden P, Piantadosi S, Lung Cancer Study Group. Peoperative chemotherapy (cisplatin and flourouracil) and radiation therapy in stage III non-small cell lung cancer: a phase II study of the lung cancer study group. J Natl Cancer Inst 1991; 83:266–272.

53. Albain KS, Rusch VW, Crowley JJ, et al. Concurrent cisplatin/etoposide plus chest radiotherapy followed by surgery for stages IIIA (N2) and IIIB non-small cell lung cancer: mature results of Southwest Oncology Group Phase II Study 8805. J Clin Oncol 1995; 13:1880–1892.

54. Rosell R, Gomez-Codina J, Camps C, et al. A randomized trial comparing preoperative chemotherapy plus surgery with surgery alone in patients with non-small cell lung cancer. N Engl J Med 1994; 330:153–158.

55. Roth JA, Fossella F, Komaki R, et al. A randomized trial comparing perioperative chemotherapy and surgery with surgery alone in resectable stage IIIA non-small cell lung cancer. J Natl Cancer Inst 1994; 86:673–680.

56. Pass HI, Pogrebnick HW, Steinberg SM, Mulshine J, Minna J. Randomized trial of neoadjuvant therapy for lung cancer: interim analysis. Ann Thorac Surg 1992; 53:992–998.

57. Elias AD, Herndon J, Kumar P, Sugarbaker D, Green MR. A phase III comparison of "best local-regional therapy" with or without chemotherapy for stage IIIA T1–3N2 non-small cell lung cancer (NSCLC): preliminary results. Proc ASCO, 1997; 16:448a (abstr. 1611).

58. Rosell A, Font A, Pitfarre A, et al. The role of induction (neoadjuvant) chemotherapy in stage IIIA NSCLC. Chest 1996; 109:102S–106S.

11

Multimodality Therapy of Stage IIIB Non-Small-Cell Lung Cancer

SCOTT J. SWANSON

Harvard Medical School
Brigham and Women's Hospital
Boston, Massachusetts

I. Introduction

The Cancer Statistics 1997 estimated there would be 178,100 new lung cancer cases in the United States in 1997 and that 160,400 deaths due to lung cancer would occur during that same period (1). The overall 5-year survival rate for lung cancer ranges from 10% to 15% (1). At least 70% of new cases will present with either regional or distant spread (1). As such, many cases require a multifaceted approach to their treatment. Many will not be appropriate for standard surgical resection alone.

Improvement in the outcome of lung cancer will occur in three ways: prevention; earlier detection; and creative, aggressive strategies for treatment of disease which has spread beyond the lung (stage III–IV). This report focuses on the last, in particular approaches to locally advanced disease (stage IIIB) that utilize a combination of chemotherapy, surgery, and radiotherapy.

II. Stage IIIB Non-Small-Cell Lung Cancer

Stage IIIB non-small-cell lung cancer (NSCLC) is defined as a tumor that invades mediastinal structures such as the trachea, heart, esophagus, and aorta, or causes a malignant pleural effusion. These tumors are designated T4 in the tumor, node, metastasis (TNM) classification system (2). Lung cancers that have spread to contralateral mediastinal nodal groups or either ipsilateral or contralateral supraclavicular nodal groups are considered to have N3 nodal involvement by the TNM system and are also considered to be stage IIIB. Stage IIIB NSCLC is, then, any tumor, without distant metastases, that has N3 nodal involvement (T1–4, N3) or a tumor that is invasive of the mediastinum or has an associated malignant pleural effusion with or without nodal involvement (T4N0–3). In contrast, stage IIIA NSCLC is defined as a tumor invasive of the chest wall, diaphragm, mediastinal pleura, or pericardium, or extending to within 2 cm of the carina (T3). Additionally, a tumor associated with atelectasis or obstructive pneumonitis of the entire lung is considered T3. An NSCLC can also be classified as stage IIIA on the basis of N2 nodal involvement defined as positive ipsilateral mediastinal or subcarinal lymph nodes.

III. Chemotherapy and Radiation Treatment for Stage IIIB Lung Cancer

The prognosis for stage IIIB lung cancer is guarded, with 5-year survival rates ranging from 5% to 10% (2). Traditionally, therapy is palliative rather than curative in intent. External beam radiation therapy is used to ameliorate respiratory symptoms associated with the primary lesion such as hemoptysis, chest pain, cough, or postobstructive pneumonia. Chemotherapy is used either alone or in combination with radiation therapy with the aim of preventing dissemination and/or as a radiosensitizer. Generally, patients with IIIB disease have a reasonable performance status and are therefore good candidates for treatment with protocol agents. Surgery is reserved for diagnosis of locally disseminated disease via mediastinoscopy, thoracotomy, or, more recently, thoracoscopy (minimally invasive technique) (3). Surgery is also employed to treat the complications of locally advanced malignancy. Drainage and sclerosis of the pleural space for a malignant pleural effusion is a standard palliative procedure (4). Occasionally, resectional therapy to palliate pain from local invasion which fails to respond to nonoperative therapy or to palliate unremitting hemoptysis is indicated.

A recent report of a randomized Phase III study from Japan examined concurrent versus sequential thoracic radiotherapy (TRT) in combination with mitomycin (M), vindesine (V), and cisplatin (P) in patients with unresectable stage IIIA and IIIB NSCLC (exclusive of T3N0 and pleural effusion) (5). Patients were all <75 years of age and had ECOG performances statuses of 0 to 2. MVP therapy consisted of P 80 mg/m^2 and M 8 mg/m^2 on days 1 and 29; V 3 mg/m^2 on days 1, 8, 29, and 36. The concurrent group (n = 156) received TRT for 3 weeks beginning on day 2 of MVP, 2 Gy/fraction 14 times (28 Gy), a rest period of 10 days, and then

28 Gy for 3 weeks. The sequential arm (n = 158) of TRT consisted of 56 Gy given after the MVP therapy in a conventional schema. The overall response rate was 84% in the concurrent group (n = 131) versus 66% in the sequential group (n = 105). The median survival in the former group was 16.5 months and 13.3 months in the latter group (*P* = .047). Three-year survival rates were 27% and 13%, respectively. There was one septic death in the concurrent group and two radiation pneumonitis deaths in the sequential group. A breakdown of the number of patients with stage IIIA versus IIIB disease was not given. This report demonstrates that in a mixed collection of stage III patients (IIIA exclusive of T3N0; IIIB exclusive of pleural effusion), a modification of the manner in which therapies are given may modestly improve survival. However, further advances are clearly needed.

Another recent report from the Southwest Oncology Group (SWOG; S9019) (6) examined concurrent cisplatin (P) and etoposide (E) plus radiotherapy (RT) for pathologic stage IIIB NSCLC in a phase II fashion. Patients with biopsy-proven NSCLC of either T4 (noneffusion) or N3 status were given two cycles of PE beginning on day 1 of RT which continued to 61 Gy followed by two more cycles of PE. There were 50 eligible patients including T4N0/1 (18 pts), T4N2 (12 pts) and T(any)N3 (20 pts). There was one treatment-related death. Five patients (10%) progressed during PE and RT. There was a 28% incidence of grade 4 neutropenia, 20% grade 3 or 4 esophagitis, 24% grade 3 or 4 anemia, and 10% grade 3 fatigue. The median survival was 13 months with a 3-year survival of 26%. The 2-year survival of the T4N0/1 subset was 33%, compared with 64% in a trial conducted by SWOG which included surgery (S8805) (7). SWOG 9019 suggests that using an aggressive combination of chemotherapy and radiotherapy that has acceptable morbidity and mortality, a 13-month median survival can be achieved in stage IIIB NSCLC exclusive of patients with pleural effusion. In their own comparison series, Albain and colleagues find surgery is important at least in the T4N0/1 subgroup (7).

Table 1 (8–12) summarizes several Phase III trials that compared radiotherapy with concurrent chemoradiotherapy for treatment of stage III NSCLC. The results are mixed, with some series showing a trend in favor of the addition of chemotherapy. Table 2 (8,13–18) displays a summary of the results of several of the larger Phase III trials which compared radiotherapy with sequential chemoradiotherapy in the treatment of stage III NSCLC. There did appear to be a benefit from chemotherapy in the two largest trials (14,18).

Newer chemotherapeutic agents, and in different combinations, are currently being examined in advanced NSCLC. Innovative treatment plans include the use of novel agents such as antiangiogenesis drugs and metalloproteinase inhibitors. Such regimens are now in Phase I human trials.

Different doses and, perhaps more importantly, different dosing schedules for radiotherapy are being investigated in stage IIIB and IV NSCLC. Hyperfrac-

Table 1 Phase III Trials of Radiotherapy Versus Concurrent Chemoradiotherapy for Stage III NSCLC

Authors	No. Pts.	Chemotherapy	Radiation therapy (Gy)	Group	Survival Median (mo)	1 yr (%)	2 yr (%)
Soresi et al. (9)	95	DDP, 15 mg/m²/wk	50.4	Chemo/RT	16	~70	~40
			50.4	RT	11	~45	~30
Ansari et al. (10)	200	DDP, 100 mg/m²/d 1, 22, 43	60	Chemo/RT	9	35?	15
			60	RT	10	40?	9
Trovo et al. (11)	180	DDP, 6 mg/m²/d	45 (C)	Chemo/RT	9.97	~40	~15
			45 (C)	RT	10.3	~40	~15
Schaake-Koning	110	DDP, 30 mg/m²/wk	55 (S)	Chemo/RT	—	44	19
et al. (12)	107	DDP, 5 mg/m²/d		Chemo/RT	—	54	26
	114			RT	—	46	13

Patients were found at resection to have either residual disease or the highest or farthest node positive for metastatic tumor.
NSCLC, non-small-cell lung cancer; Gy, gray; DDP, cisplatin; Chemo, chemotherapy; RT, radiation therapy; C, continuous-course RT; S, split-course RT.
Source: Ref. 8.

tionated radiation therapy uses twice-a-day regimens (i.e., 120 cGy BID to total dose of 69.6 Gy) (19). Continuous hyperfraction accelerated radiotherapy (CHART) typically involves three-times-a-day dosing using 140 to 150 cGy fractions to a dose of 50.4 to 54 Gy (20). Both of these techniques, particularly when combined with chemotherapy, show promise for improving survival (21).

IV. Surgical Treatment of Stage IIIB Non-Small-Cell Lung Cancer

Surgical therapy for cancer is based on the ability to remove all disease so that microscopic margins of resection are negative for tumor. The treatment of stage IIIB lung cancer has been considered nonsurgical because of the inability of surgery alone to meet this requirement and the poor results associated with surgical approaches to stage IIIB disease. Newer strategies for these difficult tumors involve either sequential or concurrent chemotherapy and radiation therapy to locally shrink tumors while also preventing systemic dissemination. Improved chemotherapeutic agents and a better understanding of the delivery of radiation therapy in combination with better supportive care have allowed more intensive neoadjuvant treatment. More aggressive surgical approaches in this setting have permitted complete resection of disease. Long-term results of such strategies are pending.

Table 2 Larger Phase III Trials of Radiotherapy Versus Sequential Chemoradiotherapy for Stage III NSCLC

Authors	No. Pts.	Chemo- therapy	Radiation therapy (Gy)	Survival Median (mo)	1 yr (%)	2 yr (%)
van Houtte et al. (13)	59	DDP/VP 16	55 (C)	11	—	—
		None		11	—	—
Dillman et al. (14,15)	180	DDF/VBL	60 (C)	13.8	55	26
		None		9.7	40	13
Mattson et al. (16)	119	CAP	55 (S)	11.0	42	19
	119	None		10.4	41	17
Morton et al. (17)	55	MACC	60 (C)	10.5	47	23
	54	None		9.7	43	12
Le Chevalier et al. (18)	353	VCPC	65 (C)	—	51	21
	None			—	41	14

NSCLC, non-small-cell lung cancer; DDP, cisplatin; VP 16, etoposide; C, continuous-course radiation therapy; VBL, vinblastine; CAP, cyclophosphamide, doxorubicin, cisplatin; S, split-course RT; MACC, methotrexate, doxorubicin, cyclophosphamide, lomustine; VCPC, vindesine, lomustine, cisplatin, cyclophosphamide.
Source: Ref. 8.

Results with surgery alone for stage IIIB NSCLC, as mentioned above, have traditionally been poor. Naruke (22) reported a 5.6% 5-year survival rate for pathologically staged IIIB NSCLC following surgical resection ($n = 159$). Broken down into subgroups, there were 55 patients with T1–3N3 disease with a 5-year survival of 0% and 104 patients with T4, any N with a survival of 8.2%. Naruke did not note a significant difference between the outcomes following surgery for patients with stage IIIB versus stage IV (7.5%; $n = 228$). This large experience underscores the problems with our current staging system. Locally advanced tumors (T4) can be completely resected in certain instances with aggressive surgical techniques. In these cases, the patient's prognosis is dependent, as with other stages of lung cancer, on the nodal status. Tumors with disseminated nodal disease involving the contralateral mediastinum or supraclavicular regions or malignant pleural effusion cannot be completely resected, and therefore patients with these tumors do not do well with primary surgical therapy.

More recently, investigators have carried out surgical resection for IIIB cancer following induction therapy in an analogous treatment strategy to that invoked in IIIA disease (23). Albain and colleagues reported the results of SWOG trial 8805 (7) in which preoperative concurrent chemotherapy (cisplatin and etoposide × two cycles) and radiation therapy (45 Gy) was followed by surgical resection in 126 patients. Seventy-five patients had biopsy-proven IIIA disease, and 51 patients had IIIB disease. These investigators reported a 3-year survival of 27% and 24% in the IIIA and IIIB groups, respectively. In a similar subgroup analysis to that reported by Naruke, Albain and her team found that the patients with T4N0-1 disease ($n = 17$) had a median survival of 28 months, whereas the patients with N3 disease ($n = 9$) were all dead within 2 years.

NSCLC associated with a malignant pleural effusion (MPE) is also defined as stage IIIB. In general, patients with MPE are excluded from aggressive chemoradiotherapy and/or surgical protocols because of their poor prognosis. A recent study looked at the effect of pleural effusion on patient prognosis in NSCLC and found that there was no difference in patient survival for stage IV and stage IIIB associated with a pleural effusion. The median survival was 5.5 months and 7.5 months, respectively (24). Stage IIIB patients, exclusive of pleural effusion, had a significantly better outlook with a median survival of 15.3 months (21).

Standard palliative surgical therapy for patients with a malignant pleural effusion employs chest tube drainage with chemical sclerosis using a number of different agents, the most common being talc. Success rates for improving shortness of breath and the prevention of fluid reaccumulation are as high as 90% (4). A Cancer and Leukemia Group B (CALGB 9334) multi-institutional study on treatment of pleural effusion is near completion. Its objective is to determine whether operative, thoracoscopic drainage of malignant pleural effusions with talc insufflation is better than current standard therapy using chest tube drainage and talc slurry at the bedside with respect to success rate, quality of life, and survival.

In contradistinction to this, several small surgical series on stage IIIB NSCLC defined by MPE have reported the results of treatment strategies that have a more curative intent. Akaogi and colleagues reported their results with pleuropulmonary resection for 23 patients with pleurally disseminated NSCLC but without distant metastases (25). Sixteen patients had a pleuropneumonectomy with mediastinal lymph node dissection, and seven patients had a partial pleuropulmonary resection with lymph node sampling. The more limited procedure was selected for elderly patients or for patients with evident mediastinal involvement by lymphogenous or direct tumor spread. All patients received intrathoracic mitomycin C (10 to 20 mg) at the time of thoracotomy closure. Three patients received postoperative radiotherapy, and four patients received postoperative intravenous chemotherapy. Seventeen patients had N2 disease on pathological evaluation of the operative specimens. Operative mortality was 8%. Median survival was 24 months for the patients who had the extended resection and no evidence of N2 disease ($n = 6$). If there were N2 nodes involved, the median survival was 13.4 months, similar to the survival of patients who had a limited resection. They found that relapse after the pleuropneumonectomy tended to be in distant sites.

A group from Roswell Park Cancer Institute reported results with pleuropneumonectomy before or after chemotherapy in 10 patients with stage IIIB NSCLC based on malignant pleural effusion without other evidence of metastatic disease (26). During that time, 10 similar patients were treated with chemotherapy with or without pleural drainage and sclerosis. The median survival in this group was 12 months, with the longest survivor living 21 months. The median survival in the group who had a pleuropneumonectomy following chemotherapy was 24 months. The operative mortality was 10% (1/10). The three patients who had an operation prior to recommended adjuvant therapy survived for 23 months (refused chemotherapy), 20 months, and 59 months (received chemotherapy).

In another report, a group from Sakai, Japan, used a novel approach combining surgical resection and intrapleural chemotherapy with radiofrequency hyperthermia in patients with lung cancer that had disseminated within the pleural space (27). Kodama and his colleagues carried out pulmonary resection in 31 patients; 17 had N2 disease. Cisplatin (50 to 100 mg) was administered via the chest tube 10 to 14 days after surgery, and radiofrequency hyperthermia was applied through the chest wall for 60 min. This was repeated every 5 to 7 days for three courses. These investigators reported no major complications and overall 3- and 5-year survival rates of 44% and 25%, respectively. Only five patients were reported to have a local recurrence. The median survival for patients with and without mediastinal lymph node metastases were 43 months and 16 months, respectively. The 5-year cumulative survival rates were 68% for those without N2 involvement and 23% for those with N2 involvement.

Aggressive surgical resection combined with innovative chemoradiotherapeutic strategies would appear to be beneficial in selected patients with locally advanced NSCLC (IIIB) heretofore thought to be unresectable. The Thoracic Oncology Program at the Brigham and Women's Hospital and Dana-Farber Cancer Institute has employed a protocol for treating patients with IIIB NSCLC on the basis of malignant pleural involvement (28). Evidence of systemic involvement is excluded radiographically, and mediastinal node involvement (N2 and N3) is excluded via surgical biopsy. Patients with adequate cardiopulmonary reserve undergo three cycles of carboplatinum and paclitaxel followed by radiographic restaging. The patients without evidence of disease progression then undergo an extrapleural pneumonectomy and node dissection to remove all gross tumor. Following an adequate period of convalescence (4 to 6 weeks), adjuvant radiation therapy is given to the ipsilateral chest to 40 Gy in cases of a complete resection (negative margin and nodes) and an incomplete resection (positive margin or nodes) to a total dose to the cone down region of 54 Gy. The early experience would suggest this is a safe and feasible treatment plan with encouraging survival data (28).

V. Conclusion

In summary, treatment for stage IIIB NSCLC traditionally utilizes chemotherapy and/or radiotherapy and has a palliative intent. Median survival is typically 9 to 12 months (8). Recently, more curative approaches are being considered in select cases because of the increased number of chemotherapeutic agents available, the ability to support patients with growth factors and other means during more intensive combination regimens, and the use of different methods/schedules of radiation therapy. The main determinant of patient survival continues to remain the nodal burden associated with the tumor. In select centers, aggressive surgical resection following induction regimens for stage IIIB NSCLC, particularly T4 lesions, permits complete removal of gross disease. Depending on the node status, a subgroup of these patients may enjoy a prolonged survival. Long-term results from such strategies have demonstrated reasonable survival in selected individuals (25,26,28). Certainly, randomized, prospective, multi-institutional studies will need to be performed to validate these data.

References

1. Parker SL, Tong T, Bolden S, Wingo PA. Cancer Statistics 1997. CA Cancer J Clin 1997; 47:5–27.
2. Mountain CF. Revisions in the international system for staging lung cancer. Chest 1997; 111:1710–1717.
3. DeCamp MM Jr, Jaklitsch MT, Mentzer SJ, Harpole DH Jr, Sugarbaker DJ. Safety and versatility of video thoracoscopy: a prospective analysis of 895 consecutive cases. J Am Coll Surg 1995; 181:113–120.
4. Reshad K, Inui K, Takeuchi Y, Takahashi Y, Hitomi S. Treatment of malignant peural effusion. Chest 1985; 88:393–397.
5. Furuse K, Fukuoka M, Takada Y, et al. A randomized phase III study of concurrent versus sequential thoracic radiotherapy (TRT) in combination with mitomycin (M), vindesine (V), and cisplatin (P) in unresectable stage III non-small-cell lung cancer (NSCLC): preliminary analysis (abstr). Proc Am Soc Clin Oncol 1997; 16:459a.
6. Albain KS, Crowley JJ, Turrisi AT III, et al. Concurrent cisplatin/etoposide plus radiotherapy (PE+RT) for pathologic stage (path TN) IIIb non-small-cell lung cancer (NSCLC): a Southwest Oncology Group (SWOG) Phase II study (S9019) (abstr). Proc Am Soc Clin Oncol 1997; 16:446a.
7. Albain KS, Rusch VW, Crowley JJ, et al. Concurrent cisplatin/etoposide plus chest radiotherapy followed by surgery for stages IIIA (N2) and IIIB non-small-cell lung cancer: mature results of Southwest Oncology Group phase II study 8805. J Clin Oncol 1995; 13:1880–1892.
8. Wagner H Jr, Ruckdeschel JC. Treatment of locally advanced and metastatic non-small-cell lung cancer. Adv Oncol 1993; 9:22–29.
9. Soresi E, Clerici M, Grilli R, et al. A randomized clinical trial comparing radiation therapy versus radiation therapy plus cis-dichlorodiammine platinum (II) in the treamtment of locally advanced non-small-cell lung cancer. Semin Oncol 1988; 15(suppl):20–25.
10. Ansari R, Tokars R, Fisher W, et al. A Phase III study of thoracic irradiation with or without concomitant cisplatin in locoregional unresectable non-small-cell lung cancer: a Hoosier Oncology Group protocol (abstr). Proc Am Soc Oncol 1991; 10:241.

11. Trovo M, Zanelli G, Minatei E, et al. Radiotherapy versus radiotherapy enhanced by cisplatin in stage III non-small-cell lung cancer. Int J Radiat Oncol Biol Phys 1992; 24:573–574.

12. Schaake-Koning C, Van Den Bogert W, Dalesio O, et al. Effects of concomitant cisplatin and radiotherapy in inoperable non-small-call lung cancer. N Engl J Med 1992; 326:524–530.

13. van Houtte P, Klastersky J, Renaud A, et al. Induction chemotherapy with cisplatin, etoposide, and vindesine before radiation therapy for non-small-cell lung cancer. Antibiot Chemother 1988; 41:131–137.

14. Dillman RO, Seagren SL, Herndon J, et al. Randomized trial of induction chemotherapy plus radiation therapy vs RT alone in stage III non-small-cell lung cancer: five-year follow up of CALGB (abstr). Proc Am Soc Clin Oncol 1993; 12:329.

15. Dillman RO, Seagren SL, Propert KJ, et al. A randomized trial of induction chemotherapy plus high-dose radiation versus radiation alone in stage III non-small-cell lung cancer. N Engl J Med 1990; 323:940–945.

16. Mattson K, Holsti L, Holsti P, et al. Inoperable non-small-cell lung cancer: radiation with or without chemotherapy. Eur J Cancer Clin Oncol 1988; 24:477–482.

17. Morton R, Jett J, Maher L, et al. Randomized trial of thoracic radiation therapy with or without chemotherapy for treatment of locally unresectable non-small-cell lung cancer (abstr). Proc Am Soc Clin Oncol 1988; 7:200.

18. Le Chevalier T, Arriagada R, Tarayre M, et al. Significant effect of adjuvant chemotherapy on survival in locally advanced non-small-cell lung cancinoma. J Natl Cancer Inst 1992; 84:58.

19. Sause WT, Scott C, Taylor S, et al. Radiation Therapy Oncology Group (RTOG) 88-08 and Eastern Cooperative Oncology Group (ECOG) 4588. Preliminary results of a Phase III trial in regionally advanced, unresectable non-small-cell lung cancer. J Natl Cancer Inst 1995; 87:198–205.

20. Saunders MI, Dische S. Continuous, hyperfractionated, accelerated radiotherapy (CHART) in non-small-cell carcinoma of the bronchus. Int J Radiat Oncol Biol Phys 1990; 19:1211–1215.

21. Shaw EG, McGinnis WL, Jett Jr, et al. Pilot study of accelerated hyperfractionated thoracic radiation therapy plus concomitant etoposide and cisplatin chemotherapy in patients with unresectable stage III non-small-cell carcinoma of the lung. J Natl Cancer Inst 1993; 85:321–323.

22. Naruke T, Goya T, Tsuchiya R, Suemasu K. Prognosis and survival in resected lung carcinoma based on the new international staging system. J Thorac Cardiovasc Surg 1988; 96:440–447.

23. Sugarbaker DJ, Herndon J, Kohman LJ, et al. Results of Cancer and Leukemia Group B protocol 8935 A multiinstitutional phase II trimodality trial for stage IIIA (N2) non-small-cell lung cancer. J Thorac Cardiovasc Surg 1995; 109:473–85.

24. Sugiura S, Ando Y, Minami H, Ando M, Sakai S, Shimokata K. Prognostic value of pleural effusion in patients with non-small-cell lung cancer. Clin Cancer Res 1997; 3:47–50.

25. Akaogi E, Mitsui K, Onizuka M, Ishikawa S, Tsukada H, Mitsui T. Pleural dissemnation in non-small-cell lung cancer: results of radiological evaluation and surgical treatment. J Surg Oncol 1994; 57:33–39.

26. Reyes L, Parvez Z, Regal A, Takita H. Neoadjuvant chemotherapy and operations in the treatment of lung cancer with pleural effusion. J Thorac Cardiovasc Surg 1991; 101:946–947.

27. Kodama K, Doi O, Higashiyama M, Yokouchi H, Tatsuta M. Long-term results of postoperative intrathoracic chemo-thermotherapy for lung cancer with pleural dissemination. Cancer 1993; 72:2.

28. Swanson SJ, Jaklitsch MT, Mentzer SJ, et al. Induction chemotherapy, surgical resection and radiation in patients with malignant pleural effusion, mediastinoscopy negative (stage IIIB) non-small-cell lung cancer (abstr). Presented at the 78th Annual Meeting of the American Association for Thoracic Surgeons, Boston, May 3–6, 1998.

12

Chemotherapy of Advanced Non-Small-Cell Lung Cancer

NAM H. DANG and ROY S. HERBST*

Dana-Farber Cancer Institute
Boston, Massachusetts

ARTHUR T. SKARIN

Harvard Medical School
Dana-Farber Cancer Institute
Brigham and Women's Hospital
Boston, Massachusetts

I. Introduction

The most lethal cancer in both men and women, lung cancer accounts for 28% of all cancer deaths, representing more than 160,000 deaths annually in the United States (Parker et al., 1997). This total is more than the combined deaths from breast, colon, and prostate cancer. In addition, it is estimated that more than 178,000 new cases of lung cancer are expected in 1997 and, to make the situation even worse, the overall cure rate for patients developing lung cancer is only approximately 13%. Most of the deaths are secondary to metastatic spread of the disease.

Lung cancer is staged according to a four-stage system described by Mountain in 1986, which was recently updated with minor revisions. By that classification, the majority of lung cancer patients present with inoperable stage III disease or with metastases to distant organs (stage IV; Mountain et al., 1986, 1987). Patients with stage IIIB or IV disease cannot be cured with current chemotherapeutic approaches, and hence all measures are aimed at prolongation of life and

---

**Present affiliation*: The University of Texas, M.D. Anderson Cancer Center, Houston, Texas.

palliation as well as improving quality of life. However, a small number of patients (20% to 40%) with advanced regional disease (stage IIIA) may be cured by combined modality approaches, including neoadjuvant or induction chemotherapy (Rosell et al., 1994; Roth et al., 1994; Skarin et al., 1989). Indeed, this number appears to be increasing with some of the more modern chemotherapy regimens initially developed in the advanced disease setting.

In this chapter, we will review major studies published over the past 20+ years in an attempt to identify established systemic cytotoxic therapies that can lead to prolonged survival and/or provide palliation in patients with advanced non-small-cell lung cancer (NSCLC), both as single agents and as combination regimens. We will also explore the newer drugs and combinations now actively under study for the treatment of this very malignant disease.

II.   Pretreatment Prognostic Factors in NSCLC Patients

No review of the chemotherapy of NSCLC would be complete without a discussion of pretreatment prognostic factors since several have reproducibly been shown in numerous studies to significantly influence patient outcomes. In a review of VA lung study group trials in the early 1970s, Zelen first demonstrated that the extent of disease (defined at that time as limited vs. extensive) and the patient's Karnofsky performance status were the most important indicators of survival (Zelen, 1973). Since then, numerous investigators have examined the importance of various factors associated with prognosis in NSCLC. Stanley evaluated 77 prognostic factors in >5000 patients with advanced NSCLC (Stanley, 1980). In this study the most important factors affecting survival were the initial Karnofsky performance status followed closely by the extent of disease involvement and the presence of weight loss. Meanwhile, in reviewing data collected from 378 patients with advanced NSCLC receiving a high-dose cisplatin-vinca alkaloid regimen (using a cisplatin dose of 120 mg/m^2), O'Connell et al. identified as important adverse prognostic factors: a Karnofsky performance status of <70%; the presence of bony metastases; metastases to two or more extrathoracic sites; an elevated serum LDH; or male sex (O'connell et al., 1986). Feld et al. issued a consensus report in 1991 which identified Karnofsky performance status, the extent or stage of disease, and the presence of weight loss as important prognostic factors (Feld et al., 1991).

The representative results from one such analysis are shown in Table 1. In this study published by Finkelstein et al. (1986), the authors reviewed 893 good performance status patients treated between 1979 and 1983 on ECOG trials, all having metastatic NSCLC and being treated with one of seven phase III combinations. The overall median survival of this patient group was 23.5 weeks with no significant differences seen among treatment groups. The etoposide-cisplatin combination had the highest proportion of 1-year survivors (25%); the mitomycin-vinblastine-cisplatin (MVP) combination had significantly fewer 1-year survivors

Table 1 Significance of Prognostic Factors by Category in 893 Patients in ECOG Randomized Trials from 1979 to 1983[a]

Characteristic, site, or symptom	Proportion who survived >1 year (%)	*P* value
Performance status		
0	64/177 (36%)	<.0001
1	89/544 (16%)	
2	15/172 (9)	
Sex		
Male	67/255 (26%)	.0005
Female	101/638 (16%)	
Prior weight loss		
None	103/391 (26%)	.001
<5%	23/200 (12%)	
5–10%	24/169 (14%)	
>10%	14/122 (11%)	
Histology		
Squamous	63/322 (20%)	.011
Adenocarcinoma	80/383 (21%)	
Large cell	30/172 (12%)	
Other	5/16 (31%)	
Liver metastases		
Yes	17/157 (11%)	.046
No	151/736 (21%)	
Bone metastases		
Yes	36/358 (10%)	<.0001
No	132/535 (25%)	
Subcutaneous metastases		
Yes	8/105 (8%)	.006
No	160/788 (20%)	
Shoulder, arm pain		
Yes	14/142 (10%)	.029
No	154/751 (21%)	

[a]Only those factors that reached statistical significance are shown.
Source: Finkelstein et al., 1986.

(12%) than any other regimen (*P* = .003), despite having the highest response rate (a fact seen repeatedly in the ECOG experience, presumably secondary to the increased toxicity of the MVP regimen). Analysis of pretreatment characteristics distinguishing patients who survived >1 year from those who did not, indicated that an initial performance status of 0; the absence of bone, liver, and subcutaneous metastases; non-large-cell histology; <5% weight loss, female sex, and lack of shoulder or arm pain symptoms all favored a better prognosis (Table 1) (Finklestein et al., 1986).

Each patient with metastatic NSCLC therefore needs a thorough assessment tailored to the specific individual before initiation of therapy. An objective determination of the extent of disease and performance status must be done, and the presence of comorbid diseases which may complicate treatment and its side effects must be considered. The physician must also be able to anticipate crises that may occur during treatment, e.g., brain metastases, obstructive pneumonia, spinal cord involvement, and impending fractures of weight-bearing bones. In addition to having predictive value for survival and probably for response to chemotherapy, performance status also appears to have important implications for treatment-related toxicity.

III. Single Agents Active in NSCLC

Given the alarming prevalence and grim prognosis of advanced NSCLC, a large number of cytotoxic agents have been investigated as potential treatments for the disease, most often in the setting of stage IV metastatic disease. The activity of these agents has been reported historically in terms of response rates. Out of more than 50+ agents tested until the last decade, only five were found to elicit objective response rates in NSCLC of >15%. These agents include cisplatin, ifosfamide, mitomycin C, vindesine, and vinblastine. Additionally, some series include etoposide on this list. Although its initial response rate was 11% overall, it has been reported to be as high as 21% in some studies (Babowski and Creech, 1983). In the meantime, carboplatin is included at times with a 9% response rate in the ECOG series and a response rate of 16% in the CALGB experience (Bonomi et al., 1989; Green et al., 1992). While the evidence for activity of these agents in NSCLC is presented in Table 2, comparisons of different drugs are difficult given the variability of studies, the disparate treatment plans, and the wide range of drug dosage, with many of these results being reported as parts of Phase I/II trials.

Although the drugs mentioned above have been shown to have modest single-agent activity in NSCLC over the past 20 years, the overall median survival of patients with advanced NSCLC treated with single-agent therapy remains disappointing, averaging about 16 to 18 weeks, with 1-year survival rates of approximately 10%.

A. Cisplatin

Among the most widely used agents for the treatment of NSCLC, cisplatin has demonstrated a response rate of about 20% in most trials in previously untreated patients (Bunn, 1986). In addition, studies have focused on the importance of cisplatin dose intensity in metastatic NSCLC, with several Phase II studies suggesting a possible increase in the efficacy of such drug dosage. Gralla et al. (1981)

Table 2 Single Agents with Significant Activity in NSCLC

Drug	Response rate	References[a]
Cisplatin	15–20%	Bunn, 1986
Carboplatin	9–20%	Bonomi, 1991; Bonomi et al., 1989
Ifosfamide	20%	Ettinger, 1989; Johnson, 1990
Etoposide	5–15%	Ruckdeschel, 1991
Mitomycin-C	20%	Kris et al., 1985, 1990
Vindesine	16–25%	Sorensen et al., 1987a
Vinblastine	16–25%	Sorensen et al., 1987a

[a]Selected references illustrating the single-agent activity of these cytotoxic agents with documented activity in NSCLC.

conducted a small randomized trial consisting of 85 patients in which a fixed dose of vindesine was given along with cisplatin at a dose of 60 mg/m^2 (low dose) or 120 mg/m^2 (high dose). Although the response rates were equivalent (at approximately 43%), median duration of response was prolonged in the high-dose group (12 vs. 5.5 months; $P = .05$), with responding patients living 21.7 months versus 10 months on the low-dose arm ($P = .02$). Myelosuppression was generally not a treatment problem; peripheral neuropathy and moderate azotemia were the major dose-limiting toxicities. Based on this trial, increased doses of cisplatin became the standard for the treatment of advanced NSCLC. Alternatively, the Southwest Oncology Group (SWOG) conducted a Phase II trial (Gandara et al., 1989, 1993) which evaluated response rate for cisplatin given at 100 mg/m^2 on days 1 and 8 every 4 weeks. This dose-intensive regimen was compared with single-agent cisplatin given in standard doses (50 mg/m^2 on days 1 and 8) for the treatment of metastatic NSCLC. There was no significant difference seen in the relative response rates (12% to 14%), with survival rates being virtually identical. However, there was an increased incidence of myelosuppression, increased ototoxicity, and greater nausea and vomiting in the higher-dose regimens. Finally, the EORTC compared low- versus high-dose cisplatin in combination with etoposide, finding no difference in the relative rates of response or survival (Klastersky, 1986). As expected, toxicity was increased in the high-dose cisplatin arm. Taken overall, these studies do not conclusively support the notion of a steep dose-response relationship for cisplatin in advanced NSCLC.

B. Carboplatin

Numerous clinical trials evaluating carboplatin as a single agent or as a component of combination regimens have been performed, and the response rates for carboplatin were shown to vary from 9% to 20% in trials testing carboplatin at a dose of 400 mg/m^2 as a single daily dose or given over 3 days (Table 2) (Bonomi, 1991;

Bonomi et al., 1989; Kreisman et al., 1987). In one of these ECOG trials (ECOG, trial 1583), carboplatin was associated with a modest but significant survival benefit when compared to five other regimens, despite having only a 9% objective response rate (Table 3) ; Bonomi et al., 1989). At the time of the study mentioned above, cisplatin in combination with etoposide was one of the most commonly used regimens of the day, with response rates of 23% to 30% and median survival values on the order of 25 weeks. Based on that experience, a randomized trial was conducted to compare the efficacy of carboplatin and etoposide to cisplatin and etoposide. There were no significant differences observed in response rates or survival duration, but there was a trend for less toxicity with the carboplatin and

Table 3 Results of Selected Randomized Trials by ECOG and SWOG During the 1980s Comparing Drug Combinations in NSCLC

Trial	Regmen randomized	No. pts.	RR %	Median survival
ECOG 2575	AFP	109	17	21.6 wk
Ruckdeschel et al., 1985	CAP	107	23 (1 CR)	23.5 wk
	CBP	112	20 (4 CR)	22.1 wk
	MVP	104	26 (5 CR)	23.7 wk
SWOG	FOMi	147	26	20 wk
Miller et al., 1986	CAP	156	17	24 wk
	FOMi/CAP	149	22	23 wk
ECOG 1581	CAMP	115	17	25.1 wk
Ruckdeschel et al., 1986	MVP	121	31	22.0 wk
	CDDP/VP16	126	20	26.0 wk
	CDDP/Vind	124	25	26.6 wk
ECOG 1583	MVP	176	20	22.7 wk
Bonomi et al., 1989	VP	175	13	25.1
	MVP/CAMP	172	13	25.0 wk
	Carbo-MVP	88	9	31.7 wk
	Ibpro-MVP	88	6	26.1 wk
SWOG	CDDP/VP16	135	16	5.3 mo
Weick et al., 1991	PVpM	136	33	4.8 mo
	CDDP/Ve	142	24	5.9 mo
	PVeMi	134	17	5.0 mo
	FOMi/CAP	133	10	5.0 mo

AFP: doxorubicin, 5-FU, cisplatin; CAP: cyclophosphamide, doxorubicin, cisplatin; CBP: cyclophosphamide, bleomycin, cisplatin; MVP: mitomycin C, vinblastine, cisplatin; FOMi: 5-FU, vincristine, mitomycin-C; CAMP: cyclophosphamide, doxorubicin, methotrexate, procarbazine; CDDP/VP16: etoposide, cisplatin; CDDP/Ve: cisplatin, vinblastine; PVeMi: cisplatin, vinblastine, mitomycin-C (alt with cisplatin, vinblastine); PVpM: cisplatin, VP16, methylglyoxal bisguanyl-hydrazone.

etoposide regimen (Klastersky et al., 1990). Other investigators have evaluated carboplatin in two drug combination therapy with vinblastine, cisplatin, or etoposide in Phase II trials. Response rates have ranged from 9% to 17%, suggesting that these combinations were not significantly more effective than carboplatin alone (Bunn, 1994; Bonomi et al., 1989).

Kreisman et al. (1987) have reviewed the CALGB experience with carboplatin by examining the effect of both carboplatin and iproplatin on advanced NSCLC. Carboplatin was found to produce a 16% response rate; however, the median survival in the carboplatin-treated patients was only 26 weeks. The Lung Cancer Working Party in Belgium conducted a randomized trial involving 162 evaluable patients with advanced NSCLC in which cisplatin (120 mg/m^2) combined with etoposide (100 mg/m^2 for 3 days) was compared to carboplatin (325 mg/m^2) combined with the same etoposide dose. Each regimen was repeated every 4 weeks. No significant differences in response rate or survival were detected, with the cisplatin regimen producing producing a 25% response rate as compared to a 20% response rate for the carboplatin regimen. The cisplatin and carboplatin regimens were associated with median survival durations of 25 and 24 weeks, respectively. Less toxicity occurred with the carboplatin regimen as there were greater degrees of granulocytopenia ($P = .005$) and a higher frequency of diarrhea ($P = .04$) in patients receiving the cisplatin treatment (Klastersky et al., 1990).

As a result of clinical pharmacokinetics studies of carboplatin, a formula for quantifying exposure to carboplatin based on renal function and dose has been proposed: area under the drug concentration $\times$ time curve (AUC) = dose/(creatinine clearance + 25). While it has been suggested that the range of AUC (carboplatin) from 5 to 7 mg/mL $\times$ minute is optimal, the individualization of carboplatin dose based on the predicted AUC should lead to safer therapy with a maximum possibility of response (Chabner and Longo, 1996).

C. Vinca Alkaloids

Among the vinca alkaloids, vinblastine and vindesine are considered active in NSCLC, with single-agent response rates ranging from 11% to 28% in most published studies (Table 2) (Sorensen et al., 1987a). Its main toxicities are neurologic and myelosuppressive in nature. While both agents have been extensively used in combination with other established agents, vinorelbine, a new vinca alkaloid, has emerged recently to be the most active (and potentially less toxic) agent in this disease and will be discussed below.

D. Ifosfamide

Another drug with single-agent activity in advanced NSCLC is ifosfamide (Table 2), with doses usually ranging from 4 to 10 g/m^2 given in 1 day or over 5 days

(Johnson, 1990). Single-agent response rates have been approximately 20% to 25%, with median survival about 9 months. Hemorrhagic cystitis is the dose-limiting toxicity of ifosfamide in the absence of mesna uroprotection. Neurotoxicity can also occur and is thought to be due to the accumulation of chloractaldehyde, a metabolite of ifosfamide that resembles chloral hydrate.

E. Etoposide

A semisynthetic derivative of podophyllotoxin whose cytotoxic effects result from the inhibition of the nuclear enzyme topoisomerase II with formation of DNA strand breaks, etoposide has a single-agent activity of about 10% in NSCLC (Babowki and Creech, 1983; Rosso et al., 1990; Ruckdeschel, 1991). Pharmacokinetic principles have guided the use of etoposide as daily oral doses in a prolonged maintenance setting, with one study revealing a response rate of 23% in 25 patients treated with a daily dose of 50 mg/m^2 for 21 days (Waits et al., 1992). However, a similar study enrolling 43 patients only demonstrated a 4% response rate (Saxman et al., 1991).

F. Mitomycin C

Utilized in NSCLC since the late 1970s, mitomycin C, administered as a single agent in doses ranging from 10 to 20 mg/m^2 every 3 to 6 weeks, has resulted in a median response rate of around 25% in 207 evaluable patients (Spain, 1993). Meanwhile, Veeder et al. conducted a randomized trial of mitomycin C versus a combination of mitomycin C, vinblastine, and cisplatin (Veeder et al., 1992). Results showed a single-agent mitomycin C response rate of 30% in patients with stage IV squamous cell tumors. Despite its relative activity in advanced NSCLC, mitomycin C results in cumulative myelotoxicity. Furthermore, rare cases of microangiopathic anemia as well as interstitial lung disease have been reported, and these features have limited its clinical utility.

IV. Development of Combination Regimens

The early history of lung cancer therapy is recorded in scores of trials employing combinations of single agents with minimal activity (i.e., adriamycin, methotrexate, procarbazine) and early studies employing combinations of these agents, which demonstrated no significant benefit as compared to treatments with these agents alone (Davis et al., 1981; Sorensen et al., 1987b). For example, Sorensen et al. conducted a randomized study of vindesine versus lomustine, cyclophosphamide, and methotrexate versus vindesine, lomustine, cyclophosphamide, and methotrexate (Sorenson et al., 1987b). Response rates (22%, 23%, and 27%) were similar, as were median durations of response (15 weeks) and survival (29 weeks).

Studies carried out in the 1970s and early 1980s, including some randomized trials, generally failed to demonstrate significant benefit for combination regimens, due primarily to the low single-agent response rates of the agents used.

In the pre-cisplatin era there were few trials with any significant evidence of measurable efficacy. Response rates of >40%, albeit in a Phase II trial, were, however, observed for two regimens: CAMP (cyclophosphamide, doxorubicin, methotrexate, and procarbazine), and MACC (methotrexate, doxorubicin, cyclophosphamide, and lomustine) (Bitran et al., 1976; Chahinian et al., 1979). In the MACC study, 41 patients with advanced bronchogenic carcinoma had an objective response rate of 46% and a median survival of 9 months. In the CAMP study, 23 patients with metastatic non–oat cell carcinoma who were treated with the chemotherapeutic combination after radiation therapy had an objective response rate of 48%.

A. CAP Chemotherapy/Emergence of Cisplatin

The availability of cisplatin opened new doors in the chemotherapeutic armamentarium for lung cancer as well as a host of other malignancies. Although the full single-agent response for cisplatin had not been clearly delineated (see above), numerous investigators proceeded with Phase II trials to examine its utility in combination regimens. One of the first combination regimens designed was CAP, which consisted of cisplatin at the dose of 40 mg/m^2, cyclophosphamide at 400 mg/m^2, and adriamycin at 40 mg/m^2 (Eagan et al., 1977). This regimen resulted in a 39% response rate in 41 previously untreated patients and a 36% response rate in 28 previously treated patients with advanced NSCLC. A subsequent study done by the same Mayo Clinic group increased cisplatin to 60 mg/m^2 and showed even better results, with a response rate of 48% (Brittell et al., 1978). Hence there does appear to be a lower limit of efficacy for this drug. These impressive results should, however, be tempered by the fact that response rates in the earlier trials were defined differently than in later studies (often less than the 50% decrease in cross-sectional area that we expect today). In addition, multiple patient selection parameters affect the response rate, varying from performance status to number and sites of metastatic disease (see above).

Based on the above results, multiple combinations involving cisplatin were employed in subsequent trials. These regimens have consistently yielded objective tumor response in 20% to 50% of patients with advanced NSCLC, with median survival durations ranging between 20 and 30 weeks in most randomized trials. Although several more promising regimens were developed, e.g., ICE and MVP (to be discussed below), no one regimen has consistently proven to be superior to others in randomized controlled trials.

Following the initial encouraging experience involving cisplatin, virtually every subsequent combination regimen that has shown promising results in Phase

II trials has contained cisplatin as a major component. The fact that cisplatin has a role as one of the most effective agents in the treatment of advanced NSCLC was proven further by a recent SWOG study (Albain et al., 1991), which reviewed 2531 lung cancer patients treated in a series of SWOG protocols. This retrospective study indicated that patients treated with cisplatin-containing regimens have a modest but significant increase in survival compared with patients who do not receive cisplatin-based chemotherapy. Multivariate analysis suggested that treatment with cisplatin is indeed associated with improved survival.

With their respective single-agent activity as described earlier, regimens of cisplatin in combination with a vinca alkaloid or an epipodophyllotoxin have been most commonly employed in the treatment of advanced NSCLC. It is interesting to note that the effects of combination chemotherapy differ only minimally in patients with squamous cell cancer, large-cell cancer, or adenocarcinoma.

B. Cisplatin + Etoposide

An early trial using the combination of cisplatin and etoposide to treat 94 patients with measurable or evaluable bronchogenic squamous cell carcinoma or adenocarcinoma reported an overall response rate of 38% with four complete remissions (CR). Additionally, in the 34 patients who did not receive any prior chemotherapy, the response rate was 56% (19/34) with three CR ($P = .02$). The overall median duration of response was 36.7 weeks, and responding patients survived significantly longer than nonresponders, with median survival being 60 weeks versus 23 weeks, respectively (Longeval and Klastersky, 1982).

A Phase I study was done to investigate ICE (ifosfamide, cisplatin, and etoposide) chemotherapy in patients with NSCLC (Shepherd et al., 1992; Shepherd, 1994). Twenty previously untreated patients with NSCLC were treated with ifofamide 4 mg/m^2 with mesna uroprotection on day 1 and cisplatin 25 mg/m$_2$ and etoposide 100 mg/m^2 on days 1 to 3 every 28 days. One patient did achieve a CR and seven patients achieved a PR, for an overall RR of 44%. As discussed above, carboplatin has been substituted in this combination with similar results and perhaps even less toxicity.

C. Cisplatin/VP16 Versus Cisplatin/Vindesine

At the beginning of the 1980s, multiple agents were found to achieve a 15% to 25% response rate in advanced NSCLC, including cisplatin, etoposide, and vindesine, and efforts were aimed at developing combination regimens containing these drugs to increase efficacy while decreasing toxicity. The combination of cisplatin with VP16 in several European studies had produced a response rate of around 40%, with the median survival in responders being between 30 and 60 weeks. Dhingra et al. subsequently conducted a randomized trial involving 167 patients to compare three cisplatin-based combinations: cisplatin with vindesine (PVD), cisplatin with

VP16 (PVP), or cisplatin with both VP16 and vindesine (PVPVD) (Dhingra et al., 1985). Efficacy was relatively identical among the three different regimens, with the observed differences in response rates not statistically significant (35% PVD, 30% PVP, and 22% PVPVD; $P = .33$). Meanwhile, response durations were 43 weeks in the PVD arm, 20 weeks in the PVP arm, and 27 weeks in the PVPVD arm, with median survival being 29 weeks in the PVD and PVP arms and 28 weeks in the PVPVD arm. As far as toxicity was concerned, the cisplatin plus VP16 arm was slightly less toxic, since more neuropathy and azotemia were seen in the vindesine-containing arms, with myelosuppression being fairly constant across all three regimens. Studies such as those mentioned above thus helped to establish the combination of cisplatin and etoposide as the standard of care for advanced NSCLC starting in the mid 1980s, with median survival around 26 weeks and the 1-year survival rates about 25% to 28% (Longeval and Klastersky, 1982).

D. Vindesine/Cisplatin Versus Vinblastine/Cisplatin

Another important early question was to address the choice of vinca alkaloid in this patient population. Vindesine and vinblastine are nearly identical in their single-agent efficacy and toxicity profiles, the former used exclusively in Europe. Kris et al. compared vindesine and cisplatin with vinblastine and cisplatin in 108 previously untreated patients randomly assigned to receive cisplatin (120 mg/m^2) and either vindesine (3 mg/m^2) or vinblastine (6 mg/m^2) (Kris et al., 1985). As one would predict, the efficacy data were relatively similar, with the response rates of 33% versus 41% (vindesine vs. vinblastine), median response durations being 8.6 versus 5.6 months (vindesine vs. vinblastine), and median survival times in responding patients 18.4 versus 16.2 months (vindesine vs. vinblastine). However, more patients receiving vinblastine plus cisplatin experienced relative neutropenia, with the absolute WBC being <2100 ($P = .003$). Perhaps there is a slight edge in favor of using vindesine (not FDA-approved in the United States), but, since etoposide became the companion drug of choice in this disease, this decision soon became moot.

A Phase II study was reported which involved treating chemotherapy-naive patients with advanced NSCLC with cisplatin 60 mg/m^2 and vindesine 3 mg/m^2 on day 1, followed by a 3-day continuous infusion of 5-FU at a dose of 800 mg/m^2/day starting on day 8 for a 14-day cycle. An overall response rate of 40% was seen in 47 evaluable patients, including one CR and 18 PRs. The median progression-free interval was 19.3 weeks, and the median survival time 41.6 weeks. Toxicity was well tolerated, with grade III or IV leukopenia and anemia occurring in 19% and 9% of patients, respectively, while only grade II thrombocytopenia was seen. Other nonhematologic toxicities were mild. This treatment program was thus observed by the authors to be similarly efficacious to other active combination chemotherapies with better toxicity profile (Nakano et al., 1996).

A randomized study by Italian investigators compared cisplatin (120 mg/m^2 day 1) + etoposide (100 mg/m^2 days 1 to 3) every 3 weeks (PE); or cisplatin (120 mg/m^2 every 4 weeks) + mitomycin-C (8 mg/m^2 days 1, 29, and 71) + vindesine (3 mg/m^2 days 1, 8, 15, and 22) (MVP); or cisplatin (120 mg/m^2 day 1) + mitomycin-C (6 mg/m^2 day 1) + ifosfamide (3 mg/m^2 day 2) every 3 weeks (MIC). Of a total of 393 consecutive, previously untreated patients with advanced NSCLC, response rates were statistically higher for both MIC (40%) and MVP (36%) than for the PE arm (23%). The MVP group had a higher estimated median survival duration (41.5 weeks) than the groups on MIC (35 weeks) or PE (25 weeks). Based on these results, the authors of this study advocated a three-drug cisplatin-based regimen (MVP; MIC) as reference treatment in advanced NSCLC (Crino et al., 1995).

E.   Large-Group Randomized Trials of Combination Regimens

In the late 1970s and early 1980s, ECOG and SWOG conducted a series of Phase III trials that systematically evaluated combination regimens that had shown response rates of 25% or greater in Phase II trials. In general, the patients enrolled in these trials were those with metastatic disease (no brain metastases, however) with good performance status, and the treatments were tested in all cell types. Besides helping to decipher the most efficacious regimen of the day, these trials also provide data on lung cancer therapeutic efficacy that are freer of the standard Phase II trial selection biases.

A study conducted by ECOG termed number 2575 (generation 5) is shown in Table 3 (Ruckdeschel et al., 1985). Between December 1979 and October 1981, four cisplatin-containing regimens with prior efficacy in Phase II trials were compared in a randomized study enrolling a total of 479 patients: CBP (cyclophosphamide, bleomycin, and cisplatin); AFP (doxorubicin, 5-FU, and cisplatin); MVP (mitomycin C, vinblastine, and cisplatin); and CAP (cyclophosphamide, doxorubicin, and cisplatin). The response rates were as follows: MVP = 26%, AFP = 17%, CBP = 20%, CAP = 23%. In this study the most active regimen was MVP with a 26% response rate, though less than the 53% observed in an earlier single-institution Phase II trial by Mason and Catalano (1980). However, there was significant toxicity associated with this regimen most specifically due to mitomycin C, which included marrow and pulmonary side effects. The CAP regimen resulted in a response rate of 23% with one CR. Although this rate was less than the original Eagan 38% response rate (Eagan et al., 1977), the earlier study counted minimal responses while the latter did not. Since there was a moderately significant difference in response rate favoring MVP with no significant difference seen for median survival, the MVP regimen was employed in the subsequent trial.

Between October 1981 and June 1983, ECOG conducted a prospective randomized trial to examine the four most active regimens for metastatic NSCLC (ECOG trial 1581; Table 3), as 486 good performance status patients were randomized to receive CAMP, MVP, VP-P (etoposide and cisplatin), or VDA-P (vindesine-cisplatin). The response rates for the regimens were as follows: CAMP 17%, MVP 31%, VP-P 20%, and VDA-P 25%, with the overall median survival time at 24.5 weeks (no significant diferences among the groups). In addition, severe toxicity and fatality rates were increased in patients with performance status of 2 or more (Ruckdeschel et al., 1986).

One of the largest modern-day trials was conducted by ECOG involving 699 eligible patients enrolled from January 1984 to July 1995 and was labeled 1583 (Table 3). This in fact represents the largest single-agent trial examining the effect of carboplatin at a dose of 400 mg/m^2 given over 15 min every 4 weeks (Table 3) (Bonomi et al., 1989). Patients who had subsequent disease progression were then treated with the combination of mitomycin/vinblastine/cisplatin (MVP). This treatment arm was compared to iproplatin at a dose of 320 mg/m^2 given every 4 weeks followed by MVP for treatment failure. These single-agent arms were compared with initial treatment with cisplatin-containing combination regimens, which included MVP, vinblastine, and cisplatin (VP) versus MVP alternating with cyclophosphamide, doxorubicin, methotrexate, procarbazine (CAMP). A total of 699 patients were treated in this trial. The following response rates were observed: MVP 20%, VP 13%, MVP/CAMP 13%, carboplatin 9%, and iproplatin 6%. MVP was associated with the highest response rate ($P = .02$), while patients receiving carboplatin or iproplatin had significantly lower response rates ($P = .03$). The overall survival in this trial was a median of 25.4 weeks with 15% of patients surviving for 1 year and 5% for 2 years. Interestingly, multivariate analysis adjusted for prognostic factors showed that carboplatin treatment was associated with significantly longer survival ($P = .008$). Also notable was the fact that the shortest median survival was observed with MVP (which had the greatest single response) as the primary treatment, yet there was a strong trend toward shorter survival (median survival = 22.7 weeks; $P = .09$). Hence, while carboplatin produced a 9% response rate in this trial, carboplatin-treated patients experienced a modest but significantly longer survival at a median of 31.7 weeks ($P = .008$) than did patients treated with other chemotherapeutic regimens. It is possible that the increased toxicity of combination regimens had an adverse effect on survival in this trial.

All the above trials demonstrated that promising regimens in Phase II studies (often from single institutions) usually prove to be less exciting when subjected to broader cooperative group Phase III studies. It is therefore critical that promising regimens be examined carefully in large cooperative trials to delineate clearly their efficacy in advanced NSCLC. These results also suggested that a number of regimens can result in clinical responses and that these responses are associated with improved survival. These studies also showed that failure to obtain a response after two or three courses of therapy should be grounds for discontinuation of treatment, since further treatment would only lead to increased toxicity with no appreciable survival effect. Another important lesson was that in three of the

ECOG trials, patients treated with MVP had the highest response rates with no appreciable improvement in the 1-year survival rate. The discordance between response rates and 1-year survival rates thus illustrates the need for well-designed trials of sufficient follow-up duration to allow for adequate survival analysis. Following this series of Phase III ECOG trials, it was concluded that most of the combination regimens that had shown promise in earlier Phase II trials have been rigorously investigated and that unfortunately none of these treatments has produced a significant improvement in survival in large randomized studies. Given these conclusions, ECOG now focuses on new drug discovery and trials of single agents. Combination regimens until recently were evaluated in limited Phase II trials, with subsequent decisions to study promising regiments in large Phase III trials to be based on survival data and response rates.

SWOG randomized 680 evaluable patients to five different cisplatin-containing regimens including cisplatin/VP-16 ± methylglyoxal bisguanylhydrazone (MGBG); cisplatin/velban; cisplatin/velban/mitomycin C or FOMi/CAP, which was CAP chemotherapy alternating with 5-FU, vincristine, or mitomycin C. The average response was 20% with 3% CR, but the duration of these responses was not statistically different by treatment regimen and varied from 2.7 to 5.0 months. Additionally, the overall median survival was 5.3 months and was not different by treatment. Hence these studies served to show that there were no discernible differences among different platin-containing treatments with etoposide, vinblastine, or MGBG, a novel agent of that time (Weick et al., 1991).

Hence the clinical application of chemotherapy for non-small-cell lung cancer should be based on the combination of agents shown to be consistently effective in properly designed clinical trials. Despite the acknowledged limitations of the drug armamentarium for metastatic lung cancer, there is cause for continued optimism. It seems clear that cisplatin-based combination regimens are the most active in the treatment of NSCLC and form the basis for comparison for new therapies. Accordingly, etoposide plus cisplatin or carboplatin has been considered, until recently, as standard therapy for metastatic NSCLC in the clinical setting. Furthermore, new data have emerged recently regarding novel uses of established agents in this disease and appear to hold promise for added therapeutic benefits. In addition to standard therapies, several new agents demonstrating activity in advanced NSCLC have also been described recently, albeit mostly in Phase II trials, and form the basis for new clinical trials involving new drugs as single agents as well as in combination with established chemotherapeutic regimens (see below).

V. Randomized Studies Comparing Chemotherapy to Supportive Care

The studies described in the preceding sections of this review spanned two decades and form the basis of the combination chemotherapy regimens of the present day in advanced NSCLC. However, even as they were being developed and were commonly used, there were scant data to demonstrate a benefit of combination chemotherapy in survival prolongation in this disease. This circumstance of course necessitated randomized studies looking at chemotherapy versus supportive care alone in patients with advanced NSCLC. Many of these studies were performed in the last decade and are reviewed below.

Although long-term management of advanced NSCLC remains unsatisfactory, there is now strong evidence from randomized controlled clinical trials and from four meta-analyses of a small but definite survival benefit when patients are treated with cisplatin-based regimens (although the absolute survival benefit is only 10% at 1 year). The past decade has seen a series of studies assessing the impact of chemotherapy on survival in advanced NSCLC. Conflicting results have been reported from studies comparing the survival benefits of chemotherapy versus supportive care alone in patients with metastatic NSCLC. A number of older studies showed no survival benefit for patients receiving chemotherapy; however, these studies employed single agents or regimens with minimal activity in NSCLC.

Eight studies were conducted from 1982 to 1993 involving over 800 patients with metastatic NSCLC (Table 4). These studies varied regarding patient selection, treatment regimens, overall number of cycles of therapy, and whether or not radiation therapy was employed. Nevertheless, several studies have reported survival benefits for chemotherapy (Rapp et al., 1988; Cormier et al., 1982; Quoix et al., 1988; Cartei et al., 1993). They are discussed below.

The National Cancer Institute of Canada (NCIC) clinical trials group conducted a prospective randomized trial, one of the first of its kind, comparing best supportive care (BSC) to two different regimens: vindesine and cisplatin (VP), and cyclophosphamide, doxorubicin, and cisplatin (CAP) (Rapp et al., 1988). A total of 251 patients from 18 centers across Canada were entered with a variable two- or three-arm schema. Altogether, 233 patients having measurable or evaluable disease with distant metastases or bulky limited disease considered inoperable or unsuitable for radical radiotherapy were eligible. The overall response rates (CR + PR) for the chemotherapy arms were 15.3% for CAP and 25.3% for VP ($P = .06$). Patients had a median survival of 32.6 weeks when treated with VP, 24.7 weeks when treated with CAP, and 17 weeks with best supportive care. The 1-year survival rate for patients treated with chemotherapy was 20% as compared with 10% for the best supportive care group. When adjusted for prognostic factors, these observed differences were found to be statistically significant ($P = .02$). Toxicity on the chemotherapy arms was significant, with leukopenia occurring in 37.8% (CAP) and 40.0% (VP), severe vomiting in 12.2% (CAP) and 23.3% (VP), and neurotoxicity in 15.6% (VP). A companion study in Canada analyzed the cost and benefits of chemotherapy and reported that polychemotherapy was less expensive than best supportive care, with longer survival in the group treated with chemotherapy (Jaakkimainen et al., 1990). The reduction in cost was due to the

Table 4   Randomized Trials in Advanced NSCLC of Chemotherapy Compared to Best
Supportive Care

Study	No. pts.	Regimen	Median survival		1-Year survival		P	RR %
			CT	BSC	CT	BSC		
Cellerino et al., 1991	128	CEPMX CCNU	34.3 wk	21.1 wk	32%	23%	.153	21
Cormier et al., 1982	39	MACC	30.5 wk	8.5 wk	15%	0	<.0005	35
Ganz et al., 1989	63	CVB	20.4 wk	13.6 wk	20%	10%	.09	22
Kaasa et al., 1991	87	CP	5 mo	3.8 mo	NA	NA	.5	NA
Quoix et al., 1988	43	Pvd	27.5 wk	9.7 wk	NA	NA	.03	NA
Rapp et al., 1988	150	CAP	24.7 wk	17 wk	22%	10%	.02	25
		VP	32.6 wk		21%			15
Cartei et al., 1993	102	CMP	8.5 mo	4 mo	38.5%	12%	<.0001	25
Woods et al., 1990	201	VP	27 wk	17 wk	25%	20%	.33	28

A summary of eight randomized trials that compare chemotherapy (CT) to best supportive care (BSC) in
NSCLC. The median and 1-year survival rates are shown when available. The specific nature of each trial and
regimen is discussed in the text.
NA, not available.

more severe symptoms experienced by patients in the supportive care group,
requiring frequent hospitalization. It was concluded that economic factors should
not adversely affect decisions regarding the use of chemotherapy in advanced
NSCLC. Those who benefited most had an ECOG performance status score of 0
to 1, weight loss of <5 kg, and limited metastatic disease. This follow-up study
showed that supportive care is associated with costs (especially hospital costs) that
may exceed those associated with the administration of chemotherapy.

Cellerino et al. in Italy randomized 128 patients with advanced NSCLC
between best supportive care or chemotherapy with cyclophosphamide, epirubicin, and cisplatin alternating every 4 weeks with methotrexate, etoposide, and
lomustine (CCNU). Median survival was 34.3 weeks in the chemotherapy arm and
21.1 weeks in the best supportive care arm. While this difference was not statistically significant ($P = .153$), high-risk subgroups did show a significant difference
in survival in favor of chemotherapy (two or more of the following: age, weight
loss, performance status >1) (Cellerino et al., 1991).

Another trial, with 48 patients, was conducted by Ganz et al (1989). Again
patients with metastatic NSCLC were randomized between best supportive care
consisting of palliative radiation, psychosocial support, analgesics, and nutritional
support, or the treatment arm consisting of supportive care plus cisplatin and vinblastine. Although the patients receiving combination therapy had a slightly
longer median survival (20.43 vs. 13.57 weeks), the observed difference was not

statistically significant ($P = .09$). In addition, the patients receiving chemotherapy experienced serious toxicity and, based on performance status analysis, experienced little if any benefit in quality of life. The authors therefore concluded that combination chemotherapy at that time provided only modest survival benefit to patients with advanced metastatic NSCLC and should not be considered standard therapy.

Another small study was performed by Cormier et al. (1982), which was a prospective randomized trial of 39 consecutive patients comparing noncisplatin combination chemotherapy with methotrexate, doxorubicin, cyclophosphamide, and lomustine (CCNU) to placebo treatment. Despite its small size, this study demonstrated a median survival benefit of 30.5 weeks for the treatment group versus 8.5 weeks for the best supportive care group ($P = .0005$).

One of the larger studies was conducted by Woods et al., which involved 201 patients with stage IIIB or IV NSCLC randomly assigned to cisplatin at a dose of 120 mg/m^2 on days 1 and 29 and vindesine at a dose of 3 mg/m^2 weekly $\times$ 6 or to supportive care alone (Woods et al., 1990). By study design, both groups were eligible to receive radiotherapy or other palliative radiotherapy as required. The overall response rate to chemotherapy was 28%, and there were no significant differences according to major prognostic criteria. Although the overall survival of the chemotherapy group (median 27 weeks) was longer than that of the supportive care group (median 17 weeks), the difference was not statistically significant ($P = .33$). Toxicity in the chemotherapy group was universal and often severe.

Cartei et al. evaluated 102 patients and conducted a study to assess possible differences regarding safety and survival of supportive care alone as compared to chemotherapy combined with supportive care in patients with metastatic NSCLC (Cartei et al., 1993). The drugs were cisplatin (75 mg/m^2), cyclophosphamide (400 mg/m^2), and mitomycin-C (10 mg/m^2) given intravenously at 3-week intervals. The main toxicities seen in those treated with chemotherapy were peripheral neuropathy and hematologic side effects. The mean survival for the supportive care group was 6.1 months (median 4.0). In the combined modality group, mean survival was 11.3 months (median 8.5 months), and the observed difference in survival was statistically significant ($P < .0001$). Survival was directly related to initial performance status in both groups ($P < .01$) and was significantly ($P < .01$) longer for patients with squamous cell carcinoma than for those with non–squamous cell carcinoma.

Quoix et al. used cisplatin/vindesine as the chemotherapy regimen in their trial of 43 patients (Quoix et al., 1988). They observed a statistically significant increase in median survival from 9.7 to 27.5 weeks ($P = .03$). Finally, Kaasa et al. studied 87 patients randomized to cisplatin/etoposide versus supportive care, which showed a median survival improvement of 5 months for the former to 3.8 months for the latter, although the difference was not statistically significance ($P = .5$) (Kaasa et al., 1991).

VI. Meta-Analyses

As described above, there are at least eight randomized studies which examined the role of chemotherapy versus best supportive care (usually defined as including radiation therapy to painful lesions) in advanced NSCLC. While these trials represent over 800 patients, only approximately half showed a statistically significant difference in favor of chemotherapy. Most of the others showed a trend in favor of the chemotherapy arm. These trials supported the use of chemotherapy in certain patients with advanced NSCLC, although the optimal chemotherapy regimen remained undefined. All trials differed regarding selection factors such as the stage of disease (IV vs. IIIB and IV), the eligibility criteria, and the exact chemotherapeutic regimens.

Given the heterogeneity of results, several meta-analyses have been performed to evaluate more precisely the role of chemotherapy in advanced NSCLC. Grilli et al. analyzed six studies and found a 24% reduction in death when compared with supportive care alone. However, this effect decreased after the first 6 months, and the mean potential gain was only on the order of 6 weeks (Grilli et al., 1993).

From a combined pool of >700 patients, Souquet et al. subsequently performed a meta-analysis of seven published randomized clinical trials of polychemotherapy versus supportive care in patients with NSCLC (Souquet et al., 1993). The numbers of deaths at 3, 6, 9, 12, and 18 months were reported, although trials employing monochemotherapy in the chemo arm were excluded. The first of its kind, this analysis included three trials which individually showed a statistically significant survival benefit (Cormier et al., 1982; Quoix et al., 1988; Rapp et al., 1988). Results showed a statistically significant odds ratio of –0.6785 in favor of chemotherapy when the analysis was performed at 3 or 6 months; however, analysis at the longer time points of 9, 12, or 18 months failed to show a statistically significant difference.

A third meta-analysis conducted by Marino et al. (1994) analyzed the same seven trials studied by Souquet while adding a trial by Buccheri et al. (1989). This meta-analysis again showed an estimated increase in median survival in favor of the chemotherapy group (from 3.9 months for BSC to 6.7 months for chemotherapy), with an absolute difference in survival at 6 months estimated at about 20% (Marino et al., 1994).

A fourth meta-analysis was recently published by Stewart et al., which included updated data from 11 randomized trials (some yet unpublished) comparing chemotherapy versus supportive care, eight of which included cisplatin-based therapy (1995). In all comparisons, results for modern regimens containing cisplatin favored chemotherapy. For cisplatin-based trials the improvement survival at 1 year was estimated at 16% for BSC as compared with 26% for patients treated with chemotherapy, with a corresponding increase of median survival from 6 to 8 months. Interestingly, for regimens containing alkalating agents (without cisplatin) the odds ratio actually trended in favor of supportive care, probably due to the toxicity of the chemotherapy.

Meta-analyses of randomized trials employing a cisplatin-based regimen compared to best supportive care have documented statistically improved survival, a benefit which is clearly modest with only a 2- to 3-month median survival increase. In the randomized study of the Canadian National Cancer Institute, for example, patients in the best supportive care arm had a median survival of 17 weeks, compared to 33 weeks for patients receiving cisplatin and vindesine. More importantly, the 1-year survival rate more than doubled, with significant symptomatic improvement in responding patients. The most active chemotherapeutic agents for NSCLC produce responses in only about 20% to 30% of patients, with complete responses being quite rare. Responding patients live longer than nonresponding patients, and nearly all have improvement in their symptoms. Because of the low response rates and minor impact on survival, better agents and combinations are thus needed.

VII.   New Agents in Lung Cancer

Given the relatively modest impact on survival in advanced NSCLC by established agents, the development of new drugs including those with novel mechanisms of action is indeed imperative. Several newer chemotherapeutic agents fitting such criteria have now been identified and have been used both as single agents and in combination with established drugs (Table 5). Some of these drugs have novel mechanisms of action (e.g., topoisomerase I inhibitors and taxanes), while others are analogs of already known active agents (gemcitabine, vinorelbine, edatrexate, and trimetrexate) (Feigal et al., 1993; Klasterky and Sculier, 1995; Giaccone et al., 1995).

A.   Paclitaxel (Taxol)

The first of a novel class of antimitotic agents, paclitaxel is derived from the bark of the pacific yew *Taxus brevifolia* (Arbuck, 1994). Its mechanism of action has been recently shown to involve the promotion of microtubule assembly and eventual inhibition of normal disassembly, leading to subsequent paralysis of the mitotic apparatus (Liebman et al., 1993). Clinical trials have demonstrated that paclitaxel has significant activity against ovarian carcinoma, melanoma, breast carcinoma, and NSCLC (Arbuck, 1994; Rowinsky et al., 1991).

Initial Phase II studies were performed on chemotherapy-naive patients with advanced NSCLC, using a 24-hour infusion at a relatively high dose of paclitaxel (200 to 250 mg/m^2). The Eastern Cooperative Oncology Group (ECOG) studied 24 patients with metastatic disease treated with 24-hour infusion of paclitaxel at 250 mg/m^2 given every 3 weeks (Chang et al., 1993). Five patients had PRs (21%),

Table 5 New Drugs with Significant Single-Agent Activity in NSCLC

Drug and schedule	Reference	No. pts. (prior Rx)	RR %	Median survival	1-Year survival
Taxol 250 mg/m^2 (24 hrs)	Chang et al., 1993	24 (none)	21	24.1 wk	41.7%
Taxol 200 mg/m^2 (24 hr)	Murphy et al., 1993	25 (none)	24	40 wk	40%
Taxotere 100 mg/m^2 (1 hr)	Cerny et al., 1994	37 (none)	23	11 mo	NA
Taxotere 100 mg/m^2 (1 hr)	Francis et al., 1994	29 (none)	38	6.3 mo	21%
Taxotere 100 mg/m^2 (1 hr)	Fossella et al., 1994	39 (none)	33	47 wk	45%
Gemcitabine 1000 mg/m^2 weekly	Anderson et al., 1994	79 (none)	20	7 mo	NA
Gemcitabine 1000 mg/m^2 weekly	Negoro et al., 1994	189 (none)	22 (3CR)	NA	NA
Gemcitabine 1250 mg/m^2 weekly	LeChevalier et al., 1993	161 (none)	22	NA	NA
Gemcitabine 1000–1250 mg/m^2 weekly	Abratt et al., 1993	76 (none)	20	9.2 mo	35%
CPT-11 100 mg/m^2 90' weekly	Fukuoka et al., 1992	72 (none)	31.9	42 wk	NA
CPT-11 100 mg/m^2 90' weekly	Negoro et al., 1991	67 (none)	0		
		26 (prior)			
Topotecan 2 mg/m^2 × 5 days	Lynch et al., 1994	20 (none)	0	NA	NA
Topotecan 0.5–1.5 mg/m^2 × 5 days	Perez-Soler et al., 1996	37 (none)	14	NA	NA
Vinorelbine 30 mg/m^2 weekly	Depierre et al., 1991	70 (none)	33	33 wk	30%
Vinorelbine 30 mg/m^2 weekly	Crawford et al., 1996	?? (none)	12	30 wk	25%
Vinorelbine 30 mg/m^2 weekly	Depierre et al., 1994	115 (none)	16	32 wk	NA
Vinorelbine 30 mg/m^2 weekly	LeChevalier et al., 1994	206 (none)	14	31 wk	30%

with a median survival time of 24.1 weeks and a 1-year survival rate of 41.7%. While no anaphylaxis was observed with premedication, leukopenia was quite significant (62.5% of patients had grade 4 and 12.5% of patients had grade 3 toxicity). Other nonhematologic toxicities, e.g., cardiotoxicity and neurotoxicity, were tolerable and reversible. In a parallel study, 25 patients with stage IIIB and stage IV NSCLC were treated at the M. D. Anderson Cancer Center with paclitaxel infusion at 200 mg/m^2 over 24 hours every 3 weeks (Murphy et al., 1993). The overall response rate was 24% with one CR and five PR. While overall median survival was 40 weeks, those with CR or PR had a median survival of 56 weeks. Neutropenia was the most significant toxicity, with the majority of patients having grade 3 or 4 granulocytopenia. While one patient had to be treated in the intensive care unit for septic shock, no toxic death occurred. While demonstrating that paclitaxel is indeed active in NSCLC, these studies also suggested the need for growth factor support to allow for greater latitude in dosage administration.

Additional work has been done to investigate the effect of dose and schedule of paclitaxel administration on NSCLC. A Phase II study involving 51 chemotherapy-naive patients with advanced NSCLC treated with 3-hour infusion of paclitaxel 175 mg/m^2 every 3 weeks for a maximum of nine cycles showed a 10% objective response rate. There were no CRs, and all responses lasted less than 5 months. Although treatment was well tolerated, with grade IV neutropenia occurring in only 16% of patients and grade III/IV myalgia/arthralgia in 22% of patients, the antitumor activity of this dose and schedule of paclitaxel was less than expected as compared to previously published trials using higher doses of paclitaxel infused over 24 hours (Milward et al., 1996). In the meantime, a Phase II study carried out by German investigators involved previously untreated patients with inoperable stage IIIB or stage IV NSCLC (Gatzemeier et al., 1995). Forty-three patients were treated with paclitaxel at a dose of 225 mg/m^2 as a 3-hour infusion every 3 weeks. Among 37 evaluable patients, early efficacy results showed eight (21.6%) PRs, and the median time of response was 8.7 weeks. Hematologic toxicities were mild, with no grade 3 or 4 leukopenia and no neutropenic fever. In addition, most nonhematologic toxicities were tolerable, consisting mainly of neuropathy or myalgias/arthralgias, with no hypersensitivity reaction or significant cardiotoxicity.

B. Docetaxel (Taxotere)

A semisynthetic paclitaxel derivative prepared from the needles of the European ewe *Taxus baccata,* docetaxel has an identical mechanism of action to paclitaxel, i.e., promoting microtubule assembly and inducing microtubule bundle formation. While being active in breast and ovarian carcinoma, a number of studies have demonstrated that docetaxel is also active in the treatment of NSCLC (Fossella et al., 1994; Cerny et al., 1994; Burris et al., 1993; Francis et al., 1994). A prospective multicenter Phase II trial conducted in Europe evaluated the objective response rate and response duration in patients with advanced NSCLC (Cerny et al., 1994). Thirty-seven chemotherapy-naive patients with advanced, nonresectable, or metastatic NSCLC were given docetaxel infusion at a dose of 100 mg/m^2 every 3 weeks. One CR and seven PRs were noted for an overall response rate of 23% (two of 37 patients did not receive the planned treatments and were inevaluable for response). The responses lasted 15 to 48 weeks with a median duration of response of 36 weeks. Dose-limiting toxicity was short-lasting leukopenia, rarely being associated with infections, although one patient died from neutropenia-related sepsis. Fluid retention, associated with edema and pleural effusions, was also observed at this dose and schedule.

A similar Phase II study was carried out by investigators at the Memorial Sloan-Kettering Cancer Center in 29 chemotherapy-naive patients with unresectable stage III or IV NSCLC. Patients received docetaxel at 100 mg/m^2 infusion over 1 hour every 3 weeks (Francis et al., 1994). Although no CRs were observed, the objective response rate was 38%, with a median response duration of 5.3 months (median survival 6 months). Neutropenia was the most common grade 4 toxicity, and fluid retention manifesting as peripheral edema and pleural effusions was also observed. Another Phase II study, at the M. D. Anderson Cancer Center, involved the treatment of 39 evaluable chemotherapy-naive patients with stage IIIB or IV with a docetaxel infusion dose of 100 mg/m^2 over 1 hour every 3 weeks (Fossella et al., 1994). An impressive response rate was noted as 13 patients (33%) achieved a PR, with a median response duration of 14 weeks, a projected median survival of 47 weeks, and an estimated 1-year survival of 45%. Most patients had grade 3 or 4 neutropenia at this dose, and there was one case of fatal neutropenic infection. A majority of patients developed fluid retention, manifesting as peripheral edema and pleural effusions. Additionally, a Phase II trial by Japanese investigators treated 75 previously untreated patients with advanced NSCLC with docetaxel at a dose of 60 mg/m^2 given over 1 to 2 hours every 3 weeks; 19% achieved a PR, and the median survival time was 297 days. While grade III/IV neutropenia was seen in 87% of patients, hypersensitivity and edema each occurred in only 4% of patients and were easily manageable with this moderate dosing of docetaxel (Kunitoh et al., 1996). Dexamethasone has proven useful in reducing hypersensitivity reactions and edema.

It is important to note that while both taxol and taxotere have shown significant activity in advanced NSCLC, no randomized trial directly comparing these two agents has been reported.

C. Vinorelbine (Navelbine)

Navelbine, an analog of vinblastine, is a semisynthetic vinca alkaloid with minimal neurotoxicity and with myelosuppression being the dose-limiting toxicity in Phase

I studies. A Phase II study (Depierre et al., 1991) involving chemotherapy-naive patients treated with infused navelbine at a dose of 30 mg/m^2 week. Seventy evaluable patients were treated, with 23 patients (33%) achieving a PR. The median response duration was 34 weeks, and the median survival for the treatment group was 33 weeks. Major toxicity was leukopenia, and neurotoxicity was rarely observed.

A subsequent multicenter Phase III trial comparing single-agent vinorelbine at 30 m^2/week with vinorelbine at the same dose and schedule plus cisplatin at 80 mg/m^2 every 3 weeks was conducted (Depierre et al., 1993), and 208 assessable patients with previously untreated stage III and IV NSCLC were enrolled. The objective response rate for those treated with vinorelbine alone was 16%, compared with a rate of 43% with the combination of vinorelbine and cisplatin. Furthermore, the time to disease progression for the group treated with the combination was 20 weeks, compared to the 10 weeks of those treated with the single agent. While the median survival time was similar in both groups (32 to 33 weeks), the 2-year survival rate for the vinorelbine patients was 5%, compared to 10% observed for the combination group. Major toxicity was leukopenia, with tolerable nonhematologic side effects.

To compare the activity of vinorelbine with a control group, a Phase III multicenter study was carried out in the United States involving patients with untreated stage IV NSCLC (Crawford et al., 1996). Patients were randomized to single-agent vinorelbine or a combination of 5-FU/leucovorin. The objective response rate for the vinorelbine group was 12%, compared to 3% rate for the 5-FU/leucovorin group (P = .03). The median survival time of the vinorelbine patients was 30 weeks, with 25% of patients alive at 1 year, compared to a median survival time of 22 weeks for the 5-FU/leucovorin group, with 16% of patients alive at 1 year. In this trial of 216 patients, vinorelbine was felt to have reasonable efficacy and acceptable toxicity, with 54% of patients experiencing grade 3 or 4 granulocytopenia versus 24% in the patients receiving 5-FU/leucovorin. There was no difference in febrile neutropenia (7%). A quality-of-life (QOL) score and symptom relief endpoint were included as secondary endpoints in this trial but, due to early dropout on the 5-FU arm, there were not enough patients for statistical significance. However, there was a trend in favor of improved symptom relief scores for the patients treated with vinorelbine. Despite a low response rate, this regimen resulted in increased survival. The most common nonhematologic toxicity was injection site reactions. The 30-week median survival is longer than all eight randomized trials of chemotherapy versus supportive care reviewed above.

The impact of vinorelbine on improved survival was again seen in a large European multicenter trial (LeChevalier et al., 1994a,b). Single-agent vinorelbine at 30 mg/m^2/week was compared with vinorelbine at the same dose and schedule plus cisplatin at 120 mg/m^2 intravenously on day 1, day 29, then every 6 weeks, compared with a third arm of vindesine at 3 mg/m^2/week and cisplatin at the same dose and schedule as described above. More than 600 patients with chemotherapy-naive stage III or IV NSCLC were enrolled. The vinorelbine-alone group had an objective response rate of 14%, with a median survival of 31 weeks, a 1-year survival rate of 30%, and 2-year survival rate of 9%. Those treated with vindesine and cisplatin had an objective response rate of 19%, a median survival time of 32 weeks, a 1-year survival rate of 27%, and a 2-year survival rate of 9%. Most notably, those treated with vinorelbine and cisplatin had an objective response rate of 28% with a median survival time of 40 weeks, a 1-year survival rate of 35%, and a 2-year survival rate of 15%. Grade 3 or 4 neutropenia was seen in 79% of the vinorelbine/cisplatin patients, compared with 53% of the vinorelbine-alone group and 48% of the vindesine/cisplatin group. Neutropenic sepsis-related mortality was 1% in all three groups. The survival advantage seen in the group treated with navelbine and cisplatin as compared to the groups treated with navelbine alone or vindesine plus cisplatin was still seen beyond 5 years of follow-up (LeChevalier et al., 1997). Given the significant improvement in survival, vinorelbine was approved in 1995 by the Food and Drug Administration as a single agent or in combination with cisplatin for the treatment of NSCLC.

A trial recently reported by the Southwest Oncology Group (Wozniak et al., 1996) compared the effect of cisplatin given at a dose of 100 mg every 4 weeks versus the combination of cisplatin plus navelbine in patients with advanced NSCLC; 432 previously untreated patients with stage IIIB or IV NSCLC were randomized to receive cisplatin at a dose of $100mg/m^2$ every 4 weeks or cisplatin every 4 weeks and navelbine at a dose of $25mg/m^2$ weekly. The response rate for those treated with cisplatin alone was 10% (with no CR) as compared to 25% for those treated with cisplatin and navelbine together. Additionally, 1-year survival for the cisplatin group was 12% and that for the combination group was 33%, a difference which was statistically significant. There was also a statistically significant advantage with regard to progression-free survival (median 2 vs. 4 months; $P = .0001$) and overall survival (median 6 vs. 7 months; $P = .001$) favoring the group treated with the combination regimen. However, more severe hematologic side effects were seen with the patients treated with cisplatin and navelbine, with 116 episodes of grade IV granulocytopenia compared to three for those treated with cisplatin alone.

D. Gemcitabine

Initially developed as an antiviral agent, gemcitabine (deoxydifluorocytidine) is a pyrimidine analog (fluorinated derivative of cytosine arabinoside) with a broad range of antitumor activity against a number of solid tumors in vitro and in vivo. Data from earlier studies demonstrated that gemcitabine may have the greatest efficacy with the lowest toxicity when given once a week for 3 out of every 4 weeks, starting at a dose of 800 mg/m^2 and increasing to a dose of 1250 mg/m^2 (Abratt et al., 1994; Anderson et al., 1994; Gatzemeier et al., 1996). Furthermore, objective responses were seen in patients with NSCLC, colon carcinoma, breast cancer, renal and bladder cancers, ovarian cancer, and pancreatic cancer. For advanced NSCLC, this drug has an aggregate response rate of 20% in patients enrolled in several published trials (Anderson et al., 1994; Abratt et al., 1994; Shepherd et al., 1993; Negoro et al., 1994; Fossella et al., 1993). A recently published Phase I study from M. D. Anderson with 32 assessable chemotherapy-naive patients treated with single-agent gemcitabine showed a PR rate of 25%, with a projected median survival duration of 49 weeks (Fossella et al., 1997). In this study, gemcitabine was administered as a 30-min intravenous infusion weekly for 3 out of every 4 weeks, with doses ranging from 1000 mg/m^2 to 2800 mg/m^2/week. The maximum tolerated dose was 2200 mg/m^2/week for 3 weeks of every 4 weeks, and dose-limiting toxicity was myelosuppression and reversible transaminase elevation, with other side effects being consistently mild.

A Phase II randomized study was recently published which evaluated the efficacy and toxicity of gemcitabine versus the combination of cisplatin and etoposide in Chinese patients with ioperable (stage III or IV) NSCLC. Patients received either gemcitabine at 1250 mg/m^2 given as a 30-min infusion on days 1, 8, and 15 of each 28-day cycle, or cisplatin 80 mg/m^2 given on day 1 and etoposide 80 mg/m^2 given on days 1, 2, and 3 of each 28-day cycle. Out of 26 assessable patients on the gemcitabine arm and 24 on the cisplatin/etoposide arm, 19% and 21%, respectively, achieved a PR, although there were no CRs on either treatment arm. The median survival times were 37 weeks on the gemcitabine arm and 48 weeks on the cisplatin/etoposide arm. Gemcitabine was better tolerated, with much less significant myelosuppression and nausea/vomiting (Perng et al., 1997). As a well-tolerated drug with few toxic side effects and with myelosuppression not being a problem at the doses described above, gemcitabine is thus a useful agent to be employed in combination with other active agents.

While it has demonstrated encouraging activity against NSCLC, gemcitabine has a relatively mild toxicity profile compared to other agents. Granulocytopenia is usually mild to moderate, with thrombocytopenia occurring occasionally. Nonhematologic side effects include nausea, vomiting, and lethargy. Abnormalities of liver transaminases have been reported in about 60% of patients; however, they are usually mild and nonprogressive, and rarely necessitate cessation of treatment. Slight proteinuria and hematuria are seen in approximately one-half of patients, although not usually associated with any change in serum creatinine or blood urea nitrogen. A reversible skin rash is also occasionally seen, as well as a flulike syndrome in about 20% of patients that is transient and rarely dose-limiting.

E. Camptothecins

Derived initially from the original plant *Camptotheca acuminata,* camptothecins inhibit the nuclear enzyme topoisomerase I, producing DNA damage through the formation of single-strand breaks (Hsiang et al., 1985; Hsiang and Liu, 1988). CPT-11 and topotecan are two semisynthetic camptothecin analogs which are active in NSCLC as well as colorectal cancer (Shimada et al., 1991), hematologic malignancies (Ohno et al., 1990), and gynecologic malignancies (Takeuchi et al., 1991) in studies pioneered by Japanese investigators.

Irinotecan (CPT-11) is a water-soluble analog of camptothecin which ironically was first under NCI development in the 1970s, but was halted due to unpredictable toxicity. More recently, initial Phase I data suggested that leukopenia and diarrhea may be dose-limiting side effects, particularly at higher levels of CPT-11 (Negoro et al., 1991). A subsequent Phase II study involved 72 chemotherapy-naive patients with inoperable NSCLC who received CPT-11 infusion at a dose of 100 mg/m^2 over 90 min once a week (Fukuoka et al., 1992). The overall partial response rate was 32% (23 out of 72 patients), with a median duration of response in patients with PRs of 15 weeks. Of the 40 patients with stage IV disease, 13 (33%) responded. The median survival duration for all patients was 42 weeks. As previously noted from Phase I data, the dose-limiting toxicities were leukopenia and diarrhea. In addition, pulmonary toxicity was seen in some patients and, although most patients responded to corticosteroid treatment, one patient died from interstitial pneumonitis.

F. Topotecan

Topotecan is another hydrophilic semisynthetic camptothecin with mixed results in NSCLC. Initial Phase I studies showed that the dose-limiting toxicity was myelosuppression while nonhematologic toxicities were tolerable (Hochster et al., 1994; Rowinsky et al., 1992). A Phase II study was terminated early as the first 20 chemotherapy-naive patients with metastatic NSCLC (out of a planned 30) showed no objective clinical response to topotecan at the dose of 2 mg/m^2/day intravenously for 5 days every 21 days for two cycles. At this dose, high-grade neutropenia was seen in the majority of patients, with three patients developing neutropenic infection and one death from presumed neutropenic sepsis (Lynch et al., 1994). On the other hand, a Phase II study examining the efficacy of single-agent topotecan involved 40 assessable patients with previously untreated, advanced NSCLC (Perez-Soler et al., 1996). With topotecan being administered at a dose of 1.5 mg/m^2/day for 5 days over 30 min every 21 days, A PR rate of 15% was noted (36% in patients with squamous cell carcinoma and 4% in those with other histologies); the overall median survival time was 38 weeks, and 1-year survival was 30%. While myelosuppression of short duration was the most common and limiting toxicity, no grade 3 or 4 nonhematologic toxicities were observed.

VIII. New Drug Combinations in NSCLC

A. Paclitaxel and Platinum-Based Agents

In view of the encouraging single-agent response rates in early studies, a number of the newer agents have been used in clinical trials in combination with previously established active agents. Although the largest experience has involved the combination of paclitaxel plus cisplatin or carboplatin, trials with other new agents in combination with platinum-based therapy have also been reported.

A Phase I/II study was completed with 32 chemotherapy-naive patients with advanced NSCLC being treated with paclitaxel and cisplatin. Paclitaxel was administered as a 3-hour infusion followed by carboplatin, with the cycles being given every 3 weeks; 38% of patients exhibited a PR, and efficacy was superior at paclitaxel doses of at least 200 mg/m^2. While hematologic toxicity was acceptable and always manageable, peripheral neurologic toxicity was dose-limiting, with its appearance being dose-dependent and cumulative after a total paclitaxel dose of approximately 1300 mg/m^2 (Belli et al., 1995).

A Phase II study by investigators at the Fox Chase Cancer Center involved 53 chemotherapy-naive patients with stage IV or stage IIIB with malignant pleural effusion NSCLC treated with paclitaxel at an dose of 135 mg/m^2/day and carboplatin using the Calvert area under the curve (AUC) formula of 7.5 (Langer et al., 1995). The treatment was repeated at 3-week intervals for a total of six cycles with GCSF support. The objective response rate was 62% with 28 partial responses and five complete responses, the median progression-free survival was 28 weeks, and the median survival time was 53 weeks. Myelosuppression was the principal toxicity, although neutropenia was modulated with growth factor support. Seven episodes of fever/neutropenia occurred, all during the first cycle, but no septic deaths were reported. Neuropathy, myalgias, arthralgias, and thrombocytopenia were generally mild, albeit cumulative.

Another Phase II study from Vanderbilt involved 51 previously untreated patients with stage IIIB or stage IV NSCLC treated with paclitaxel (135 or 175 mg/m^2) administered by 24-hour intravenous infusion on day 1 and 1-hour infusion of carboplatin (300 mg/m^2 or dosed to AUC of 6) on day 2 (Johnson et al., 1996). Treatment was repeated every 28 days for a total of six cycles, and hematopoietic growth factors were not routinely used. There were no complete and 14 partial responses, for an overall response rate of 27%. The medium progression-free survival time was 23.8 weeks with a median survival time of 38 weeks and a survival rate at 1 year of 32%. While nonhematologic toxicity was modest, the major toxicity was neutropenia requiring GCSF support in some patients, particularly those treated at the higher paclitaxel dose. There were two treatment-related deaths due to neutropenic sepsis. The relatively lower response rate seen in this study compared to the trial reported by Langer et al. (1995) may be due to study population heterogeneity as well as relative differences in drug dose and dose intensity.

Rowinsky et al. combined carboplatin and paclitaxel given over 3 hours in a Phase I/II trial involving chemotherapy-naive patients with stage IV NSCLC (Rowinsky et al., 1995). Paclitaxel is given from a range of 175 mg/m^2 to 225 mg/m^2 while carboplatin is dosed from AUC of 7 to 9. The activity of paclitaxel employed in this manner does not appear to be compromised while there was less hematologic toxicity. Out of 10 evaluable patients with NSCLC there were five PRs.

In another Phase I study, Vafai et al. enrolled patients with advanced NSCLC with taxol infusion over 3 hours in combination with carboplatin at an AUC dose of 6 (1995). The MTD was 250 mg/m^2 with dose-limiting toxicity of grade 3 osteo/arthralgias or sensory neuropathy. Although this regimen is published only in abstract form, the initial overall response rate was 63% in 30 evaluable patients with two CRs and 15 PRs. While median survival was 10 months, 1-year survival rate was 38% with a trend for longer survival at higher taxol doses. An advantage with this regimen is the ease of administration, which allows outpatient therapy. However, there are no randomized Phase III data available to compare its efficiency to other known regimens.

The optimal infusion schedule for paclitaxel remains unknown. Preclinical and early Phase I studies suggested an increased activity of taxol from a longer infusion time (Arbuck, 1994; Liebman et al., 1993). Georgiadis et al. have evaluated a 4-day continuous infusion of taxol from a range of 100 to 120 mg/m^2 in combination with cisplatin from 60 to 80 mg/m^2 (1995); 16 patients with advanced NSCLC have been treated at the MTD of 120 mg/m^2 with anRR of 56% (one CR and eight PRs). More recently, several studies have evaluated the administration of taxol over a 1-hour infusion time (Evans et al., 1997; Hainsworth et al., 1995), with response rates being similar to those observed with longer infusions. Hence, 1-hour infusion of taxol appears to be a safe schedule, with severe hypersensitivity reactions seen in <1% of >2000 infusions when used as a single agent or with other chemotherapeutic agents (Greco, personal communication, 1997).

B. Recent ECOG Trial

A recent ECOG study randomized patients into three treatment arms—cisplatin plus etoposide, taxol at a dose of 250 mg/m^2 plus cisplatin with GCSF support, and taxol at 135 mg/m^2 with cisplatin, with close to 200 patients enrolled in each arm and with taxol being infused over a period of 3 hours (Table 6) (Bonomi et al., 1996). The primary endpoints were response rate, median survival, and toxicity. Time to disease progression, pharmacokinetics, and quality-of-life data were collected but have not yet been analyzed. Patients with stage IIIB or IV NSCLC who demonstrated a performance status of 0 or 1 and who did not have brain metastases were eligible. The response rate for etoposide and cisplatin was 12%, taxol 135/cisplatin 26%, and taxol 250/GCSF/cisplatin 32% ($P = .001$). Improved survival was observed in patients receiving either taxol combination with median and 1-year survival, respectively, of 7.7 months and 32% for the control, 9.6 and 37% for taxol, at 135 mg/m^2, and 10.0 and 39% for taxol at 250 mg/m^2 ($P = .016$).

Table 6 Response and Survival Data from ECOG Study 5592

Regimen	Response rate (%)	Median survival (months)	1-Year survival (%)
Etoposide + cisplatin[a]	12	7.7	32
Taxol 135 mg/m^2 + cisplatin[b]	26[d]	9.6[e]	37
Taxol 250 mg/m^2 + cisplatin[c] + GCSF	32[d]	10.0[e]	39

[a](Control.) Cisplatin 75 mg/m^2 IV (day 1) + etoposide 100 mg/m^2 IV on days 1–3. Eligible patients had stage IIIB or IV NSCLC. There were 560 patients randomized equally among the three groups.
[b]Taxol injection 250 mg/m^2 IV infused over 24 hours (day 1) followed by cisplatin 75 mg/m^2 (day 2) + GCSG 5 μg/kg/d SC (starting on day 3).
[c]Taxol 135 mg/m^2 IV infused over 24 hours (day 1) followed by cisplatin 75 mg/m^2 (day 2).
[d]P = <.001 for both taxol groups compared to etoposide/cisplatin. There was no statistically significant difference between the taxol 135 mg/m^2 and taxol 250 mg/m^2 groups.
[e]P = .016 for each of the taxol groups compared to etoposide/cisplatin. There was no statistically significant difference between the taxol 135 mg/m^2 and taxol 250 mg/m^2 groups.
Source: Bonomi et al., 1996.

However, there was no statistically significant difference between the two taxol arms. Toxicities included grade 3 to 4 neutropenia, with the highest rate of toxicity in the group treated with the higher taxol dose. There were 7% to 9% occurrences of neutropenic sepsis, with a 1% to 3% rate of septic death. Other nonhematologic side effects included neurotoxicity and myalgias. Of note, the toxicities were not different among the three arms of the trial.

C. ICE-T

At DFCI we have recently completed a Phase I study of iosfamide, carboplatin, etoposide, and paclitaxel in advanced lung cancer (ICE-T), with placitaxel being administered as a 24-hour continuous infusion in conjunction with growth factor support (Strauss et al., 1995). The dosage of paclitaxel was escalated from an initial dose of 75 mg/m^2 to a target dose of 225 mg/m^2;34 patients have been accrued. Substantial hematologic toxicity was observed with 26% developing fever and neutropenia, 56% grade 4 neutropenia, and 26% grade 4 thrombocytopenia. Among the 22 patients with NSCLC, 27% achieved an objective response (with two having a complete response). Further follow-up of this study utilizing administration of taxol over 3 hours with an additional 11 patients with NSCLC reveals a PR of 36% and stable disease in 41% of 33 patients with a median survival of 13.6 months and 1-year survival of 52% (Strauss et al., 1997).

D. Other New Combination Regimens

As might be expected, many investigators have begun to explore new doublet and now even triplet combinations of agents in non-small-cell lung cancer. There have been several Phase I/II studies that have examined the combination of cisplatin and taxotere which have revealed response rates of 46% and 53% each in 25 patients (Cole et al., 1995). In addition, Belani et al. recently reported a Phase II trial in which 47 patients with advanced NSCLC were treated with docetaxel 75 mg/m^2 plus cisplatin 75 mg/m^2 every 21 days (Belani et al., 1997). The overall response rate was 21% (one CR, nine PRs); median survival was 11.5 months. The major toxicities encountered with this regimen included febrile neutropenia (8.5%), grade 4 pulmonary toxicity (4.3%), grade 4 neuromotor toxicity (2.1%), severe asthenia (12.8%), and severe fluid retention (2.1%).

Camptothecin-based combinations have also been explored, as a Japanese Phase II study involving the treatment of 26 chemotherapy-naive patients with stage IIIB or stage IV NSCLC with cisplatin and CPT-11 was reported (Masuda et al., 1992). There were 14 partial responses (54%), and significant toxicity was infrequent; the major toxic effects were leukopenia and diarrhea, although no treatment-related infections or treatment-related deaths occurred.

A Phase I study was done to determine the maximum tolerated doses of gemcitabine and cisplatin, each given weekly for 3 weeks with a 1-week rest, with the starting doses for gemcitabine and cisplatin being 1000 mg/m^2 week and 25 mg/m^2/week, respectively. Out of 47 assessable chemotherapy-naive patients with advanced NSCLC, 14 achieved a PR (30%); the median duration of response was 16 weeks, and the median survival time was 24 weeks. Based on mathematical modeling, the authors recommended Phase II doses of this active regimen of cisplatin and gemcitabine to be 30 mg/m^2 and 1500 mg/m^2 weekly for 3 weeks, respectively (Shepherd et al., 1996).

The combination of gemcitabine and cisplatin was examined in a study involving 50 assessable chemotherapy-naive patients with advanced NSCLC given gemcitabine on days 1, 8, and 15 at a dose of 1000 mg/m^2 and cisplatin on day 15 at 100 mg/m^2, with chemotherapy being administered in 28-day cycles. The overall response rate was 52% with two CRs (4%) and 24 PRs (48%). The median survival duration was 13 months and the 1-year survival rate was 61%. While grade 3 and 4 neutropenia occurred in 39% and 19% of patients, respectively, and grade 3 and 4 thrombocytopenia occurred in 13% and 8% of patients, respectively, relatively few patients required dose modifications for any of the three weekly doses of chemotherapy (Abratt et al., 1997). Crino et al. reported a Phase II study involving 46 previously untreated patients treated with gemcitabine at a dose of 1000 mg/m^2 given weekly on days 1, 8, and 15, and cisplatin at a dose of 100 mg/m^2 on day 2 of each 28-day cycle (1997). One CR and 26 PRs were observed for an overall response rate of 58%. Thrombocytopenia was the main side effect, with 51% of patients having grade III to IV toxicity.

Furthermore, Lopez-Cabrerizo ct al. recently reported a trial in which 136 chemonaive patients with advanced NSCLC were randomized to receive either gemcitabine 1250 mg/m^2 on days 1 and 8 with cisplatin 100 mg/m^2 on day 1, or etoposide 100 mg/m^2 on days 1 to 3 plus cisplatin 100 mg/m^2 on day 1 (1997). For the gemcitabine group, response rate was 49% (one CR, 32 PRs), while the etoposide group had anobjective response rate of 28% (0 CR, 15 PRs). While there was a higher response rate in the gemcitabine plus cisplatin group, grade 3 or 4 thrombocytopenia was observed in 21% in the gemcitabine plus cisplatin group and in 7% of the etoposide plus cisplatin group.

Novel ifosfamide-based combination chemotherapy has also been recently reported. Previously untreated patients with advanced NSCLC were treated with ifosfamide plus paclitaxel or ifosfamide plus vinorelbine in two Phase I studies, with both regimens being given mesna and granulocyte colony-stimulating factor support. The dose-limiting toxicity for both regimens was neutropenia, with other toxicities being generally mild. A PR rate of 27% was noted among those treated with ifosfamide/paclitaxel, and while final analysis is still pending for the ifosfamide/vinorelbine group, the authors noted that responses have so far been encouraging (Hoffman et al., 1996).

Finally, a Phase I study of vinorelbine and ifosfamide with GCSF support was recently published. Forty-two chemotherapy-naive patients with advanced NSCLC received vinorelbine starting at 15 mg/m^2 on days 1, 2, and 3, and ifosfamide starting at 2 g/m^2 on days 1, 2, and 3, with GCSF support for all patients and cycles being repeated every 21 days. The overall response rate was 40%, and the median survival duration was 50 weeks, with a 1-year survival rate of 48%. The dose-limiting toxicity was neutropenia and sepsis at a maximum administered vinorelbine dose of 35 mg/m^2 for 3 days. The recommended Phase II dose was vinorelbine 30 mg/m^2 with ifosfamide 1.6 g/m^2, both given on 3 consecutive days (Masters et al., 1997).

IX. Second-Line Therapy for NSCLC

As is obvious from even a cursory review of the available literature regarding the treatment of advanced NSCLC, many patients with relatively good prognostic factors (e.g., good performance status, minimal weight loss) have heretofore incurable disease with relatively chemoresistant tumors. For many of these patients, the impact of treatment with first-line chemotherapy is minimal. Not surprisingly, data regarding second-line therapy for progressive disease are quite scarce. While many tumors are inherently resistant to available treatments, it is theoretically possible that others may become more refractory to additional treatments due to an acquired resistance. For many patients with progressive disease after first-line chemotherapy, the decision to attempt additional treatments versus the option of best supportive care for symptomatic relief must be made judiciously and must be tailored for each individual patient. However, a subset of patients may benefit from additional treatments, and several groups have attempted to identify the optimal regimens to be employed in the setting of second-line therapy.

While docetaxel has an impressive single-agent response rate in untreated advanced NSCLC, it has also been shown to be active in patients with previously treated disease. A Phase II study conducted at the M. D. Anderson Cancer Center involved 42 assessable patients with stage IIIb or IV platinum-refractory NSCLC (Fossella et al., 1995). Docetaxel was administered intravenously at 100 mg/m^2 over 1 hour every 3 weeks; nine patients (21%) achieved a PR, with the median response duration being 17 weeks. As noted previously, dose-limiting grade 3 to 4 neutropenia was seen in most patients, and there was one case of fatal neutropenic infection. In addition, fluid retention was a significant side effect in the majority of patients, although such edema would respond to steroid administration.

Given the fact that taxol demonstrated significant activity in chemotherapy-naive patients with advanced NSCLC, investigators were naturally interested in its role as a second-line agent to be used in refractory disease. A number of trials have been reported; however, they consisted mostly of small patient populations with varied doses and schedules. A report by Roa et al. involved 18 previously treated NSCLC patients being treated with taxol infusion at 200 mg/m^2 over 1 to 3 hours and carboplatin at an AUC dose of 5 every 21 days (Roa et al., 1996). Discouragingly, there was 0 out of 18 response seen in this study. Another group also used taxol to treat 14 patients with metastatic NSCLC who had failed previous chemotherapy. Taxol was given at a dose of 250 mg/m^2 over 24 hours (or 200 mg/m^2 for those receiving extensive prior irradiation). Two PRs lasting 70 and 73 days respectively were seen, and median survival was 120 days. Of note is the fact that no significant anemia, thrombocytopenia, or cardiac toxicity was reported (Ruckdeschel et al., 1994)

Given the heterogeneity of data reported so far in trials enrolling relatively few patients, it is quite difficult to make a definite conclusion regarding the role of taxol as second-line therapy. There is thus an urgent need for well-controlled randomized trials to investigate the effect of taxol as a second-line therapy on survival and overall quality of life in previously treated patients with advanced NSCLC. In addition, it will be important to explore new drug treatment regimens for good performance status and relapsed patients, especially as taxol gets moved up more frequently to first-line therapy. Novel Phase I agents including angiogenesis inhibitors and matrix metalloproteinase inhibitors are being actively studied by various groups at this time as potential new treatment regimens.

X. Quality of Life

As documented in this chapter, while the traditional endpoints used for cytotoxic therapy have improved for NSCLC (i.e., response rate, median survival, and 1-

year survival), the benefits remain marginal. Therefore decisions regarding treatment must be made within the context of each individual patient. However, in order to guide patients with their decisions, the question of quality of life (QOL) must be addressed. In several studies the rate of subjective response is higher than the objective response would ordinarily predict. Furthermore, chemotherapy regimens that produce a response rate of only 20% to 30% can relieve symptoms in 60% to 70% of patients (Ellis et al., 1995; Fernandez et al., 1989; Kris et al., 1990). In addition, many studies showed increasing numbers of patients with "stable disease." Three randomized trials were recently published which documented the beneficial effect of combination chemotherapy on the QOL of patients suffering from advanced NSCLC. Helsing and Bergman randomized 48 patients to receive best supporting care (BSC) only or BSC plus a chemotherapy regimen of carboplatin 300 mg/m^2 IV and etoposide 120 mg/m^2 × 5 PO every 4 weeks for a maximum of eight cycles (Helsing and Bergman, 1997). Median survival times were 29 weeks and 11 weeks for those randomized to chemotherapy versus BSC, respectively, with 1-year survival rate for the former being 28% and 8% for the latter. Importantly, patients who were treated with chemotherapy experienced significantly less dyspnea and cough, less fatigue, and better overall physical functioning than those treated with BSC alone. Furthermore, while group differences were smaller for emotional and social functioning and global QOL, the authors noted that trends were seen to favor those treated with chemotherapy.

Another study enrolled 300 symptomatic patients with advanced NSCLC and randomized them to receive either BSC alone or gemcitabine 1000 mg/m^2 administered on days 1, 8, and 15 of a 28-day schedule (Anderson et al., 1997). While patients requiring immediate palliative radiotherapy were excluded from the study, 42.3% of those in the BSC arm needed radiotherapy within the first 2 months on study versus 7.3% of those treated with gemcitabine. An overall response rate of 17.4% was noted for the gemcitabine arm, and chemotherapy was well tolerated, with transient myelosuppression being the major toxicity. Further proof of the beneficial effect of chemotherapy was seen as Billingham et al. found that patients with advanced NSCLC treated with up to four courses of MIC (mitomycin 6 mg/m^2, ifosfamide 3 g/m^2, cisplatin 50 mg/m^2 IV q21 days) have a superior QOL as compared to those treated with supportive care alone (Billingham et al., 1997). These and other reports therefore strongly suggest that chemotherapy indeed does have a positive effect on palliation and the QOL of patients with advanced NSCLC.

The measurement of quality of life of course necessitates a functional instrument to reliably evaluate the efficacy of treatment methods, and numerous attempts to devise such an instrument have been made. For example, Cella et al. described the FACT-L scale (Functional Assement of Cancer Therapy—Lung) as a QOL instrument, which is a 44-item self-report instrument measuring multiple facets of the QOL issue (Cella et al., 1993). Available in eight languages with its reliability and validity having been assessed, it is currently being used in several Phase II and III lung cancer clinical trials.

Finally, it must be realized that quality of life is a subjective measure. An informative survey was done in Canada to asses the opinions of physicians in regard to lung cancer treatment (Mackillop et al., 1987). One hundred eighteen Canadian physicians who treat patients with lung cancer on a regular basis were polled regarding their own treatment preference if they themselves were diagnosed with advanced NSCLC. Only 15% of the physicians in the survey expressed a desire for chemotherapy in the setting of symptomatic metastatic disease.

XI. Conclusion

While the new drugs are exciting, one must not lose sight of the fact that aside from the navelbine studies and the recent ECOG trial with cisplatin/taxol, to date there are no other mature randomized trials which address a comparison of these combinations. Hence, at the time of this writing, carboplatin plus taxol (owing to its ease of administration, tolerability, and Phase II data alone) is among the most commonly used chemotherapeutic regimens in the practice of oncology. However, in a research setting it is the authors' belief that all suitable patients should be placed on a clinical research study, either with novel agents or new combinations or randomized Phase III comparison protocols.

The cooperative groups have recently designed trials which will begin to address some of these questions (Table 7). A SWOG trial will evaluate navelbine/cisplatin versus taxol/carboplatin. A CALGB proposed study will evaluate taxol versus taxol/carboplatin; and an ECOG trial will evaluate cisplatin/taxol (24 hours) versus cisplatin/gemcitabine versus cisplatin/taxotere versus carbopatin/ taxol (3 hours) All new trials will study response and survival, palliation of symptoms and QOL issues, or cost-effectiveness, or a combination of all these parameters.

Despite numerous efforts to produce efficacious treatments, the outcome of patients with advanced NSCLC remains poor. While there are responses in 20% to

Table 7   Large Cooperative Trials Planned or Under Way for Advanced Stage NSCLC in the United States

CALGB	Taxol vs. taxol/carboplatin
SWOG	Taxol/carboplatin vs. vinorelbine/cisplatin
ECOG	Taxol vs. taxol/cisplatin vs. docetaxel/cisplatin vs. gemcitabine/cisplatin

In all the trials taxol is planned to be given over 3 hours.

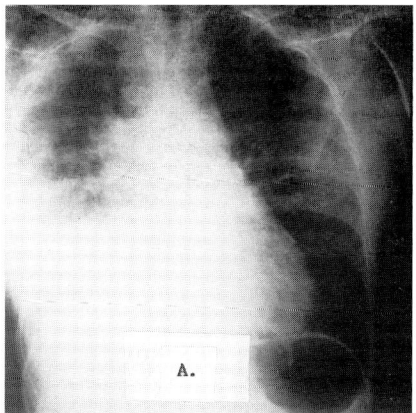

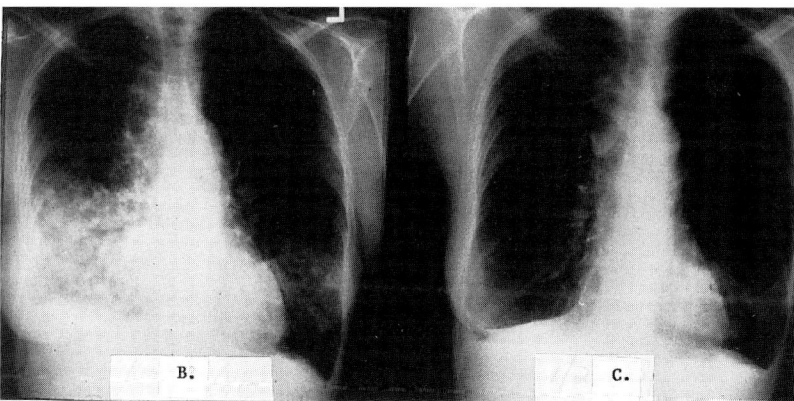

Figure 1 A 57-year-old woman presented with NSCLC extensively involving the right lung with parenchymal, mediastinal, and pleural disease. Metastases were also present in the left lung. (A) Baseline chest film. (B) Chest film 3 weeks after the first cycle of cisplatin-based chemotherapy. Marked regression of tumor has occurred. (C) Follow-up chest film 4 months after start of chemotherapy, showing a clinical complete remission. Isolated brain metastases were fatal 3 years later.

40% of patients with CR rates <5% (Fig. 1), with occasional published reports of complete spontaneous remission in patients with metastatic NSCLC (Kappauf et al., 1997), >15 years after cisplatin was introduced into the treatment of patients with advanced NSCLC, drug therapy remains controversial despite the multiple randomized trials and meta-analyses that have been described here and that have demonstrated a positive benefit in terms of absolute survival. However, this benefit is small, and the cost (both physical and economic) is only now being more carefully assessed. Active regimens, however, can be utilized in the multimodality therapy of earlier-stage lung cancer, where the tumor burden is much less and the results including improved cure rates are more substantial. Hence chemotherapy of metastatic disease is only now beginning to be incorporated into standard treatments for advanced NSCLC. Outside of a trial, the criteria for administering chemotherapy must therefore remain conservative since, while proven, the survival benefits are relatively small. Quality-of-life issues and the patient's individual performance characteristics are paramount in the decision process regarding various treatment options. It is also imperative that the physician be convinced of the patient's full understanding of the risks and benefits associated with treatment after thorough discussions prior to the administration of chemotherapy. For those patients who are actively treated, assessable tumor lesions should be present and measurable, and continous monitoring of these markers would allow for the decision regarding continuation or stoppage of treatment to be made. Generally, current treatment should be discontinued after two to three cycles if there is no measurable response or in the presence of disease progression. Indeed, responses to effective treatment usually occur after two cycles, and the effective chemotherapy regimen may be continued for as many as four to six cycles. After this period of time, benefit may be minimal since cumulative toxicity may become more evident along with drug resistance and progressive disease.

The possibility of interobserver variability in judging response rate accuracy in published oncology trials should also be considered when reading the available literature. A recent study showed that an independent evaluation committee may significantly disagree with the investigators of a large multicenter trial in oncology when evaluating objective response based on medical imaging, with major disagreements occurring in 40% and minor disagreements in 10.5% of the reviewed files. The number of significant tumor response was reduced by 23.2% after review by the evaluation committee; reasons for disagreements included errors in tumor measurements, errors in selection of measurable targets, intercurrent diseases, and radiologic technical problems (Thiesse et al., 1997).

Finally, although it is likely that only a subset of NSCLC patients will benefit from currently available chemotherapeutic regimens, intensive search for possible predictors of response to chemotherapy using the techniques of molecular medicine is ongoing. Molecular markers, such as p53, RAS, Bcl-2, and HER2/NEU, may yield clues regarding the biologic properties of various subsets of NSCLC and may direct future disease-specific therapies. In addition, identification of such molecular markers may allow the practicing physician to correlate markers with clinical outcomes following treatments, hence serving as guideposts for future decision making regarding the treatments of advanced NSCLC.

References

1. Abratt R, Bezwoda W, Falkson G, et al. (1994). Efficacy and safety profile of gemcitabine in non-small-lung cancer: a Phase II study. J Clin Oncol 12:1535–1540.
2. Abratt R, Bezwoda W, Goedhals L, Hacking D (1997). Weekly gemcitabine with monthly cisplatin: effective chemotherapy for advanced non-small-cell lung cancer. J Clin Oncol 15(2):744–749.
3. Albain K, Crowley J, LeBlanc M, et al. (1991). Survival determinants in extensive non-small cell lung cancer: the Southwest Oncology Group Experience. J Clin Oncol 9:1618–1625.
4. Anderson H, Lund B, Bach F, et al. (1994). Single-agent activity of weekly gemcitabine in advanced non-small-cell lung cancer: a Phase II study. J Clin Oncol 12:1821–1826.
5. Anderson H, Cottier B, Nicolson M, et al. (1997). Phase III study of gemcitabine versus best supportive care in advanced non-small cell lung cancer. Lung Cancer 18(suppl 1):9.
6. Arbuck S (1994). Paclitaxel. What schedule? What dose? J Clin Oncol 12:233–236.
7. Babowski M, Creech J (1983). Chemotherapy of non-small cell lung cancer: a reappraisal and look to the future. Cancer Treat Rep 10:159.
8. Belani C, Bonomi P, Dobbs T, et al. (1997). Docetaxel and cisplatin combination in patients with non-small cell lung cancer. A multicenter Phase II trial. Lung Cancer 18(suppl 1):12–13.
9. Belli L, LeChevalier T, Gottfried M, et al. (1995). Phase I/II study of paclitaxel plus cisplatin as first-line chemotherapy for advanced non-small cell lung cancer: preliminary results. Semin Oncol 22(suppl 15):29–33.
10. Billingham L, Cullen M, Woods J, et al. (1997). Mitomycin, ifosfamide and cisplatin (MIC) in non-small cell lung cancer: 3. Results of a randomised trial evaluating palliation and quality of life. Lung Cancer 18(suppl 1):9.
11. Bitran J, Desser R, Meester T, et al. (1976). Cyclosphosphamide, adriamycin methotrexate and procarbazine (CAMP)—effective four-drug combination chemotherapy for metastatic non–oat cell bronchogenic carcinoma. Cancer Treat Rep 60:225.
12. Bonomi P, Finkelstein D, Ruckedschel J (1989). Combination chemotherapy versus single agents followed by a combination chemotherapy in stable IV non-small-cell lung cancer. A study of Eastern Cooperative Oncology Group. J Clin Oncol 7:1602–1613.
13. Bonomi P (1991). Carboplatin in non-small cell lung cancer: review of the Eastern Cooperative Oncoly Group trial and comparison with carboplatin trials. Semin Oncol 18:2–7.
14. Bonomi P, Kim K, Chang A (1996). Phase III trial comparing etopside, cisplatin vs. taxol with cisplatin-GCSF vs. taxol/cisplatin in advanced non-small cell lung cancer, an ECOG trial. Proc Am Soc Clin Oncol 15:382.
15. Brittell J, Eagan T, Ingle N (1978). cis-Dichlorodiammineplatinum alone followed by adriamycin plus cyclophosphamide in combination for adenocarcinoma of the lung. Cancer Treat Rep 62:1207–1210.

16. Buccheri G, Ferrigno D, Curcio A, et al. (1989). Continuation of chemotherapy vs supportive care alone in patients with inoperable non-small cell lung cancer and stable disease after two or three cycles of MACC. Cancer 63:428–432.

17. Bunn PJ (1986). The expanding role of cisplatin in the treatment of non-small cell lung cancer. Semin Onocol 16(suppl 6):1–11.

18. Bunn P Jr (1994). New drug combinations in the treatment of advanced non-small cell (NSCLC) and small cell (SCLC) lung cancer.

19. Burris H, Eckhardt J, Fields S (1993). Phase II trials of taxotere in patients with non-small cell lung cancer. Proc Am Soc Clin Oncol 12:335 (Abstr 1116).

20. Cartei G, Cartei F, Cantone A, et al. (1993). Cisplatin-cyclophosphamide-mitomycin combination chemotherapy with supportive care versus supportive care alone for treatment of metastatic non-small cell lung cancer. J Natl Cancer Inst 85:794–800.

21. Cella D, Tulsky D, et al. (1993). The functional assessment of cancer therapy scale: development and validation of the general measure. J Clin Oncol 11:570.

22. Cellerino R, Tummarello D, Guidi F, et al. (1991) A randomized trial of alternating chemotherapy versus best supportive care in advanced non-small cell lung cancer. J Clin Oncol 9:1453–1461.

23. Cerny T, Kaplan S, Pavlidis N, et al. (1994). Docetaxel (taxotere) is active in non-small-cell lung cancer: a Phase II trial of the EORTC early clinical trials group (ECTG). Br J Cancer 70:328.

24. Chabner B, Longo D (1996). Cancer Chemotherapy and Biotherapy: Principles and Practice. Lippencott-Raven, Philadelphia. 367.

25. Chahinian A, Mandel E, Holland J, et al. (1979). MACC (methotrexate, adriamycin, cyclosphosphamide and CCNU) in advanced lung cancer. Cancer 43:1590–1597.

26. Chang A, Kim K, Glick J (1993). Phase II study of taxol, merbarone and piroxantrone in stage IV non-small-cell lung cancer: the Eastern Oncology Group results. J Natl Cancer Inst 85:388.

27. Cole J, Gralla R, Marques C, et al. (1995). Phase II study of cisplatin + docetaxel (taxotere) in non-small-cell lung cancer (NSCLC). Proc Am Soc Clin Oncol 14:357.

28. Cormier Y, Bergeron D, LaForge J, et al. (1982). Benefits of polychemotherapy in advanced non-small cell bronchogenic carcinoma. Cancer 50:845–849.

29. Crawford J, O'Rourke M, Schiller J, et al. (1996). Randomized trial of vinorelbine compared with fluorouracil plus leucovorin in patients with stage IV non-small-cell lung cancer. J Clin Oncol 14:2774–2780.

30. Crino L, Clerici M, Figoli F, et al. (1995). Chemotherapy of advanced non-small-cell lung cancer: a comparison of three active regimens. A randomized trial of the Italian Oncology Group for Clinical Research (G.O.I.R.C.). Ann Oncol 6:347–353.

31. Crino L, Scagliotti G, Marangolo M, et al. (1997). Cisplatin-gemcitabine combination in non-small cell lung cancer. A Phase II study. J Clin Oncol 15:297–303.

32. Davis S, Rambotti P, Park Y (1981). Combination cyclophosphamide, doxorubicin, and cisplatin (CAP) chemotherapy for extensive non-small cell carcinoma of the lung. Cancer Treat Rep 65:958–958.

33. Depierre A, Lemarie E, Dabouis G (1991). A Phase II study of navelbine in the treatment of non-small-cell lung cancer. Am J Clin Oncol 14:115.

34. Depierre A, LeBeau B, Chasting C (1993). Reslts of a Phase II randomized study of vinorelbine-cisplatin in non-small cell lung cancer. Proc Am Soc Clin Oncol 12:340.

35. Dhingra H, Valdivieso M, Carr D (1985). Randomized trial of three combinations of cisplatin with vindesine and/or VP-16213 in the treatment of lung cancer. J Clin Oncol 3:176–183.

36. Eagan R, Ingle J, Frytak S, et al. (1977). Platinum based polychemotherapy versus dianhdrogalactitol in advanced non-small cell lung cancer. Cancer Treat Rep 61:1339–1345.

37. Ellis P, Smith I, Hardy J, et al. (1995). Symptom relief with MVP (mitomycin C, vinblastine and cisplatin) chemotherapy in advanced non-small-cell lung cancer. Br J Cancer 71:366–370.

38. Evans W, Earle C, Stewart D, et al. (1997). Phase II study of a one hour paclitaxel infusion in combination with carboplatin for advanced non-small cell lung cancer. Lung Cancer 18:83–94.

39. Feigal E, Christian M, Cheson B (1993). New chemotherapeutic agents in non-small-cell lung cancer. Semin Oncol 20:185.

40. Feld R, Arriagada R, Ball D (1991). Prognostic factors in non-small cell lung cancer: a consensus report. Lung Cancer 8:3–5.

41. Fernandez C, Rossell R, Abad-Esteve A (1989). Quality of life during chemotherapy in non-small cell lung cancer patients. Acta Oncol 28:129–133.

42. Finkelstein D, Ettinger D, Ruckdeshel J, et al. (1986). Long-term survivors in metastatic non-small cell lung carcinoma: an Eastern Cooperative Oncology Group study. J Clin Oncol 4:702–709.

43. Fossella F, Lippman S, Pang A (1993). Phase I gemcitabine by 30 minute weekly intravenous infusion 3 weeks every 4 wks for non-small cell lung cancer. Proc Am Soc Clin Oncol 12:326.

44. Fossella F, Soo Lee J, Murphy W, et al. (1994). Phase II study of docetaxel for recurrent or metastatic non-small cell lung cancer. J Clin Oncol 12:1238–1244.

45. Fossella F, Soo Lee J, Shin D, et al. (1995). Phase II study of docetaxel for advanced or metastatic platinum-refractory non-small-cell lung cancer. J Clin Oncol 13:645–651.

46. Fossella F, Lippman S, Shin D, et al. (1997). Maximum-tolerated dose defined for single-agent gemcitabine: a Phase I dose escalation study in chemotherapy-naive patients with advanced non-small cell lung cancer. J Clin Oncol 15(1):310–316.

47. Francis P, Rigas J, Kris M, et al. (1994). Phase II trial of docetaxel in patients with stage III and IV non-small-cell lung cancer. J Clin Oncol 12:1232.

48. Fukuoka M, Nitani H, Suzuki A, et al. (1992). A Phase II study fo CPT-11, a new derivative of camptothecin, for previously untreated non-small-cell lung cancer. J Clin Oncol 10:16–20.

49. Gandara D, Wold H, Perez E (1989). Cisplatin dose intensity in non-small cell lung cancer: Phase II results of a day 1 and day 8 high-dose regimen. J Natl Cancer Inst 81:790–794.

50. Gandara D, Crowley J, Livingston R (1993). Evaluation of cisplatin intensity in metastatic non-small cell lung cancer: a Phase III study of the Southwest Oncology Group. J Clin Oncol 11:873–878.

51. Ganz P, Figlin R, Haskel C, (1989). Supportive care versus supportive care and combination chemotherapy in metastic non-small cell lung cancer. Does chemotherapy make a difference? Cancer 63:1271–1278.

52. Gatzemeier U, Heckmayr M, Newhauss R (1995). Phase II study with paclitaxel for the treatment of advanced inoperable non-small cell lung cancer. Lung Cancer 12(suppl 2):S101–S106.

53. Gatzemeier U, Shepherd F, LeChevalier T, et al. (1996). Activity of gemcitabine in patients with non-small cell lung cancer: a multicenter extended Phase II study. Eur J Cancer 32:243–248.

54. Georgiadis M, Brown J Schinler B (1995). Phase I study of a four day continuous infusion of paclitaxel followed by cisplatin in patients with advanced lung cancer. Proc ASCO 14:353.

55. Giaccone G, Huizing M, Postmus P (1995). Dose-finding and sequencing study of paclitaxel and carboplatin in non-small cell lung cancer. Semin Oncol 22(suppl 9):78–82.

56. Gralla R, Casper E, Kelsen D (1981). Cisplatin and vindesine combination chemotherapy for advanced carcinoma of the lung: a randomized trial investigating two dosage schedules. Ann Intern Med 95:414.

57. Green M, Kreisman H, Doll D (1992). Carboplatin in non-small cell lung cancer: an update on the Cancer and Leukemia Group B experience. Semin Oncol 19(S):44–49.

58. Grilli R, Oxman A, Julian J (1993). Chemotherapy for advanced non-small-cell lung cancer: how much benefit is enough? J Clin Oncol 11:1866–1872.

59. Hainsworth J, Thompson D, Greco F (1995). Paclitaxel by 1-hour infusion: an active drug in metastatic non-small cell lung cancer. J Clin Oncol 13:1609–1614.

60. Helsing M, Bergman B (1997). Chemotherapy with carboplatin and etoposide improves quality of life and survival in patients with advanced non-small cell lung cancer. Lung Cancer 18(suppl 1):8.

61. Hochster H, Liebes L, Speyer J (1994). Phase I trial of low-dose continuous topotecan infusion in patients with cancer: an active and well tolerated regimen. J Clin Oncol 12:553–559.

62. Hoffman C, Masters G, Drinkard L, et al. (1996). Ifosfamide-based combination chemotherapy in advanced non-small cell lung cancer: Two Phase I studies. Semin Oncol 23 No(3 suppl 6):11–15.

63. Hsiang Y-H, Hertzberg R, Hecht S, Liu L (1985). Camptothecin induces protein-linked DNA breaks via mammalian DNA topoisomerase I. J Biol Chem 260:14873–14878.

64. Hsiang Y-H, Liu L (1988). Identification of mammalian DNA topoisomerase I as an intracellular target of the anticancer drug camptothecin. Cancer Res 48:1722–1726.

65. Jaakkimainen L, Goodwin P, Pater J (1990). Counting the cost of chemotherapy in a National Cancer Institute of Canada randomized trial in non-small cell lung cancer (NSCLC). J Clin Oncol 8:1301.

66. Johnson D (1990). Overview of ifosfamide in small cell and non-small cell lung cancer. Semin Oncol 17(S4):24–30.

67. Johnson D, Paul D, Hande K, et al. (1996). Paclitaxel plus carboplatin in advanced non-small cell lung cancer: A Phase II trial. J Clin Oncol 14:2054–2060.

68. Kaasa S, Lund E, Thorud E, et al. (1991). Symptomatic treatment versus combination chemotherapy for patients with extensive non-small cell lung cancer. Cancer 67:2443–2447.

69. Kappauf H, Gallmeier W, Wunsch P, et al. (1997). Complete spontaneous remission in a patient with metastatic non-small-cell lung cancer. Ann Oncol 8:1031–1039.

70. Klastersky J (1986). Therapy with cisplatin and etoposide for NSCLS. Semin Oncol 13:104–114.

71. Klatersky J, Sculier J, Lacroix H (1990). A randomized study comparing cisplatin or carboplatin plus etoposide in patients with advanced non-small cell lung cancer: European Organization for Research and Treatment of Cancer protocol 17861. J Clin Oncol 8:1556–1562.

72. Klatersky J, Sculier J (1995). Dose-finding study of paclitaxel (taxol) plus cisplatin in patients with non-small cell lung cancer. Lung Cancer 12(suppl 2):S117–S125.

73. Kreisman H, Ginsberg S, Propert K, et al. (1987). Carboplatin or iproplatin in advanced non-small cell lung cancer: a Cancer and Leukemia Group study. Cancer Treat Rep 71:1049.

74. Kris M, Gralla R, Kalman L, et al. (1985). A randomized trial comparing vindesine plus cisplatin with vinblastine plus cisplatin in patients with non-small cell lung cancer, with an analysis of methods of response assessment. Cancer Treat Rep 69:387–395.

75. Kris M, Gralla R, Potanovich L, et al. (1990). Assessment of pre-treatment symptoms and improvement after EDAM + mitomycin + vinblastine in patients with inoperable non-small cell lung cancer. Proc Am Soc Clin Oncol 9:229.

76. Kunitoh H, Watanabe K, Onoshi T, Furuese K, Niitani H, Taguchi T (1996). Phase II trial of docetaxel in previously untreated advanced non-small-cell lung cancer—a Japanese cooperative study. J Clin Oncol 14(5):1649–1655.

77. Langer C, Leighton J, Comis R, et al. (1995). Paclitaxel and carboplatin in combination in the treatment of advanced-non-small cell lung cancer: a Phase II toxicity, response, and survival analysis. J Clin Oncol 13:1860–1870.

78. LeChevalier T, Brisgand D, Douillard J, et al. (1994a). Randomized study of vinorelbine and cisplatin versus vindesine and cisplatin versus vinorelbine alone in advanced non-small-cell lung cancer: Results of a European multicenter trial including 612 patients. J Clin Oncol 12:360.

79. LeChevalier T, Pujol J, Douillard J, et al. (1994b). A three-arm trial of vinorelbine (navelbine) plus cisplatin, vindesine plus cisplatin, and single-agent vinorelbine in the teatment of non-small cell lung cancer: an expanded analysis. Semin Oncol 21(suppl 10):28–34.

80. LeChevalier T, Pujol J, Douillard J, et al. (1997). Six year follow up of the European Multicentre Randomised Study comparing navelbine (NVB) alone vs NVB + cisplatin (CDDP) vs vindesine (VDS) + CDDP in 612 patients with advanced non-small cell lung cancer. Lung Cancer 18(suppl 1):13.

81. Liebmann J, Cook J, Lipschultz C (1993). Cytotoxic studies of paclitaxel (taxol) in human tumor cell lines. Br J Cancer 68:1104–1109.

82. Longeval E, Klastersky J (1982). Combination chemotherapy with cisplatin and etoposide in bronchogenic squamous cell carcinoma and adenocarcinoma. Cancer 50:2751–2756.

83. Lopez-Cabrerizo M, Cardenal F, Artal A, et al. (1997). Gemcitabine plus cisplatin versus etoposide plus cisplatin in advanced non-small cell lung cancer: a randomized trial by the Spanish lung cancer group. Lung Cancer 18(suppl 1):10.

84. Lynch T, Kalish L, Strauss G (1994). Phase II study of topotecan in metastatic non-small-cell lung cancer. J Clin Oncol 12:347.

85. Mackillop W, O'Sullivan B, Ward G (1987). Non-small-cell lung cancer: how oncologists want to be treated. Int J Radiat Oncol Biol Phys 13:929.

86. Marino P, Pampallona S, Preatoni A (1994). Chemotherapy vs supportive care in advanced non-small-cell lung cancer. Results of a meta analysis of the literature. Chest 106:861–865.

87. Mason B, Catalano R (1980). Mitomycin, vinblastine and cisplatin combination chemotherapy in non small cell lung cancer. Proc Am Soc Clin Oncol 21:447.

88. Masters G, Hoffman P, Hsieh A, et al. (1997). Phase I study of vinorelbine and ifosfamide in advanced non-small cell lung cancer. J Clin Oncol 15:884–892.

89. Masuda N, Fukuoka M, Kudoh S, et al. (1992). CPT-11 in combination with cisplatin for advanced non-small cell lung cancer. J Clin Oncol 10:1775–1780.

90. Milward M, Bishop J, Friedlander M, et al. (1996). Phase II trial of a 3-hour infusion of paclitaxel in previously untreated patients with advanced non-small-cell lung cancer. J Clin Oncol 14:142–148.

91. Mountain C (1986). A new international staging system for lung cancer. Chest 89(suppl):225S–233S.

92. Mountain C (1987). The new international staging system for lung cancer. Surg Clin North Am 67:925.

93. Murphy W, Fossella F, Winn R (1993). Phase II study of taxol in patients with untreated advanced non-small-cell lung cancer. J Natl Cancer Inst 8:384.

94. Nakano T, Ikegamis H, Nakamurai S, et al. (1996). A Phase II study of cisplatin, vindesine and continuously infused 5-fluorouracil in the treatment of advanced non-small-cell lung cancer. Br J Cancer 73:1096–1100.

95. Negoro S, Fukuoka M, Masuda N, et al. (1991). Phase I study of weekly intravenous infusion of CPT-11, a new derivative of camptothecin, in the treatment of advanced non-small-cell lung cancer. J Natl Cancer Inst 83:1164.

96. Negoro S, Fukuoka M, Kurita Y, et al. (1994). Results of Phase II studies of gemcitabine in non-small cell lung cancer (abstr). Proc Am Soc Clin Oncol 13:367.

97. O'Connell J, Kris M, Grall R (1986). Frequency and prognostic importance of pretreatment clinical characteristics in patients with advanced non-small lung cancer treated with combination chemotherapy. J Clin Oncol 4:1604–1614.

98. Ohno R, Okada K, Masaoka T, et al. (1990). An early Phase II study of CPT-11: a new derivative of camptothecin, for the treatment of leukemia and lymphoma. J Clin Oncol 8:1907–1912.

99. Parker S, Tong T, Bolden S, Wingo P (1997). Cancer statistics, 1997. CA Cancer J Clin 47:5–27.

100. Perez-Soler R, Fosella F, Gilsson B, et al. (1996). Phase II study of topotecan in patients with advanced non-small cell lung cancer previously untreated with chemotherapy. J Clin Oncol 14:503–513.

101. Perng R, Chen Y, Ming-Liu J, et al. (1997). Gemcitabine versus the combination of cisplatin and etoposide in patients with inoperable non-small cell lung cancer in a Phase II randomized study. J Clin Oncol 15:2097–2102.

102. Quoix E, Dieterman A, Charbonneau J (1988). Disseminated non-small cell lung cancer: a randomized trial of chemotherapy versus palliative care. Lung Cancer 4:A181.

103. Rapp E, Pater J, Willan A (1988). Chemotherapy can prolong survival in patients with advanced non-small-cell lung cancer—report of a Canadian multicenter randomized trial. J Clin Oncol 6:633.

104. Roa V, Conner A, Mitchell R (1996). Carboplatin and paclitaxel for advanced non-small cell lung cancer in previously treated patients. Proc Am Soc Clin Oncol 15:403.

105. Rosell R, Gomea-Codina J, Camps C (1994). A randomized trial comparing pre-operative chemotherapy plus surgery with surgery alone in patients with non-small cell lung cancer. N Engl J Med 330:153.

106. Rosso R, Salvati F, Ardizzoni A (1990). Etoposide versus etoposide plus high-dose cisplatin in the management of advanced non-small cell lung cancer. Cancer 66:130.

107. Roth J, Fossella F, Komaki R (1994). A randomized trial comparing pre-operative chemotherapy and surgery with surgery alone in resectable stage IIIA non-small-cell lung cancer. J Natl Cancer Inst 88:673.

108. Rowinsky E, Gilbert M, McGuire W, et al. (1991). Sequences of taxol and cisplatin: a Phase I and pharmacologic study. J Clin Oncol 9:1692–1703.

109. Rowinsky E, Grochow L, Hendricks C, et al. (1992). Phase I and pharmacologic study of topotecan: a novel topoisomerase inhibitor. J Clin Oncol 10:647–656.

110. Rowinsky E, Sartorious S, Bowling M, et al. (1995). Paclitaxel on a 3-hour schedule and carboplatin in non-small cell lung cancer, use of maximally tolerated and clinically relevant single-agent doses in combination is feasible. Proc Am Soc Clin Oncol 14:354.

111. Ruckdeschel J (1991). Etoposide in the management of non-small cell lung cancer. Cancer 67:250–253.

112. Ruckdeschel J, Finkelstein D, et al. (1985). Chemotherapy for metastatic non-small cell bronchogenic carcinoma: EST:2575, generation V—a randomized comparison of four cisplatin-containing regimens. J Clin Oncol 3:72–79.

113. Ruckdeschel J, Finkelstein D, Ettinger D, et al. (1986). A randomized trial of the four most active regimens for metastatic non-small cell lung cancer. J Clin Oncol 4:14–22.

114. Ruckdeschel J, Wagner H, Williams C, et al. (1994). Second-line chemotherapy for resistant, metastatic non-small cell lung cancer: the role of taxol. Proc Am Soc Clin Oncol 13:357.

115. Saxman S, Loehrer SP, Logie K (1991). Phase II trial of daily oral etoposide in patients with advanced non-small-cell lung cancer. Invest New Drugs 9:253–259.

116. Shepherd F (1994). Treatment of advanced non-small cell lung cancer. Semin Oncol 21(suppl 7):7–18.

117. Shepherd F, Evans W, Goss P, et al. (1992). Ifosfamide, cisplatin and etoposide (ICE) in the treatment of advanced non-small cell lung cancer. Semin Oncol 19(suppl 1):54–58.

118. Shepherd F, Gatzemeier W, Gatfried M, et al. (1993). An extended Phase II study of gemcitabine in non-small cell lung cancer (NSCLC). Proc Am Soc Clin Oncol 12:330.

119. Shepherd F, Burkes R, Cormier Y, et al. (1996). Phase I dose-escalation trial of gemcitabine and cisplatin for advanced non-small cell lung cancer: usefulness of mathematic modeling to determine maximum-tolerable dose. J Clin Oncol 14:1656–1662.

120. Shimada Y, Yostino M, Wakui A, et al. (1991). Phase II study of CPT-11, a new camptothecin derivative, in patients with metastatic colorectal cancer. Proc Am Soc Clin Oncol 10:135.

121. Skarin A, Jochelson M, Sheldon T, et al. (1989). Neoadjuvant chemotherapy in marginally resectable stage III non-small cell lung cancer: long-term follow-up in 41 patients. J Surg Oncol 40:266–274.

122. Sorensen J, Osterlind K, Hansen H (1987a). Vinca alkaloids in the treatment of non-small cell lung cancer. Cancer Treat Rep 14:29–41.

123. Sorensen J, Hansen H, Dombernowsky P, et al. (1987b). Chemotherapy for adenocarcinoma of the lung: a randomized study of vindesine versus lomustine, cyclophosphamide, and methotrexate versus all four drugs. J Clin Oncol 5:1169–1177.

124. Souquet P, Chauvin F, Boissel J, et al. (1993). Polychemotherapy in advanced non-small cell lung cancer: a meta-analysis. Lancet 342:19–21.

125. Spain R (1993). The case for mitomycin in non-small cell lung cancer. Oncology 50(suppl):35–52.

126. Stanley K (1980). Prognostic factors for survival in patients with inoperable lung cancer. J Natl Cancer Inst 65:25–32.

127. Stewart L, Pignon J, Parmar M, et al. (1995). Chemotherapy in non-small cell lung cancer: a meta-analysis using updated data on individual patients from 52 randomized clinical trials. Br Med J 311:899.

128. Strauss G, Lynch T, Elias A, et al. (1995). A Phase I study of ifosfamide/carboplatin/etoposide/paclitaxel in advanced lung cancer. Semin Oncol 22(suppl 9):70–74.

129. Strauss G, Lynch T, Elias A, et al. (1997). Ifosfamide/carboplatin/etoposide/paclitaxel in advanced lung cancer: update and preliminary survival analysis. Semin Oncol 24 (suppl 12):S73–S80.

130. Takeuchi S, Takamizawa H, Takeda Y, et al. (1991). Clinical study of CPT-11, a camptothecin derivative, on gynecological malignancy. Proc Am Soc Clin Oncol 10:189.

131. Thiesse P, Ollivier L, DiStefano-Louineau D, et al. (1997). Response rate accuracy in oncology trials: reasons for interobserver variability. J Clin Oncol 15:3507–3514.

132. Vafai D, Israel V, Zaretsky S, et al. (1995). Phase I/II trial of combination carboplatin and taxol in non-small cell lung cancer (NSCLC). Proc Am Soc Clin Oncol 14:352.

133. Veeder M, Jett J, JQ S (1992). A Phase III trial of mitomycin C alone versus mitomycin C, vinblastine, and cisplatin for metastatic squamous cell lung carcinoma. Cancer 70:2281–2287.

134. Waits T, Johnson D, Hainsworth J (1992). Prolonged administration of oral etoposide in non-small cell lung cancer: a Phase II trial. J Clin Oncol 10:292–296.

135. Weick J, Crowley J, Natale R, et al. (1991). A randomized trial of five cisplatin-containing treatments in patients with metastatic non-small cell lung cancer. A Southwest Oncology Group study. J Clin Oncol 9:1157–1162.

136. Woods R, Williams C, Levi J, et al. (1990). A randomized trial of cisplatin and vindesine versus supportive care only in advanced non-small cell lung cancer. Br J Cancer 61:608–611.

137. Wozniak A, Crowley J, Balcerzak S (1996). Randomized Phase III trial of cisplatin

(CDDP) vs CDDP plus navelbine (NVB) in treatment of advanced non-small cell lung cancer (NSCLC): report of a Southwest Oncology Group study (SWOG-9038) (abstr 1110). Proc Am Soc Clin Oncol 15:374.

138. Zelen M (1973). Keynote address on biostatistics and date retrieval. Cancer Chemother Rep 4:31.

13

Multimodality Therapy for Non-Small-Cell Cancer Metastases to the Brain

RODOLFO HAKIM

Fundación Santa Fe de Bogotá
Bogotá, Columbia

**EBEN ALEXANDER III and
PETER McL. BLACK**

Brigham and Women's Hospital
The Children's Hospital
Boston, Massachusetts

JAY S. LOEFFLER

Harvard Medical School
Massachusetts General Hospital
Boston, Massachusetts

I. Introduction

Within the past few years, significant advances have occurred in the diagnosis and treatment of non-small-cell lung cancer (NSCLC) metastases to the brain. With currently available treatments, most lung cancer patients do not die of their brain metastases; instead, they usually experience effective palliation of neurological symptoms and meaningful extension of life. Future advances in the use of surgery, chemotherapy, radiosurgery, and newer cancer therapy techniques may lead to further increases in the efficacy of treatment for brain metastases.

Surgical excision has been performed in patients with NSCLC brain metastases since the turn of the last century. Results were often discouraging due to the crude techniques available at the time for localization and surgical removal. With improvement in imaging and localization techniques and operative procedures, complication rates have fallen dramatically and survival times have risen. Currently, surgery is accepted as an important part of the management of select patients with brain metastases. Recent series examining heterogeneous groups of patients report survival times of 10 to 14 months (1–4).

For nearly 40 years, radiation therapy has been the mainstay of the treatment of patients with NSCLC brain metastases. Its role has been greatly influenced by improved brain imaging techniques such as CT and MRI. Even though its major goal is the palliation of neurological signs and symptoms, there are selected patients for whom radiotherapy also significantly improves overall survival. Our knowledge of optimal dose fractionation schedules for patients with brain metastases has largely been determined by randomized trials conducted by the Radiation Therapy Oncology Group (RTOG).

This chapter will review how, in patients with solitary NSCLC brain metastases, aggressive CNS therapy prolongs survival and quality of life.

II. Frequency

In the past, brain metastases were believed to occur relatively infrequently. Many previous estimates, based on historical neurosurgical series, suggested that metastases made up only about 10% of the total number of intracranial tumors (5). However, because of the past reluctance of surgeons to operate on patients with known systemic cancer, these older neurosurgical series grossly underestimated the actual occurrence of brain metastases.

Modern neuroimaging techniques and more careful autopsy studies of cancer patients have shown that metastases to the brain, as a group, are actually the most common intracranial tumors in the adult population; they are 10 times more frequent than primary tumors (6–9). At present, brain metastases are estimated to occur in 20% to 40% of cancer patients (6,10); 15% to 30% of these are from NSCLC (11,12). As many as 170,000 new cases of brain metastases occur per year in the United States (13), and these numbers may increase in the future as the ability to detect small tumors with magnetic resonance imaging (MRI) improves and as a result of the longer survival of cancer patients in general.

III. Method of Spread and Distribution from the Lungs

The most common mechanism of metastasis to the brain is by hematogenous spread, usually through the arterial circulation. More than 60% of patients who develop brain metastases also have evidence of either primary lung cancers or known metastases to the lung from a primary tumor located elsewhere (14–17). Intracranial metastases may involve the brain parenchyma, the cranial nerves, the blood vessels (including the dural sinuses), the dura, the leptomeninges, and the inner table of the skull. Of the intracranial metastases of NSCLC, the most common are intraparenchymal metastases, and these will be the main focus of this chapter.

NSCLC metastases, as well as other metastases in the brain, are most commonly found in the area directly beneath the gray-white matter junction (14). The predominance of metastases at this site is due to a change in the diameter of the blood vessels at this point; the narrowed vessels act as a trap for emboli. Brain metastases also tend to be more common at the terminal "watershed areas" of arterial circulation (the zones on the border of or between the territories of the major cerebral vessels). The distribution of metastases among the large subdivisions of the central nervous system follows roughly the relative weight and blood flow to each area. Approximately 80% of brain metastases from lung cancer are located in the cerebral hemispheres, 15% in the cerebellum, and 5% in the brainstem (6,14).

Brain metastases may be single or multiple. The phrase *single brain metastasis* refers to an apparent single cerebral lesion; no implication is made regarding the extent of cancer elsewhere in the body. On the other hand, the phrase *solitary brain metastasis* is properly used to describe the relatively rare occurrence of a single brain metastasis that is the only known site of metastatic cancer in the body. It is not unusual for a patient with a resected lung cancer at a later point in time to develop a solitary brain metastasis.

Whereas in some cancers metastases are often single, NSCLC has a greater tendency to produce multiple cerebral lesions (14,18). Older studies using computed tomography (CT) scan data suggested that brain metastases were single in slightly less than 50% of lung cancer patients (6,14). However, recent studies using MRI have shown that single metastases occur in only one-third to one-fourth of the patients with cerebral metastases (19).

IV. Clinical Manifestations

Brain metastases may be detected before the primary tumor is found (precocious presentation) or at the same time (synchronous presentation), but more commonly the diagnosis of the primary tumor antedates the development of the brain metastasis (metachronous presentation). More than 80% of metastases to the brain from NSCLC are discovered *after* the diagnosis of the primary lung tumor has been made (13).

Since the signs and symptoms related to cerebral lesions resulting from metastases vary, the presence of brain metastases should be suspected in all patients with known systemic cancer who develop new neurological findings. More than two-thirds of patients with cerebral metastases have some neurological symptoms during the course of their illness (6,7,20). Whether gradual or acute in onset, the symptoms are seldom specific enough to allow a definitive diagnosis. Progressive neurological dysfunction is usually related to the gradually expanding tumor mass with associated edema and/or to the development of obstructive hydrocephalus. Occasionally, a more acute onset may occur after a seizure, a hemorrhage into a metastasis, or a stroke (caused by embolization and/or invasion of an artery by tumor cells), or from compression (6,21).

The clinical presentation of NSCLC brain metastases is similar to that of other mass lesions in the brain (Table 1). The four most common symptoms are headaches, cognitive dysfunction, focal weakness, and seizures. Less commonly, gait, speech, or vision disturbances may be the sole complaints.

Table 1 Symptoms (A) and Signs (B) of Brain Metastases in 392 Patients

(A)

Symptom	No. patients	Percent
Headache	163	42
Mental change	121	31
Focal weakness	107	27
Seizure	80	20
Gait ataxia	65	17
Speech problems	40	10
Sensory disturbance	24	6

(B)

Sign	No. patients	Percent
Hemiparesis	174	44
Altered mental status	139	35
Gait ataxia	49	13
Hemisensory loss	36	9
Papilledema	36	9

Source: Pooled data from Refs. 53, 54.

Headaches occur in approximately half of patients with brain metastases; these are often mild, diffuse, or bifrontal, therefore having no localizing value. However, when focal, the headache may be localized at the site of the lesion in as many as 70% of cases. Early-morning headache, believed to be associated with increased intracranial pressure, occurs in less than half of tumor patients with headaches (20). Headaches are more common in patients with multiple metastases and with metastases in the posterior fossa. In the case of posterior fossa metastases, the headache is caused by increased intracranial pressure as the result of brain edema or hydrocephalus stimulating pain-sensitive structures such as the venous sinuses and the dura at the base or back of the skull. The headaches may become more intense upon postural changes (the lower the level of the head is with respect to the level of the heart, the higher the intracranial pressure will be) or straining, and may be associated with other symptoms characteristic of increased intracranial pressure, such as vomiting, visual blurring, confusion, and, rarely, syncope. Papilledema, the classic hallmark of raised intracranial pressure, is now present in <10% percent of patients when they are first diagnosed with cerebral metastases due to the fact that an earlier diagnosis is permitted by readily available neuroimaging.

Memory problems and mood or personality changes are reported by one-third of patients, whereas cognitive dysfunction as detected by standard tests of mental status may be present in as many as 75%. The discrepancy in the frequency of signs and symptoms may be explained by the slowness with which the signs develop, by frank denial, or by neglect when the symptoms involve the nondominant hemisphere.

Focal weakness is the presenting symptom of 20% to 40% of patients. Usually gradual in onset, a hemiparesis may be subtle and may go unnoticed by the patient.

Seizures occur in approximately 10% of patients as the first sign of metastases. However, as many as 40% of patients develop seizures during the course of their disease.

V. Diagnosis

The best diagnostic test for NSCLC brain metastases is contrast-enhanced MRI. This tool is even more sensitive than double-dose delayed-contrast CT scanning (19,22–24).

Imaging findings that favor a diagnosis of metastases include a gray-white junction location, a lesser degree of margin irregularity, and a small tumor nidus with a large amount of associated vasogenic edema (25). Although T2-weighted sequences in MRI are sensitive in showing vasogenic edema as areas of increased signal intensity, not all NSCL metastatic tumors have sufficient edema to be identified (26). Such lesions are typically <5 mm in diameter, may lie next to a larger metastatic lesion, and may be located in the temporal lobes or in the cortical and subcortical areas.

Not all brain lesions found in patients with systemic cancer are metastases. The differential diagnosis includes primary brain tumors (benign or malignant), abscesses, cerebral infarcts, hemorrhages, and demyelinating disease. Contrast-enhanced MRI can usually differentiate among these possibilities, and the finding of multiple lesions is strongly suggestive of metastases. In a recent study of patients with known systemic cancer and single lesions demonstrated by contrast MRI, 11% had lesions other than brain metastases when tissue was obtained (1); half of the nonmetastatic lesions were primary brain tumors while the other half were infections. The false-positive rate for diagnosis of multiple metastases is unknown but is certainly less than the 11% quoted for single metastases. Biopsy is the only truly reliable method of establishing the diagnosis, if any doubt remains after contrast-enhanced imaging studies.

VI. Treatment

Therapeutic decisions require careful evaluation of numerous factors such as: the size, location, and histological features of the tumor; the patient's age, neurological status, and general condition; the likelihood of occult intracranial metastases; the extent of the systemic cancer, as well as its past or potential response to therapy; and possible damage to other organ systems from previous treatment. For surgical candidates, the extent of the systemic disease is the most important variable since its progression is the major cause of death (27); other considerations are neurological status prior to surgery, whether the patient has single or multiple metastases, and the interval between diagnosis of the primary neoplasm and the brain metastasis.

A. Surgery

Surgical excision of a tumor(s) serves three main purposes: first, tissue diagnosis; second, decreasing the mass effect on normal tissue and therefore decreasing elevated intracranial pressure and local irritation; and third, removal of as many tumor cells as possible and therefore prolongation of survival.

Surgery has been used for patients with a single brain metastasis for many years. It has been proven useful in selected patients since 1947, when Flavell resected a symptomatic right temporal lobe metastasis from a patient with a lung mass. The patient underwent a pneumonectomy 8 weeks later (T2N0 squamous carcinoma) and lived >2 years (28). Since that time, several single-institution, retrospective series have documented an improved survival after surgical resection compared to observation alone. Table 2 summarizes several large series published after 1985. Unfortunately, it is difficult to compare different series in the literature for the following reasons: first, many span decades include small cell lung cancer and do not include contrast-enhanced spiral computed tomography or MRI scans to rule out widespread CNS disease; second, several series measure survival from the thoracotomy point of view, which lengthens survival in patients with metachronous lesions; and finally, most series contain small numbers of patients treated with a variety of therapies and therefore make statistical analysis difficult.

1.   Management Determinations for Brain Metastases in General

Even though the advantage of surgical resection in immediately relieving neurological signs and symptoms secondary to tumor mass effect is undeniable, uncontrolled retrospective studies of the overall benefit of surgical resection have shown conflicting results. Some of these studies suggested an advantage in local control and quality of life for patients undergoing surgery and whole-brain radiotherapy when compared to treatment with whole-brain radiotherapy alone.

The publication of Patchell et al. (1) from the University of Kentucky Medical Center was the first study to address this issue in a prospective randomized study with 48 patients. Their results demonstrated that patients with or without active systemic cancer and a single brain metastasis treated with surgical resection (documented by a postoperative enhanced CT scan) combined with whole-brain

Table 2 Literature Review: Isolated Brain Metastases from NSCLC

Location (author)	Inclusion dates	(n)	Median survival (months)	Long-term survival (5-year)	Significance
Henry Ford (Magilligan)	1960–1985	41	13	21% ± 6.5%	Pulmonary wedge resection
Little Rock, AK (Read)	1968–1988	92	24	21%	Combined surgery: craniotomy and thoracotomy
Pisa, Italy (Mussi)	1975–1988	45	19	16%	Pulmonary lobectomy; nodal stage of primary: N0
Sondato, Italy (Rizzi)	1983–1988	21	11	—	Timing: complete resection of primary after craniotomy
Fukuoka, Japan (Ide)	1978–1989	25	6.5	—	Resection of primary
Osaka, Japan (Nakagawa)	1978–1990	89	11.6	—	Resection of primary, histology, Karnofsky >80
Taipei, Taiwan randomized (Chang)	1984–1990	32 / 19 supportive care	7 prospective, 2 $P < .01$		—
Memorial Sloan (Wronski/Arbit)	1976–1991	231	11	12.5%	High Karnofsky, younger age, complete resection of primary, supratentorial location of mets
Univ. Maryland (Hankins)	1964–1994	19	20	45% ± 11.1%	Complete resection of primary; nodal stage: N0 or N1; age: <55 yrs
Brain Tumor Ctr. (Harpole)	1986–1995	113	11	8%	Complete resection of primary; stage of primary: I–II; nodal stage: N0

Source: Pooled data from Refs. 52, 55–65.

radiotherapy (36 Gy/12 fractions) lived longer (40 versus 15 weeks), had fewer local recurrences in the CNS (20% versus 52%), and had a better quality of life than patients treated with the same dose of whole-brain radiotherapy alone. The median time to recurrence for the group treated with surgery plus radiotherapy was 59 weeks, compared to 21 weeks for the group treated with whole-brain radiotherapy alone. In a multivariate analysis, the factors significant for increased survival were surgical treatment of the metastasis, the absence of extracranial disease, longer time to the development of the brain metastasis, and younger age. All patients who were randomized to radiotherapy alone underwent stereotactic biopsy to confirm the diagnosis of cancer (of note, 6/54 or 11% of patients at surgical resection or biopsy had a diagnosis other than metastatic disease and were excluded from the study). Most investigators would have anticipated an advantage in local control in the CNS for those patients treated with complete surgical resection plus whole-brain radiotherapy compared to patients treated with the same dose of whole-brain radiotherapy alone. This study has led to a substantial degree of debate in the neuro-oncology community regarding the appropriate therapy for patients with a single brain metastasis (29); some have interpreted the data as an indication to recommend surgery for all patients; others have argued that, by using higher doses of radiotherapy, results similar to those achieved with surgery and radiotherapy could be obtained.

A recently published series by Noordijk and associates from Holland (30) also randomized patients ($n = 66$) to surgery and whole-brain radiotherapy versus whole-brain radiotherapy alone. The total radiotherapy was 40 Gy in 20 fractions (200 cGy b.i.d.) for a total of 2 weeks of therapy. The major endpoint of this study was, like Patchell's, overall survival with an advantage being demonstrated for those patients undergoing surgical resection and whole-brain radiotherapy as compared with whole-brain radiotherapy alone (median 10 vs. 6 months; $P = .04$). The largest difference in survival was found in the patients with inactive extracranial disease, with a median survivals of 12 and 7 months for combined treatment and radiotherapy alone, respectively. In a subset analysis (accepting the potential pitfalls of this statistical method), older patients (>60 years) and patients with active extracranial disease did not appear to benefit from the addition of surgery. It is not surprising that older patients had decreased survival rates compared to their younger counterparts since it is well known that older age is one of the most important adverse prognostic factors for patients with a wide variety of intracranial histologies both primary and metastatic.

A factor that greatly influences determining the viability of resectability is the number of metastases. As late as 1990, most neuro-oncologists and neurosurgeons considered surgery for multiple metastases justified in only rare instances. Indeed, the consensus was that the presence of multiple lesions strongly contraindicated surgery and that the circumstances precipitating the rare decisions to operate on multiple metastases were limited to a life-threatening mass effect on the brainstem, an unknown diagnosis, or two or more lesions that could be removed through a single cranial opening (31). However, surgical benefits have been considerably expanded with the technical advances that have occurred in the past few years.

Our recent evaluation of the efficacy of surgery for patients with multiple lesions revealed that surgery offers an important option for managing these patients (4). Fifty-six patients who underwent surgery for multiple brain metastases were divided into two groups: group A, those who had one or more lesions remaining after surgery ($N = 30$); and group B, those who had all lesions removed ($N = 26$). Patients in group B were matched by type of primary tumor, presence or absence of systemic disease, and time from first diagnosis of cancer to diagnosis of brain metastases, to a group of patients undergoing surgery for a single lesion (group C; $N = 26$). Median survivals were 6, 14, and 14 months for patients in groups A, B, and C, respectively. Besides the significant difference in survival rates between groups A and B and groups A and C, there was a significant correspondence in recurrence or neurologic improvement rates between groups B and C, indicating that surgery for patients with multiple metastatic lesions that can all be removed is as effective as surgery for a single lesion. Patients in whom all lesions cannot be surgically excised may also be surgical candidates of resection of one or more highly symptomatic, debilitating, or life-threatening lesions can produce greater and more rapid palliation of symptoms than might be achieved by radiation alone.

2. Reoperation for Recurrent Metastatic Brain Tumors

Unfortunately, 31% to 48% of surgically treated patients will develop recurrence in the brain. Treatment for recurrence following surgical resection and radiation therapy must be carefully considered, and the options are limited. In 1988, Sundaresan et al. (32) evaluated the value of reextirpation and found that neurologic improvement was accomplished in 66% of the patients, with a median duration of 6 months, no mortality, and only one instance (5%) of increased deficit. Repeat resection was recommended as an important therapeutic option in symptomatic patients with accessible lesions before using other experimental treatments.

In 1992, Kaye suggested that the considerations for deciding on reoperation should include the length of time since the initial operation, the intracerebral location of the recurrence, radiosensitivity of the tumor, systemic spread of the tumor, and age and performance status of the patient. He noted that the shorter the tumor-free interval, the less likelihood of a successful period of palliation following further resection (33).

3. Complications

Operative complications must always be considered in a discussion of surgical therapy. Causes of operative mortality (death within 30 days of operation) are often related to herniation due to edema and increased intracranial pressure, hemorrhage in the operative site or in other metastatic foci, uncontrolled systemic cancer, or thromboembolic phenomena such as pulmonary embolism. Complications such as hematomas, infections, and pseudomeningocele formation occur in 8% to 9% of all craniotomies for brain metastases (4). An estimated 10% of patients will develop clinically evident thromboembolic complications such as deep vein thrombosis or pulmonary embolism (34). Because death from uncontrolled systemic NSCLC is not related to the brain, the rate of postoperative mortality is not entirely due to the neurosurgical operation.

Almost all studies of patients treated after the mid-1970s show an operative mortality of <10%. Recent studies report an operative mortality rate of 3% or less. Surgical mortality has been reported to vary with the extent of removal of the brain metastasis: gross total removal of a metastasis gives a lower rate of operative mortality than partial resection. Patients undergoing partial resection may have a doubled 30-day mortality risk (35). Therefore, the goal of any operation should be gross total tumor removal whenever possible.

Surgical morbidity (increased postoperative neurologic deficits) is more difficult to quantify than surgical mortality due to the somewhat subjective nature of determination. Recent reports indicate that morbidity is generally 5% or lower (1,2,4,36).

B. Radiation Therapy

The major result of radiation is the improvement of specific neurological symptoms. The overall published response rate is symptom-dependent, but ranges from 70% to 90% (37). Over half the patients with headaches, seizures, or symptoms of increased intracranial pressure have a complete response to whole-brain radiotherapy, although the duration of response continues for 1 year in only 65% of patients. Cranial nerve deficits will improve in approximately 40% of patients, but the potential for improvement is directly related to the interval from diagnosis to radiotherapy (37). Patients with known systemic NSCLC with new cranial nerve(s) deficits should undergo contrast-enhanced MRI within 24 hours if possible. The expected improvement of neurological function is dependent on the function class at the time of initiation of whole-brain radiotherapy (38).

1. Postoperative Radiotherapy

Even in 1997, the ultimate role of postoperative whole-brain radiation therapy as an adjuvant treatment to surgery has not been clearly defined. Theoretically, postoperative radiotherapy is expected to destroy microscopic residual NSCLC cells at the site of resection and at other locations in the brain if they exist, therefore reducing the recurrence rate and prolonging survival.

Although most authors recommend postoperative whole-brain radiotherapy for intracranial metastases in general, only four retrospective studies have specifically examined this question (39–42). Three of these studies have demonstrated that recurrence rate is, indeed, reduced by adjuvant whole-brain radiotherapy (41,42). Only one of these studies indicated that survival was also significantly extended for patients receiving whole-brain radiotherapy (42). The patients in this study were operated on between 1972 and 1982, and it is unclear whether all patients were evaluated with CT scan. Without such evaluation, it is obvious that many patients suspected of having had a single metastasis would, in fact, harbor multiple lesions. In such patients there would be an obvious advantage to receiving adjuvant whole-brain radiotherapy.

Survival is not always extended since the status of the systemic disease is its most important indicator in surgically treated patients. It is interesting to note that the only study that failed to detect any beneficial effect of radiotherapy (40), either in reducing recurrence or extending survival, also examined patients with no evidence of systemic disease at the time of craniotomy.

The most important argument against the routine use of postoperative whole-brain radiotherapy involves the significant risk of radiation-induced cognitive changes and other long-term neurotoxicity. One of the most important benefits of surgical excision of brain metastasis is the significant chance some patients have of becoming long-term survivors. If these patients are rendered neurocognitively impaired by whole-brain radiotherapy given at the time of craniotomy, the value of surgery is greatly diminished.

2. Reirradiation

Occasionally, patients are reirradiated with whole-brain or partial-brain radiotherapy at the time of recurrence. The percentage of patients who undergo reirradiation is quite small since most patients who recur within the CNS also have progressive extracranial disease and are treated with supportive measures only. A review of three series with a combined experience involving 189 patients was recently published (37). The overall clinical response rate ranged from 42% to 75% with a median survival from the time of reirradiation of between 3.5 and 5 months. Although there is no consensus on reirradiation with conventional techniques (43), some investigators have argued that reirradiation should be considered for patients who remain in good general condition but experience neurological deterioration 4 or more months after a satisfactory response to the initial course of whole-brain radiotherapy (44). Even though brain tolerance is probably exceeded by reirradiation (45), few clinical data exist documenting the effects of this approach since the expected survival is so limited. If reirradiation is being considered, radiosurgery (see below) is probably the best radiotherapeutic approach since the amount of normal brain reirradiated is significantly reduced with these highly sophisticated radiation delivery systems.

3. Radiosurgery

Radiosurgery is a technique of external irradiation that utilizes multiple collimated convergent beams to deliver stereotactically a high single dose of radiation to a small target volume (46). The hallmark of this technique is the rapid dose fall-off at the target edges. The radiobiologic effects of radiosurgery are associated with small blood vessel thrombosis, reproductive cell death, or growth arrest (47). The development of pathological and/or clinical radionecrosis is not a required outcome for radiosurgery to be successful (48).

It is clear that a more aggressive treatment than standard whole-brain radiotherapy is warranted in younger patients who present with a single NSCLC brain lesion without evidence of progressive extracranial disease. Some investigators believe that radiosurgery can serve as a surgical alternative (49,50). The biological and physical characteristics of metastases (radiographically discrete, small, spherical, and noninvasive) appear to make them ideal radiosurgery targets (51). Results obtained by treating metastases with radiosurgery indicate local control is obtained in 73% to 98% of patients, with median follow-up of 5 to 26 months (46). In multi-institutional trial involving 116 patients treated with radiosurgery for single brain metastases using a mean dose of 17.5 Gy, local tumor control was obtained in 99 patients (85%) (50). The 2-year actuarial tumor control rates for the whole group was 67% ± 8% with a plateau in the curve at 18 months. In a multivariate analysis, better local control was obtained in patients who received whole-brain radiotherapy in addition to radiosurgery, and in patients with "radioresistant" histologies (melanoma and renal cell carcinoma).

VII.   Solitary NSCLC Brain Metastases—Brigham and Women's Hospital Experience (52)

The tumor database of patients treated for brain metastases from NSCLC at the Brain Tumor Center at Brigham and Women's Hospital and Dana-Farber Institute was searched from October 15, 1986, to June 8, 1995. There were 260 patients with NSCLC treated for brain metastases, of whom 113 (43.46%) had isolated brain metastases (documented radiologically). There were 63 females (56%) and 50 males (44%) with a mean age of 57 ± 9 years (range, 36 to 75 years). The histopathological diagnosis and stage of the lung cancer primary is shown in Table 3.

Of the 113 patients with isolated brain metastases, 63 patients had a single lesion and 50 patients had multiple lesions (two to seven); for the entire group the median was two (range, one to seven). Sixty patients (53.10%) had a metachronous presentation of the brain metastases diagnosed at a median time of 20 months (range, 6 to 180 months) posttreatment of the lung primary, while 53 patients (46.90%) had a synchronous presentation. Sixty-four (57%) of the 113 patients

Table 3 Histopathology and Stage of the
NSCLC Primary

Histology	n	%
Adenocarcinoma	67	59%
Squamous	24	21%
Large cell undifferentiated	13	12%
Non-small-cell, not typed	9	8%
Stage		
I (T1–2N0)	43	38%
II (T1–2N1)	13	12%
IIIA (T3N0–2, T1–2N2)	44	38%
IIIB (T3Nx, T1–2N3)	13	12%

had a clinical presentation with one or more of the following neurological symptoms: headache (45 patients, 40%); dizziness and/or ataxia (23 patients, 20%); and seizures (18 patients, 16%).

A. Treatment and Outcome

As the initial treatment, all patients underwent whole-brain radiation therapy (WBRT) in fraction sizes of 150 to 200 cGy for a median total of 3000 cGy (range, 2400 to 5000 cGy). For the second part of the treatment, 52 patients (46%) had surgical resection to a median of one lesion (range, one to seven), and the remaining 61 patients (54%) received stereotactic radiosurgery with a median dose of 1800 cGy (range, 1330 to 2494 cGy). The lesion sizes treated with either surgical resection or radiosurgery were 2.3 ± 1.3 cm in diameter (range, 0.5 to 7.0 cm). Clinical and radiological (head MRI) follow-up was obtained every 3 to 4 months in the multidisciplinary Brain Tumor Clinic or through referring physicians.

There were two perioperative deaths: one patient died from aspiration pneumonia and sepsis on postoperative day 23, and the second patient died from aspiration pneumonia and myocardial infarction on day 24. The median follow-up interval for the remaining 111 patients was 26 months (range, 14 to 101 months). Nineteen patients (16.8%) were alive at the last follow-up: 13 patients (11.5%) were disease-free, and six patients (5.3%) had a recurrence (five in the brain and one elsewhere). Ninety-two patients (81.4%) were dead: 91 patients (80.5%) died from recurrent NSCLC (75% of these were in the brain), and one patient (0.9%) died of a myocardial infarction without evidence of active disease.

Survival time was calculated from the date of surgery (craniotomy or SRS) until the date of death or last follow-up. The 2-year overall survival after the brain metastases treatment was 33% (median 11 months) (Fig. 1). Univariate and multi-variate survival analyses (Table 4) (1,2) demonstrated a survival benefit for patients who had a complete resection of the lung primary ($n = 86$, median 16 months; $P = .001$) (Fig. 2a), for those with a stage I or II lung tumor ($n = 56$, median 18 months; $P = .004$) (Fig. 2b), and also for the patients with negative intrathoracic lymph nodes ($n = 50$, median 18 months; $P = 0.01$) (Fig. 2c). Survival was unaffected by: timing of presentation of brain metastases and the primary (synchronous versus metachronous), the number of brain metastases treated, the type of therapy utilized (surgical resection vs. radiosurgery), and histology (adenocarcinoma, squamous, and large cell). These data may suggest that systemic disease rather than metastases is the crucial determinant of survival.

VIII. Summary

In summary, there is compelling evidence to suggest that aggressive local therapy for patients with isolated NSCLC brain metastases improves survival and quality of life. One of the most important factors for an extended survival is the stage of the lung primary (stage I or II) and therefore its resectability. The results from the Brigham and Women's Hospital conclude that patients with a low-stage non-small-cell lung primary and isolated brain metastases (single or multiple) should be treated aggressively with a total resection of the lung primary; whole-brain radiation therapy plus surgical resection or radiosurgery is the treatment of choice for the metastatic brain lesion(s).

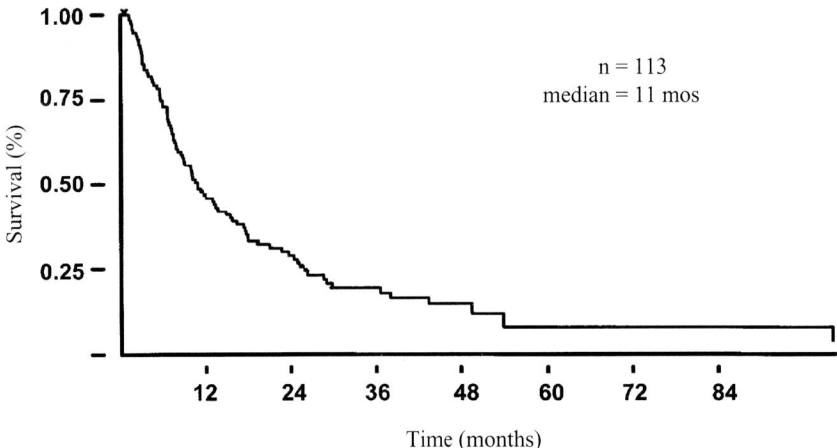

Figure 1   Kaplan-Meier of overall cancer-specific survival for the 113 patients.

Table 4 Survival Analysis

(A) Univariate Analysis Variable	n	Median survival (months)	P value
Resection			
Complete	86	14	
Biopsy	27	6	.0010
Stage			
I or II	56	17	
III	57	7	.0011
Nodal status			
Negative	50	16	
Positive	63	7	.0013
Vascular invasion at resection			
Absent	26	16	
Present	31	13	.12
Number of metastases			
1	63	12	
2–7	50	10	.2
Presentation			
Synchronous	53	11	
Metachronous	60	10	.2
Brain therapy type			
Resection	52	11	
Radiosurgery	61	12	.2

(B) Multivariate Analysis Variable	Risk ratio	Confidence interval	P value
Stage I or II	1.32	1.02–1.69	.040
No positive nodes	1.54	0.98–2.58	.070

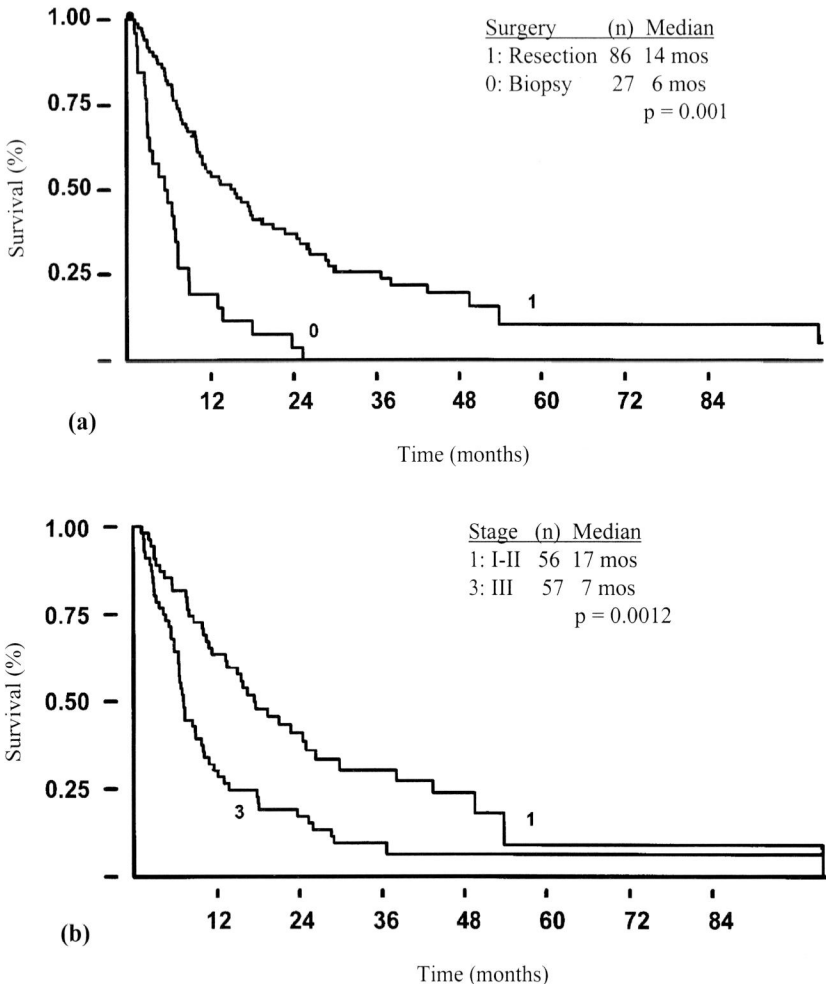

Figure 2 Actuarial graphs demonstrating an improvement in survival for the patients who (a) underwent a complete resection of the lung primary, (b) had a stage I–II lung tumor, and/or (c) had negative lymph nodes.

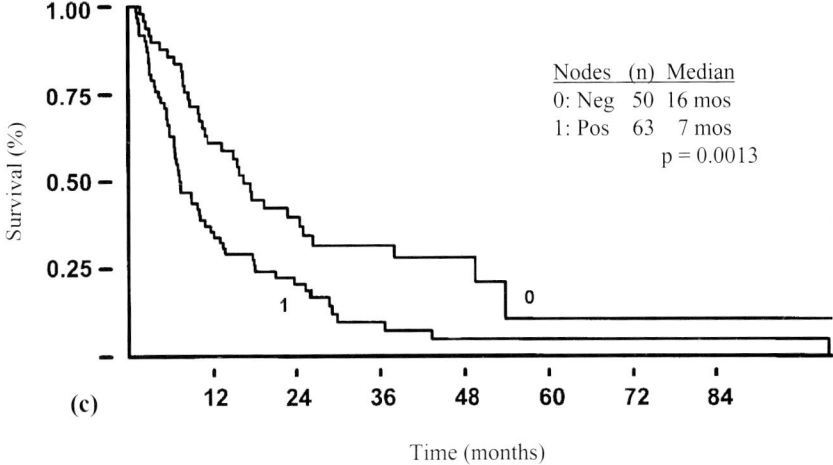

(c)

Time (months)

References

1. Patchell RA, Tibbs PA, Walsh JW, et al. A randomized trial of surgery in the treatment of single metastases to the brain (see comments). N Engl J Med 1990; 322:494–500.

2. Sundaresan N, Galicich JH. Surgical treatment of brain metastases. Clinical and computerized tomography evaluation of the results of treatment. Cancer 1985; 55:1382–1388.

3. Ferrara M, Bizzozzero L, Talamonti G, D'Angelo VA. Surgical treatment of 100 single brain metastases. Analysis of the results. J Neurosurg Sci 1990; 34:303–308.

4. Bindal RK, Sawaya R, Leavens ME, Lee JJ. Surgical treatment of multiple brain metastases. J Neurosurg 1993; 79:210–216.

5. Earle K. Metastatic and primary intracranial tumors of the adult male. J Neuropathol Exp Neurol 1954; 13:448–454.

6. Cairncross JG, Posner JB. The management of brain metastases. In: MD Walker, ed. Oncology of the Nervous System. Boston: Nijhoff, 1983:341–377.

7. Posner JB. Diagnosis and treatment of metastases to the brain. Clin Bull 1974; 4:47–57.

8. Takakura K, Sano K, Hojo S, Hirano A. Metastatic Tumors of the Central Nervous System. Tokyo: Igaku Shoin, 1982.

9. Walker AE, Robins M, Weinfeld FD. Epidemiology of brain tumors: the national survey of intracranial neoplasms. Neurology 1985; 35:219–226.

10. Posner J. Neurologic complications of cancer. Philadelphia: F. A. Davis Company, 1995.

11. Ochsner H, DeBakey M. Significance of metastasis in primary carcinoma of the lungs: report of two cases with unusual site of metastasis. J Thorac Surg 1942; 11:357–387.

12. Olson KB. Primary carcinoma of the lung. Am J Pathol 1935; 11:449–468.
13. Posner JB. Management of brain metastases. Rev Neurol 1992; 148:477–487.
14. Delattre JY, Krol G, Thaler HT, Posner JB. Distribution of brain metastases. Arch Neurol 1988; 45:741–744.
15. Galluzzi S, Payne P. Brain metastases from primary bronchial carcinoma: a statistical study of 741 necropsies. Br J Cancer 1956; 10:408–414.
16. Benton J, Steckel R, Kagan A. Diagnostic imaging in clinical cancer management: brain metastases. Invest Radiol 1988; 23:335–341.
17. Saphner T, Gallion HH, Van Nagell JR, Kryscio R, Patchell RA. Neurologic complications of cervical cancer. A review of 2261 cases. Cancer 1989; 64:1147–1151.
18. Dropcho EJ. Management of multiple brain metastases. In: VC Hachinski, ed. Challenges in Neurology. Philadelphia: F. A. Davis Company, 1992:269–281.
19. Sze G, Milano E, Johnson C, Heier L. Detection of brain metastases: comparison of contrast-enhanced MR with unenhanced MR and enhanced CT. Am J Neuroradiol 1990; 11:785–791.
20. Posner JB. Clinical manifestations of brain metastasis. In: Weiss LGH, Posner JB, eds. Brain Metastases. Boston: G. K. Hall and Company, 1980:189–207.
21. Nutt SH, Patchell RA. Intracranial hemorrhage associated with primary and secondary tumors. Neurosurg Clin North Am 1992; 3:591–599.
22. Yuh WT, Engelken JD, Muhonen MG, Mayr NA, Fisher DJ, Ehrhardt JC. Experience with high-dose gadolinium MR imaging in the evaluation of brain metastases. Am J Neuroradiol 1992; 13:335–345.
23. Davis PC, Hudgins PA, Peterman SB, Hoffman J Jr. Diagnosis of cerebral metastases: double-dose delayed CT vs contrast-enhanced MR imaging. Am J Neuroradiol 1991; 12:293–300.
24. Runge VM, Kirsch JE, Burke VJ, et al. High-dose gadoteridol in MR imaging of intracranial neoplasms. J Magn Reson Imaging 1992; 2:9–18.
25. Williams AL. Tumors. In: Williams AL, Haughton VM, eds. Cranial Computed Tomography: A Comprehensive Text. St. Louis: C. V. Mosby, 1985:17–29.
26. Price AC, Runge VM, Babigian GV. Brain; neoplastic disease. In: Runge VM, ed. Clinical Magnetic Resonance Imaging. Philadelphia: Lippincott, 1990:113–175.
27. Galicich JH, Sundaresan N, Arbit E, Passe S. Surgical treatment of single brain metastasis: factors associated with survival. Cancer 1980; 45:381–386.
28. Flavell G. Solitary cerebral metastases from bronchial carcinomata: their incidence in case of successful removal. Br Med J 1949; 2:736–737.
29. Loeffler JS, Shrieve DC. What is appropriate therapy for a patient with a single brain metastasis? (editorial; comment) (see comments). Int J Radiat Oncol Biol Phys 1994; 29:915–917; discussion 920.
30. Noordijk EM, Vecht CJ, Haaxma-Reiche H, et al. The choice of treatment of single brain metastasis should be based on extracranial tumor activity and age (see comments). Int J Radiat Oncol Biol Phys 1994; 29:711–717.
31. Patchell RA. Brain metastases. Neurol Clin 1991; 9:817–824.
32. Sundaresan N, Sachdev V, DiGiacinto G. Reoperation for brain metastasis. J Clin Oncol 1988; 6:1625–1629.
33. Kaye A. Malignant brain tumors. In: Little J, Awad I, eds. Reoperative Neurosurgery. Baltimore: Williams and Wilkins, 1992:49–76.

34. Constantini S, Kornowski R, Pomeranz S, Rappaport ZH. Thromboembolic phenomena in neurosurgical patients operated upon for primary and metastatic brain tumors. Acta Neurochir 1991; 109:93–97.
35. Haar F, Patterson RH. Surgery for metastatic intracranial neoplasms. Cancer 1972; 30:1241–1245.
36. Brega K, Robinson WA, Winston K, Wittenberg W. Surgical treatment of brain metastases in malignant melanoma. Cancer 1990; 66:2105–2110.
37. Coia LR. The role of radiation therapy in the treatment of brain metastases. Int J Radiat Oncol Biol Phys 1992; 23:229–238.
38. Borgelt B, Gelber R, Kramer S, et al. The palliation of brain metastases: final results of the first two studies by the Radiation Therapy Oncology Group. Int J Radiat Oncol Biol Phys 1980; 6:1–9.
39. DeAngelis LM, Mandell LR, Thaler HT, et al. The role of postoperative radiotherapy after resection of single brain metastases. Neurosurgery 1989; 24:798–805.
40. Dosoretz DE, Blitzer PH, Russell AH, Wang CC. Management of solitary metastasis to the brain: the role of elective brain irradiation following complete surgical resection. Int J Radiat Oncol Biol Phys 1980; 6:1727–1730.
41. Hagen NA, Cirrincione C, Thaler HT, DeAngelis LM. The role of radiation therapy following resection of single brain metastasis from melanoma. Neurology 1990; 40:158–160.
42. Smalley SR, Schray MF, Laws E Jr, O'Fallon JR. Adjuvant radiation therapy after surgical resection of solitary brain metastasis: association with pattern of failure and survival. Int J Radiat Oncol Biol Phys 1987; 13:1611–1616.
43. Coia LR, Aaronson N, Linggood R, Loeffler J, Priestman TJ. A report of the consensus workshop panel on the treatment of brain metastases. Int J Radiat Oncol Biol Phys 1992; 23:223–227.
44. Cooper JS, Steinfeld AD, Lerch IA. Cerebral metastases: value of reirradiation in selected patients. Radiology 1990; 174:883–885.
45. Schultheiss TE, Kun LE, Ang KK, Stephens LC. Radiation response of the central nervous system (see comments) (published erratum appears in Int J Radiat Oncol Biol Phys 1995; 32(4):1269). Int J Radiat Oncol Biol Phys 1995; 31:1093–1112.
46. Loeffler JS, Flickinger JC, Shrieve DC, et al. Radiosurgery for the treatment of intracranial lesions. In: Devita VT, Hellman S, Rosemberg SA, eds. Important Advances in Oncology. Philadelphia: JP Lippincott, 1995:141–156.
47. Larson DA, Flickinger JC, Loeffler JS. The radiobiology of radiosurgery (editorial; comment). Int J Radiat Oncol Biol Phys 1993; 25:557–561.
48. Loeffler JS, Larson DA. Radiosurgery in the management of intracranial lesions: a radiation oncology perspective. In: Dewey WC, Edington M, Fry RJM, Hall EJ, Whitmore GF, eds. Radiation Research: A Twentieth-Century Perspective. San Diego, CA: Harcourt Brace Jovanovich, 1992:535–540.
49. Mehta MP, Rozental JM, Levin AB, et al. Defining the role of radiosurgery in the management of brain metastases. Int J Radiat Oncol Biol Phys 1992; 24:619–625.
50. Flickinger JC, Kondziolka D, Lunsford LD, et al. A multi-institutional experience with stereotactic radiosurgery for solitary brain metastasis (see comments). Int J Radiat Oncol Biol Phys 1994; 28:797–802.

51. Loeffler JS, Kooy HM, Wen PY, et al. The treatment of recurrent brain metastases with stereotactic radiosurgery (see comments). J Clin Oncol 1990; 8:576–582.

52. Harpole D, Amos A, Alexander E III, et al. Stage of the primary is important when treating isolated brain metastases from lung cancer (meeting abstract). Proc Annu Meet Am Soc Clin Oncol 1996; 15:A1143.

53. Cairncross JG, Kim JH, Posner JB. Radiation therapy for brain metastases. Ann Neurol 1980; 7:529–541.

54. Zimm S, Wampler GL, Stablein D, Hazra T, Young HF. Intracerebral metastases in solid-tumor patients: natural history and results of treatment. Cancer 1981; 48:384–394.

55. Hankins JR, Miller JE, Salcman M, et al. Surgical management of lung cancer with solitary cerebral metastasis. Ann Thorac Surg 1988; 46:24–28.

56. Magilligan D Jr, Duvernoy C, Malik G, Lewis J Jr, Knighton R, Ausman JI. Surgical approach to lung cancer with solitary cerebral metastasis: twenty-five years' experience. Ann Thorac Surg 1986; 42:360–364.

57. Read RC, Boop WC, Yoder G, Schaefer R. Management of non-small cell lung carcinoma with solitary brain metastasis (see comments). J Thorac Cardiovasc Surg 1989; 98:884–890; discussion 890–891.

58. Rizzi A, Tondini M, Rocco G, et al. Lung cancer with a single brain metastasis: therapeutic options. Tumori 1990; 76:579–581.

59. Ide Y, Oka K, Tsuchimochi H, Mizoguchi T, Fukushima T, Tomonaga M, Shirakusa T. Surgical results of brain metastasis from lung cancer—prognostic factors. Neurol Med Chir 1991; 31:18–23.

60. Chang D, Yang RC, Luh K, Kuo SH, Hong R, Lee LN. Late survival of non-small cell lung cancer patients with brain metastases. Chest 1992; 101:1293–1297.

61. Wronski M, Burt M. Results and prognostic factors of surgery in the management of non-small cell lung cancer with solitary brain metastasis (letter; comment). Cancer 1992; 70:2021–2023.

62. Nakagawa H, Miyawaki Y, Fujita T, et al. Surgical treatment of brain metastases of lung cancer: retrospective analysis of 89 cases. J Neurol Neurosurg Psychiatry 1994; 57:950–956.

63. Mussi A, Pistolesi M, Lucchi M, et al. Resection of single brain metastasis in non-small-cell lung cancer: prognostic factors. J Thorac Cardiovasc Surg 1996; 112:146–153.

64. Arbit E, Wronski M, Burt M, Galicich JH. The treatment of patients with recurrent brain metastases. A retrospective analysis of 109 patients with non-small cell lung cancer. Cancer 1995; 76:765–773.

65. Alexander E III, Moriarty TM, Davis RB, et al. Stereotactic radiosurgery for the definitive, noninvasive treatment of brain metastases. J Natl Cancer Inst 1995; 87:34–40.

14

Laboratory Models to Evaluate New Agents for the Systemic Treatment of Lung Cancer

BEVERLY A. TEICHER*

Lilly Research Laboratories
Indianapolis, Indiana

EMIL FREI III

Dana-Farber Cancer Institute and the
Joint Center for Radiation Therapy
Harvard Medical School
Boston, Massachusetts

I. Introduction

Lung cancer is among the most commonly occurring malignancies in the world. Lung cancers may grow at the primary site for some time before invading the vascular and lymphatic channels, allowing spread to lymph nodes and distant metastatic sites. The most frequent sites of metastases are bone, liver, adrenals, and brain; however, autopsy studies have found lung cancer metastases in every organ system (1). For many years lung cancer was treated primarily with surgery and/or radiation therapy to local sites of disease. Since the 1980s, however, the treatment of lung cancer has seen increasing use of combined-modality approaches to therapy directed toward specific stage disease with combination chemotherapy being administered prior to and/or after surgery or prior to, during, and/or after radiation therapy. These newer approaches to treatment have resulted in improving survival rates in these very difficult malignancies, and have opened up lung cancer as a disease suitable for investigative approaches.

In the laboratory, as in the clinic, lung cancer is very difficult to cure with current therapies. The model systems available for preclinical studies of lung cancer may be categorized as cell lines grown in culture and tumor lines grown in a host organism. However, for the purpose of this review, a more useful characterization of the models for lung cancer is:

---

*Formerly at Dana-Farber Cancer Institute and the Joint Center for Radiation Therapy, Boston, Massachusetts.

1. Syngeneic systems in which a tumor is grown in the host in which the tumor arose. Syngeneic model systems are usually fully functional immunologically and allow the process of metastasis to proceed, as occurs in patients.

2. Xenograft systems in which human lung cancer is grown in cell culture or in an immune-deficient animal, usually a nude or SCID mouse. Xenograft model systems allow human lung cancer tumor cells to be studied in isolation in culture or in an immunocompromised murine host where tumor nodules will grow but rarely metastasize.

II. Syngeneic Models: Lewis Lung Carcinoma

This tumor originated spontaneously as a carcinoma of the lung of a C57BL mouse in 1951 in the laboratory of Dr. Margaret R. Lewis at the Wistar Institute. The Lewis lung carcinoma was among the earliest transplantable tumors used to identify new anticancer agents. Sugiura and Stock found that the Lewis lung carcinoma produced tumors 100% of the time, producing a very malignant carcinoma. These investigators at the Sloan-Kettering Institute for Cancer Research used the Lewis lung carcinoma along with several other transplantable tumors to determine the antitumor activity of a series of phosphoramides from which the antitumor alkylating agent thiotepa emerged (2–4). Twenty years later, DeWys, working at the Strong Memorial Hospital of the University of Rochester School of Medicine, standardized techniques for following primary tumor growth by tumor volume measurements and for assessing the response of lung metastases to a therapeutic intervention (5). DeWys observed the Gompersian pattern of primary tumor growth, effects of tumor burden on therapeutic efficacy, and effects of the presence of the primary tumor on the growth rate of the lung metastases (6). Dr. G. Gordon Steel and coinvestigators continued working with the Lewis lung carcinoma and in the mid- and late 1970s developed culture colony formation techniques, lung colony formation techniques, and limiting dilution techniques to assess tumor response to new anticancer drugs and radiation therapy (7,8).

This syngeneic tumor system mimics the human disease in that from the primary tumor it metastasizes to lungs, bone, and liver. It is nonimmunogenic and is grown in a host with a fully functional immune system. The rate of tumor growth is relatively rapid with a tumor volume doubling time of 2.5 days and is lethal in 21 to 25 days. Although this growth rate is rapid, it is in line with the life span of the host, which is about 2 years.

The following sections will illustrate the value of the Lewis lung carcinoma model to assess new anticancer drugs and combinations (gemcitabine and navelbine), new therapeutic approaches (antiangiogenic therapy), and immunotherapy (interleukin-12).

A. Gemcitabine and Navelbine

Gemcitabine (LY18801; 2′,2′-difluorodeoxycytidine) is an analog of the natural pyrimidine. The mechanism of action and metabolism of gemcitabine has been well characterized (9,10). Deoxycytidine kinase activates gemcitabine to gemcitabine monophosphate, gemcitabine diphosphate, and gemcitabine triphosphate. The triphosphate competes with deoxycytidine triphosphate for incorporation into DNA and results in chain termination 1 bp beyond the point of insertion (10,11). The addition of a base pair after gemcitabine triphosphate protects this lesion from excision by exonucleases. Gemcitabine cytotoxicity is proportional to the intracellular concentration of gemcitabine triphosphate and its incorporation into DNA. The diphosphate of gemcitabine exerts a time- and concentration-dependent inhibition of the enzyme ribonucleotide reductase, thereby diminishing intracellular deoxycytidine triphosphate and enhancing the incorporation of gemcitabine triphosphate into DNA (9). In cell culture, gemcitabine causes accumulation of cells in the S phase of the cell cycle (9,12,13). Gemcitabine is active against a number of solid tumors in vitro and has demonstrated activity against many solid tumor models including the CX-1 human colon cancer xenograft and the LX-1 human lung carcinoma xenograft in nude mice (11–14). In Phase I human trials, gemcitabine has been evaluated in a variety of schedules. The greatest efficacy with the least toxicity has been demonstrated with a weekly schedule (9). In Phase II human trials, gemcitabine has demonstrated activity against small-cell lung, non-small-cell lung, breast, ovarian, pancreatic, myeloma, prostatic, renal, and bladder cancer (15,16). Gemcitabine has demonstrated a 22% objective tumor response rate in a database of 331 patients diagnosed with non-small-cell lung cancer receiving drug on a weekly schedule in a dose range of 800 mg/m^2 to 1250 mg/m^2.

Vinorelbine (navelbine) is a new, semisynthetic vinca alkaloid whose antitumor activity is related to its ability to depolymerize microtubules which dissolve the mitotic spindles (17–22). Its activity in cell culture was equal to or greater than other vinca alkaloids (22). Vinorelbine was as effective as vinblastine against A2780 human ovarian carcinoma cell lines and was more cytotoxic than other vinca alkaloids against a human bronchial epidermoid carcinoma (19). In a variety of human tumor cell lines (leukemia, non-small-cell lung cancer, small-cell lung cancer, colon, breast, melanoma, and brain), vinorelbine was cytostatic at nanomolar concentrations that are significantly below achievable plasma levels (19,22). In a number of in vivo studies exploring activity in rodent tumor models and human tumor xenografts in athymic mice, vinorelbine demonstrated efficacy against P388, L1210, B16, and M5076 in vivo in murine models and in animals with human tumor xenografts. Phase I human trials have shown that in a weekly intravenous administration, the maximum tolerated dose of vinorelbine was 30 mg/m^2; this dose was the recommended dosage to be used in subsequent Phase II human trials employing a weekly schedule (20,23,24). Phase II human trials employing weekly schedules of vinorelbine have demonstrated activity against small-cell lung cancer, non-small-cell lung cancer, and ovarian and breast cancers (22). Vinorelbine as a single agent was studied in nonrandomized Phase II human trials as first-line therapy in non-small-cell lung cancer using a weekly schedule and has shown good activity, with 23 responders out of 70 evaluable patients producing a response rate of 32.8%. The median duration of response was 34 weeks (22,23,25).

Gemcitabine was an active anticancer agent in animals bearing the Lewis lung carcinoma. Gemcitabine was well tolerated by the animals over the dosage range from 40 mg/kg × 3 to 80 mg/kg × 3 (Table 1). Navelbine was administered in three different well-tolerated regimens with total doses of 10, 15, and 22.5 mg/kg. Both gemcitabine and navelbine produced increasing tumor growth delay with increasing dose of the drug. To assess the efficacy of the drug combination, the intermediate dosage regimen of navelbine was combined with each dosage level of gemcitabine. These combination regimens were tolerated and the tumor growth delay increased with increasing dose of gemcitabine. Isobologram methodology (26) was used to determine whether the combinations of gemcitabine and navelbine achieved additive antitumor activity (Fig. 1). At gem-

Table 1 Growth Delay of the Lewis Lung Carcinoma and Number of Lung Metastases on Day 20 After Treatment of the Tumor-Bearing Animals with Gemcitabine With or Without Navelbine[a]

Treatment group[b]	Tumor growth delay, days	Number of lung metastases
Controls	—	35
Gemcitabine		
40 mg/kg, days 7, 10, 13	3.2 ± 0.3	1.5
60 mg/kg, days 7, 10, 13	6.6 ± 0.5	1
80 mg/kg, days 7, 10, 13	9.2 ± 0.7	1
Navelbine		
10 mg/kg, day 7	1.5 ± 0.3	11
10 mg/kg, day 7 + 5 mg/kg, day 13	3.1 ± 0.3	10.5
7.5 mg/kg, days 7, 10, 13	4.9 ± 0.5	11
Navelbine (10 mg/kg) day 7+ (5 mg/kg) day 13 + gemcitabine		
40 mg/kg, days 7, 10, 13	6.6 ± 0.6	0.8
60 mg/kg, days 7, 10, 13	10.2 ± 0.9	0.5
80 mg/kg, days 7, 10, 13	11.1 ± 1.2	0

[a]Mean days ± SEM for treated tumors to reach 500 mm^3 compared with untreated controls. Control tumors reached 500 mm^3 in 12.4 ± 1.2 days
[b]All drugs were administered by intraperitoneal injection.

citabine doses of 40 mg/kg and 60 mg/kg, the combination regimens achieved additivity, with the experimental tumor growth delay falling within the calculated envelope of additivity. At the highest dose of gemcitabine, the combination regimen produced less than additive tumor growth delay.

The untreated control animals in this study had a mean number of 35 lung metastases on day 20 (Table 1). Gemcitabine was highly effective against disease metastatic to the lungs such that the mean number of lung metastases on day 20 was decreased to 1.0 to 1.5 or to 3% to 4% of the number found in the untreated controls. Each of the navelbine regimens decreased the number of lung metastases on day 20 to 10 or 11 or to about 30% of the number found in the untreated control animals. The combination regimens were highly effective against Lewis lung carcinoma metastatic to the lungs, with a mean number of <1–0 metastases found on day 20. These results support the notion that gemcitabine and navelbine can be an effective anticancer drug combination against non-small-cell lung cancer.

B. Antiangiogenic Therapy

Tumors are dynamic, complex, living tissues undergoing the varied processes of tissue growth under the guidance of aberrant malignant cells. Cytotoxic anticancer therapies have focused solely on the eradication of the malignant cell, which is an

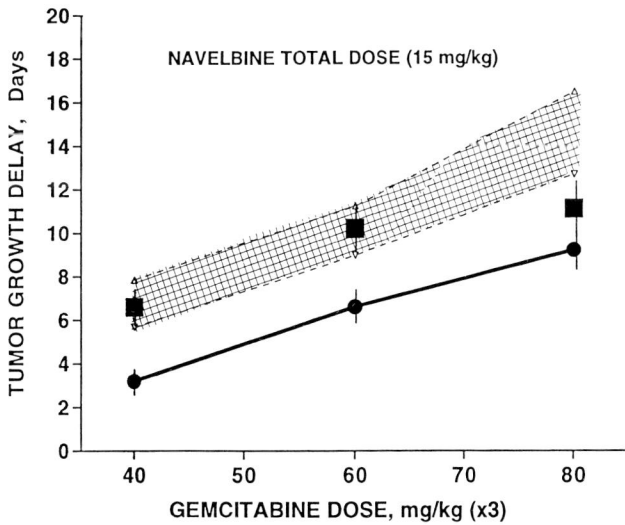

Figure 1 Growth delay of the Lewis lung carcinoma produced by a range of doses of gemcitabine alone (●) or along with navelbine (15 mg/kg total dose) (■). The shaded area is the envelope of additivity determined by isobologram analysis. The bars are SEM.

absolute necessity in cancer therapy. The growth processes of tumors are normal processes, and the invasion processes of tumors are normal processes; it is the inappropriate activation of these processes that comprises the morbidity of malignant disease. These normal processes involving normal cells are valid therapeutic targets. A systems approach to cancer therapy involves choosing multiple targets in malignant and normal cells for therapeutic attack to develop more effective therapeutic regimens (27).

Potentiation of the efficacy of cytotoxic anticancer therapies by administration of antiangiogenic agents has been demonstrated in several in vivo experimental systems (28–34). Among the most promising of the antiangiogenic agents is TNP-470, a synthetic analog of the fungal antibiotic fumagillin. TNP-470 is a potent inhibitor of endothelial cell migration (35), endothelial cell proliferation (36–39), and capillary tube formation (40). TNP-470 also inhibits angiogenesis, as demonstrated in the chick chorioallantoic membrane (CAM) assay, the rabbit, and the rodent cornea (40). TNP-470 has been shown to inhibit the growth of certain primary and metastatic murine tumors as well as human tumor xenografts (41–48). TNP-470 undergoes a rapid metabolism in vivo (49).

The combination of TNP-470 and minocycline along with cytotoxic anticancer therapies formed particularly effective treatments for the Lewis lung carcinoma (31). Minocycline is a tetracycline and a matrix metalloproteinase inhibitor, specifically a collagenase inhibitor which has demonstrated antiangiogenic activity (28,30–34,50). The characteristics of minocycline as a modulator of cytotoxic therapies in Lewis lung carcinoma have been described (28,30). Although exposure to TNP-470/minocycline along with cytotoxic anticancer agents in cell culture did not markedly increase cell killing by the cytotoxic agents (33), treatment of tumor-bearing animals with the same combination regimens markedly increased tumor growth delay, and when Lewis lung carcinoma–bearing mice were treated with TNP-470/minocycline and cyclophosphamide, 40% to 50% of the animals were cured (31). In vivo increased levels of drugs, cyclophosphamide, and cisplatin were detected in the tumors of animals treated with TNP-470/minocycline (33).

When administered to animals bearing the Lewis lung carcinoma subcutaneously on alternate days beginning on day 4 and continuing until day 18, TNP-470 was a moderately effective modulator of the cytotoxic therapies (Table 2). TNP-470 was most effective with melphalan, BCNU, and radiation, increasing the tumor growth delay produced by these treatments 1.8- to 2.4-fold. TNP-470 along with minocycline administered intraperitoneally daily on days 4 to 18 comprised a highly effective antiangiogenic agent combination. The increases in tumor growth delay produced by the modulator combination TNP-470/minocycline along with the cytotoxic therapies ranged from two- to fourfold. In the treatment group receiving TNP-470/minocycline and cyclophosphamide, approximately 40% of the animals were long-term (>120 days) survivors. Each of the cytotoxic therapies

Table 2 Growth Delay of the Lewis Lung Tumor Produced by Various Anticancer Treatments Alone or in Combination with Potential Antiangiogenic Modulators

Treatment group	Tumor growth delay, days[a]			
	Alone	+ Minocycline[b]	+TNP-470	+TNP-470/ MINO
—	—	1.2 ± 0.4	2.1 ± 0.4	1.8 ± 0.4
CDDP (10 mg/kg)	4.5 ± 0.3	5.0 ± 0.3	6.0 ± 0.5	10.9 ± 0.8
Cyclophosphamide (3 × 150 mg/kg)	21.5 ± 1.7	32.4 ± 1.8	25.3 ± 2.2	44.8 ± 2.8[c]
Melphalan (10 mg/kg)	2.7 ± 0.3	4.3 ± 0.3	6.0 ± 0.5	8.5 ± 0.6
BCNU (3 × 15 mg/kg)	3.6 ± 0.4	5.2 ± 0.4	6.3 ± 0.5	14.6 ± 1.0
X-rays (5 × 3 Gy)	4.4 ± 0.3	7.8 ± 0.6	10.6 ± 1.1	15.3 ± 1.2

[a]Tumor growth delay is the difference in days for treated tumors to reach 500 mm^3 compared with untreated control tumors. Untreated control tumors reach 500 mm^3 in about 14 days. Mean ± SE of 15 animals.
[b]Minocycline (10 mg/kg) was administered IP daily on days 4–18. TNP-470 (30 mg/kg) was administered SC on alternate days for 8 injections beginning on day 4. CDDP and melphalan were administered IP on day 7. Cyclophosphamide and BCNU were administered IP on days 7, 9, and 11. X-rays were delivered daily on days 7–11 locally to the tumor-bearing limb.
[c]Five out of 12 long-term survivors (> 180 days).

(including radiation, which was delivered locally to the tumor-bearing limb) produced a reduction in the number of lung metastases found on day 20 (Table 3). Neither TNP-470, minocycline, nor the combination of antiangiogenic agents altered the number of lung metastases or the percentage of large (vascularized) lung metastases on day 20. The modulators did not alter the number of lung metastases from those obtained with the cytotoxic therapies except in the case of cyclophosphamide, where many animals treated with the drug and antiangiogenic agent combination had very few metastases on day 20, and most of those were very small.

To determine the efficacy of the modulator combination against established disease, TNP-470 and minocycline were administered on different schedules while the cytotoxic treatments remained as previously described (Table 4). The antiangiogenic agent administration schedule (days 4 to 11) began when the tumors were palpable and extended through the cytotoxic treatments; the second antiangiogenic agent schedule (days 7 to 11) allowed modulator administration during the same period as the cytotoxic therapies, and the third antiangiogenic agent schedule (days 7 to 18) allowed initiation of modulator administration at the same time as initiation of the cytotoxic therapy and extended the modulators for 1 week after com-

Table 3 Number of Lung Metastases on Day 20 from SC Lewis Lung Tumors After Various Anticancer Therapies Alone or in Combination with Potential Antiangiogenic Modulators

Treatment group	Mean number of lung metastases (% large)			
	Alone	+Minocycline	+TNP-470	+TNP-470/ MINO
—	20 (62)	20 (50)	21 (51)	18 (54)
CDDP (10 mg/kg)	13 (58)	11 (48)	14.5 (34)	14 (50)
Cyclophosphamide (3 × 150 mg/kg)	12 (40)	6 (33)	6 (30)	2 (25)
Melphalan (10 mg/kg)	13 (48)	11 (50)	15 (47)	15 (45)
BCNU (3 × 15 mg/kg)	16 (53)	15 (38)	15.5 (45)	13 (38)
X-rays (5 × 3 Gy)	15 (40)	13 (30)	10 (40)	12 (42)

Table 4 Growth Delay of the Lewis Lung Tumor Produced by Various Anticancer Treatments Alone or in Combination with TNP-470 and Minocycline Administered on Various Schedules

Treatment group	Tumor growth delay, days				
		TNP-470 + minocycline			
	Alone	Days 4–11	Days 7–11	Days 7–18	Days 4–18
—	—	1.4 ± 0.3	0.6 ± 0.3	0.9 ± 0.3	1.8 ± 0.4
Cyclophosphamide (3 × 150 mg/kg)	21.5 ± 1.7	37.1 ± 2.7	28.8 ± 2.4	32.1 ± 2.9	44.8 ± 2.8
BCNU (3 × 15 mg/kg)	3.6 ± 0.4	11.8 ± 1.4	10.4 ± 1.7	10.6 ± 1.5	14.6 ± 1.6
X-rays (5 × 3 Gy)	4.4 ± 0.3	10.4 ± 1.6	6.6 ± 1.2	6.7 ± 1.0	15.3 ± 1.7

pletion of the cytotoxic therapies. As would be expected, the most effective therapies were those begun on day 4, when the tumor burden was smallest. However, both the day 7–11 and day 7–18 modulator treatment schedules resulted in enhanced tumor growth delays compared with the cytotoxic therapies alone. In combination with cyclophosphamide, the antiangiogenic agent schedules beginning on day 4 resulted in 1.7- and 2.1-fold increased tumor growth delay, and the antiangiogenic agent schedules beginning on day 7 resulted in 1.3- and 1.5-fold increased tumor growth delay compared with cyclophosphamide alone. BCNU on days, 7, 9, and 11 along with the antiangiogenic agent schedules beginning on day

4 produced 3.3- and 4-fold increases in tumor growth delay, while the antiangiogenic agent schedules beginning on day 7 produced a 2.9-fold increase in tumor growth delay. Finally, the antiangiogenic agent schedules beginning on day 4 resulted in 2.4- and 3.5-fold increases in tumor growth delay, while the antiangiogenic agent schedules beginning on day 7 resulted in a 1.5-fold increase in tumor growth delay. Varying the modulator administration schedules did not appear to affect response of the metastatic disease to the therapies (Table 5). Only in the case of cyclophosphamide was it evident that beginning the antiangiogenic agent administration on day 7 led to decreased efficacy of the therapy against metastatic disease.

Based on the results of several positive Phase II human trials, paclitaxel and carboplatin are commonly being used to treat advanced non-small-cell lung cancer. Recently, a study was carried out to determine whether TNP-470 and minocycline would interact positively with that drug combination. Paclitaxel (36 mg/kg) administered by intravenous injection on days 7 through 11 after tumor cell implantation produced 4.6 days of tumor growth delay, which was increased 1.4-fold to 6.4 days of tumor growth delay when administered along with TNP-470 and minocycline (Table 6). A single intraperitoneal injection of carboplatin (50 mg/kg) on day 7 after tumor cell implantation produced a tumor growth delay of 4.2 days. When carboplatin was administered along with TNP-470 and minocycline, a tumor growth delay of 7.8 days resulted, a 1.9-fold increase compared with carboplatin alone. The combination of the cytotoxic anticancer drugs, paclitaxel and carboplatin, was well tolerated by the animals and produced a tumor growth delay of 6.6 days. The complete regimen including TNP-470 and minocycline along with paclitaxel and carboplatin produced a tumor growth delay of 10.5 days, a 1.6-fold increase compared with the cytotoxic drug combination alone.

Treatment with the antiangiogenic agent combination decreased the number

Table 5 Number of Lung Metastases on Day 20 from SC Lewis Lung Tumors After Various Anticancer Therapies Alone or in Combination with TNP-470 and Minocycline Administered on Various Schedules

Treatment group	Mean number of lung metastases (% large) TNP-470 + Minocycline				
	Alone	Days 4–11	Days 7–11	Days 7–18	Days 4–18
—	20 (62)	17 (57)	20 (52)	20 (48)	18 (54)
Cyclophosphamide 3 × 150 mg/kg	12 (40)	2 (25)	4 (18)	4 (28)	2 (25)
BCNU (3 × 15 mg/kg)	16 (53)	17 (41)	12 (42)	14 (25)	15 (45)
X-rays (5 × 3 Gy)	15 (40)	15 (38)	17 (34)	15 (38)	12 (42)

Table 6 Growth Delay of the Lewis Lung Carcinoma and Number of Lung Metastases on Day 20 After Treatment of the Animals with Paclitaxel and/or Carboplatin With or Without Antiangiogenic Agents

Treatment group	Tumor growth delay[a] (days)	Number of lung metastases
Controls	—	40 ± 7
TNP-470 (30 mg/kg), SC, alt d 4–18 + minocycline (10 mg/kg) IP, d 4–18	1.0 ± 0.3	27 ± 5
Paclitaxel (36 mg/kg) IV d 7–11	4.6 ± 0.3	22 ± 4
TNP/MINO/Paclitaxel	6.4 ± 0.4[b]	20 ± 4
Carboplatin (50 mg/kg) IP, d 7	4.2 ± 0.3	25 ± 4
TNP/MINO/carboplatin	7.8 ± 0.5[c]	21 ± 3
Paclitaxel/carboplatin	6.6 ± 0.4	13 ± 2
TNP/MINO/paclitaxel/carboplatin	10.5 ± 0.6[b]	8 ± 1

[a]Tumor growth delay is the difference in days for treated tumors to reach 500 mm^3 compared with untreated control tumors. Untreated control tumors reach 500 mm^3 in about 12.4 ± 0.3 days. Mean ± SE of 15 animals.
[b]Significantly increased tumor growth delay compared with the cytotoxic therapy alone—$P < .01$.
[c]$P < .005$.

of lung metastases on day 20 to 68% of the number found in untreated control animals. Both of the cytotoxic chemotherapeutic agents also decreased the number of lung metastases on day 20. Paclitaxel administration decreased the number of lung metastases to 55% of controls, which was not significantly altered by the addition of coadministration of TNP-470/minocycline. Treatment with carboplatin decreased the number of lung metastases to 63% of the number in the untreated control animals. Addition of TNP-470/minocycline administration to treatment with carboplatin did not significantly alter the number of lung metastases compared with carboplatin alone. The combination of the cytotoxic drugs reduced the number of lung metastases to 33% of the number in the control animals. With the addition of treatment with TNP-470/minocycline to the combination of cytotoxic anticancer drugs, the number of lung metastases was reduced to 20% of the number in the untreated control animals.

The antiangiogenic combination of TNP-470 and minocycline administered for 2 weeks did not alter the growth of the Lewis lung carcinoma, the EMT-6 mammary carcinoma, the 9L gliosarcoma, or the FSaII fibrosarcoma (29,31–34,51,52). However, when TNP-470 and minocycline were added to treatment with cytotoxic anticancer therapies, tumor response was markedly increased.

When C3H mice bearing the FSaIIC fibrosarcoma were treated with TNP-470/minocycline for 5 days prior to intravenous injection of the fluorescent dye Hoechst 33342, there was a shift toward greater brightness of the entire tumor cell population, so that the 10% brightest and the 20% dimmest cell subpopulations were composed of cells containing much more dye than the same subpopulations in the control tumor (Fig. 2) (31). The TNP-470 and minocycline–treated tumors were more easily penetrated by the lipophilic dye (31). This was the first indication that TNP-470 and minocycline treatment might allow greater distribution of small molecules into tumors. Subsequent studies showed that this same TNP-470/minocycline regimen increased the levels of [^{14}C]cyclophosphamide, cisplatin, and molecular oxygen in the Lewis lung tumor.

To determine the effects of TNP-470/minocycline on paclitaxel and carboplatin distribution into the Lewis lung carcinoma, [^{14}C]paclitaxel was administered to Lewis lung carcinoma–bearing animals pretreated with TNP-470/minocycline or not pretreated on day 8 after tumor implantation, and tissues were collected over a 24-hour time course (Fig. 3). At early time points (1 min and 15 min) after intravenous administration of the [^{14}C]paclitaxel, there was a fivefold higher concentration of the drug of the tumors of animals that had been pretreated with TNP-470/minocycline. At the intermediate time points the [^{14}C]paclitaxel levels were similar in both the pretreated animals and those that had not been treated with TNP-470/minocycline; however, by 24 hours there was a twofold

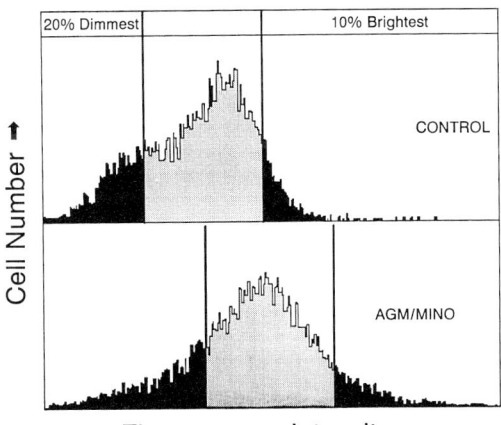

Figure 2 Fluorescence distribution in FSaIIC tumor cells after IV injection of tumor-bearing animals with Hoechst 33342 (2 mg/kg). The data shown are for an untreated control tumor and a tumor treated with TNP-470 (3 × 30 mg/kg, SC) and minocycline (5 × 10 mg/kg, IP).

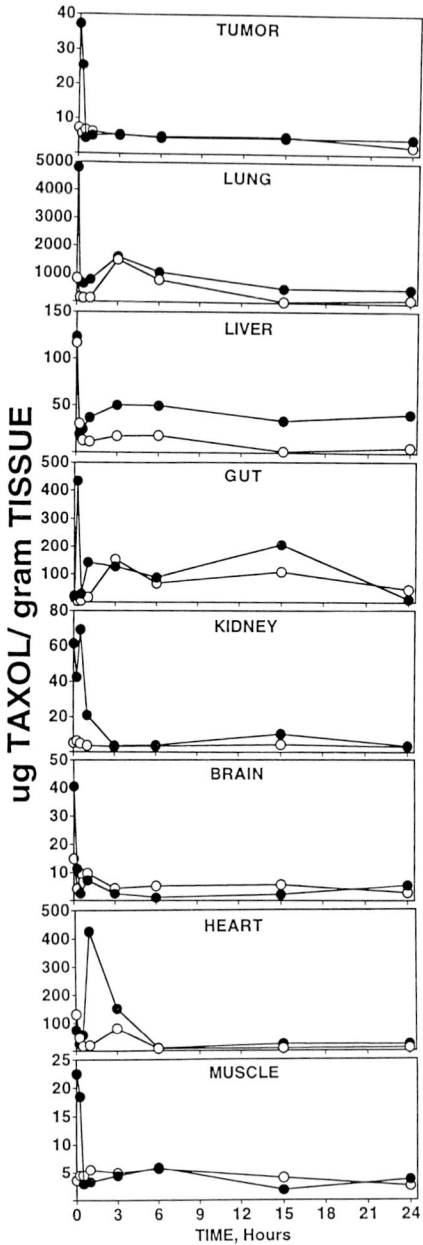

Figure 3 Tissue levels of ^{14}C from [^{14}C]paclitaxel in C57BL mice bearing Lewis lung tumors SC in the hind leg over a time course after IV injection of 36 mg/kg of the drug alone on day 8 (○) or after administration of the drug to animals treated with TNP-470 (30 mg/kg, SC) days 4, 6, and 8, and minocycline (10 mg/kg, IP) daily days 4–8 after tumor cell implantation (●).

greater concentration of [^{14}C]paclitaxel in the tumors of the animals pretreated with TNP-470/minocycline compared with those that had not received the antiangiogenic therapy. The pattern of [^{14}C]paclitaxel distribution into the other tissues was similar, with greater peak levels of [^{14}C]paclitaxel in the tissues of animals pretreated with TNP-470/minocycline. In the liver, however, there was a prolonged increased level of [^{14}C]paclitaxel in the livers of the pretreated animals. By far the highest levels of [^{14}C]paclitaxel were found in the lungs of the animals where the peak level in the pretreated animals reached 4800 μg/g tissue. Other tissues with relatively high paclitaxel concentrations were gut and heart.

Concentrations of platinum from carboplatin were two- and threefold higher in the tumors of animals pretreated with TNP-470/minocycline at 15 min and 30 min after drug administration, respectively (Fig. 4). Between 6 hours and 24 hours after carboplatin administration, platinum levels in the tumors of pretreated animals remained about twofold greater than in animals that did not receive the antiangiogenic therapy. Overall, the tissues of the animals pretreated with TNP-470/minocycline had higher platinum levels, with the greatest differentials being in kidney, brain, muscle, and liver. The highest platinum levels overall were in kidney, gut, liver, and brain.

To determine whether pretreatment with TNP-470/minocycline might also alter the tissue distribution of large molecules into tumors and tissues, [^{14}C]albumin was administered to TNP-470/minocycline pretreated and nonpretreated Lewis lung carcinoma–bearing animals (Fig. 5). There was a two- to threefold higher concentration of [^{14}C]albumin in the tumor over the first hour after protein injection and a concentration differential with higher concentrations in the tumors of the pretreated animals persisting over the 24 hours examined. A similar pattern pertained for the other tissues with TNP-470/minocycline-pretreated animals having higher tissue concentrations of [^{14}C]albumin than the tissues of nonpretreated animals. The highest peak levels of [^{14}C]albumin were in liver and lung. The uptake of each of these molecules into the Lewis lung tumor was increased, yet the number of intratumoral vessels in these tumors visualized by CD31 or factor VIII staining to 30% to 50% of the number in the untreated control tumors (53).

Administration of TNP-470/minocycline decreased the hypoxia in the Lewis lung carcinoma; therefore a study was undertaken to determine whether this antiangiogenic regimen would increase the response of the tumor to fractionated radiation therapy. Tumor growth delay experiments were performed in animals treated similarly to those in the oxygen studies, using fractionated radiation therapy as the oxygen-dependent cytotoxic modality (Fig. 6). Administration of TNP-470 and minocycline on days 4 through 18 along with fractionated radiation on days 7 through 11 resulted in increased tumor growth delay by the radiation therapy such that 6 days of growth delay required about 5×3.8 Gy under normal conditions and about 5×2.9 Gy in the TNP-470/minocycline-treated animals. When the TNP-470/minocycline-treated animals were allowed to breathe carbogen for

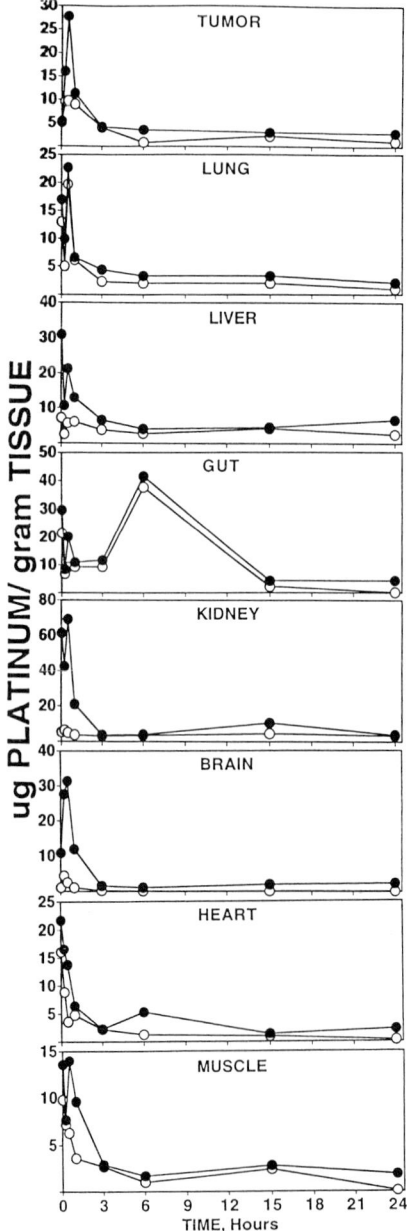

Figure 4   Tissue levels of platinum (Pt) from carboplatin in C57BL mice bearing Lewis lung tumors SC in the hind leg over a time course after IV injection of 300 mg/kg of the drug alone on day 8 (○) or after administration of TNP-470 (30 mg/kg, SC) days 4, 6, and 8, and minocycline (10 mg/kg, IP) daily days 4–8 after tumor cell implantation (●).

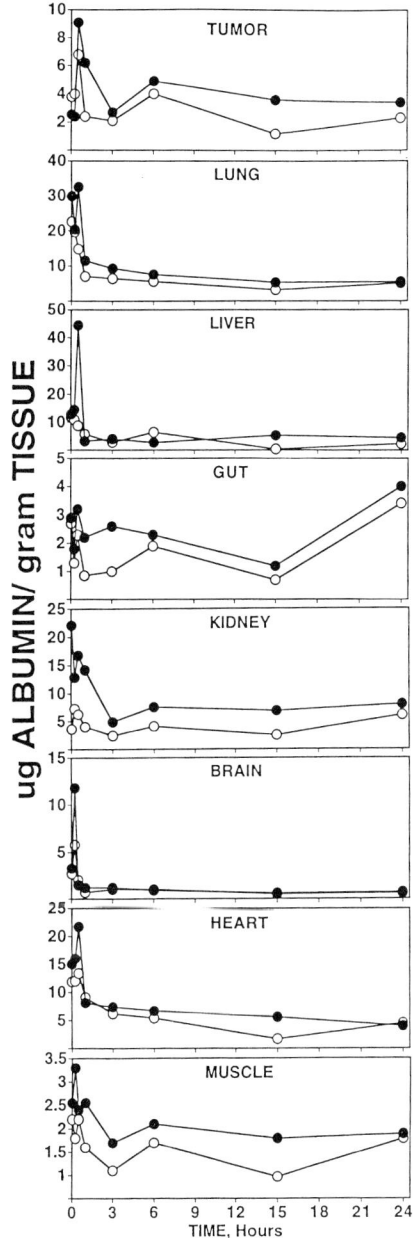

Figure 5 Tissue levels of ^{14}C from $[^{14}C]$albumin in C57BL mice bearing Lewis lung tumors SC in the hind leg over a time course after IV injection of 10 mg/kg of the protein alone on day 8 (○) or after administration of the protein to animals treated with TNP-470 (30 mg/kg, SC) days 4, 6, and 8, and minocycline (10 mg/kg, IP) daily days 4–8 after tumor cell implantation (●).

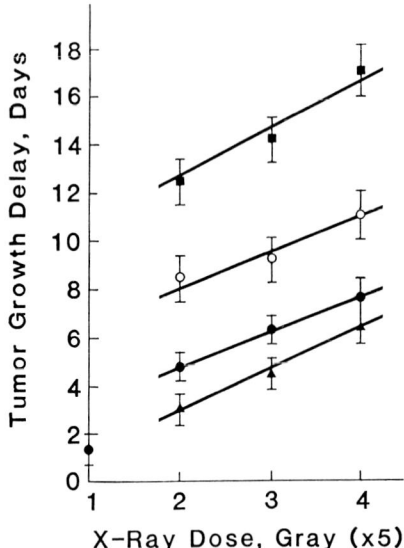

Figure 6 Growth delay of the Lewis lung carcinoma produced by daily fractionated radiation delivered in fractions of 2, 3, or 4 Gy locally to the tumor-bearing limb for 5 days on days 7–11 alone (▲); in animals treated with TNP-470 (30 mg/kg, SC) on alternate days and minocycline (10 mg/kg, IP) daily on days 4–18 (●); in animals treated with TNP-470/minocycline (as above) and allowed to breathe carbogen for 1 hour prior to and during radiation delivery (○); and in animals treated with TNP-470/minocycline as above) and injected IV with the perflubron emulsion (8 mL/kg) and then allowed to breathe carbogen for 1 hour prior to and during radiation delivery (■). The points are the means of 15 animals. Bars are SEM.

1 hour prior to and during radiation delivery, there was an overall 2.2-fold increase in tumor growth delay compared with the growth delay obtained in air-breathing animals. Administration of the perflubron emulsion (8 mL/kg) along with carbogen breathing resulted in a further increase in tumor growth delay in the TNP-470/minocycline-treated animals, which was a 3.4-fold increase over that obtained in the air-breathing animals.

There was a linear relationship between the decrease in the percent of pO_2 readings ≤5 mm Hg and the tumor growth delay achieved with each fractionated radiation regimen (Fig. 7). At radiation doses of 2 Gy and 3 Gy there was a 2.5-day increase in tumor growth delay for each 10% decrease in the pO_2 readings ≤5 mm Hg, and at the radiation dose of 4 Gy there was a 3.1-day increase in tumor growth delay for each 10% decrease in the pO_2 readings ≤5 mm Hg (34).

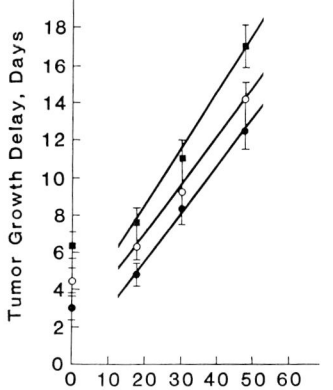

Figure 7   Relationship between decrease in the percent of tumor pO_2 readings ≤ 5 mm Hg and tumor growth delay at each radiation dose: 5×2 Gy ($\bullet$), 5×3 Gy ($\bigcirc$), and 5×4 Gy ($\blacksquare$). Points are the means of 10 tumors. Bars = SEM.

C. Immunotherapy: Interleukin-12

Interleukin-12 (IL-12) is a naturally occurring cytokine which serves as a link between the innate and the cognate cellular immune systems (54–57). IL-12 has the ability to act as a natural killer (NK) cell and a T-cell growth factor (58–60), to enhance NK/LAK cell cytolytic activity (60–62), to augment cytolytic T-cell responses (61), and to induce secretion of cytokines, particularly interferon gamma (IFN-γ) from T and NK cells (63).

IL-12 has been shown to induce tumor regression and rejection in a variety of murine tumor models when administered as a single agent (64–68). This tumor regression results from activation of immune mechanisms that involve IFN-γ, CD4+, and CD8+ cells (64,65). IL-12 has also been described as an antiangiogenic agent through the induction of IFN-γ (69).

Both T and NK cells have been implicated as antitumor effector cells (70), and IFN-γ has been shown to have antitumor activity in animals (71,72). IL-12 has the potential to be used as an immunomodulatory cytokine in the therapy of malignancies (71,73,74), as well as in gene therapy (75,76). Brunda et al. (64) have shown that systemic administration of murine IL-12 can slow, and in some cases inhibit, the growth of both established subcutaneous tumors in mice and experimental pulmonary or hepatic metastases of B16F10 murine melanoma, M5076 reticulum cell sarcoma, or RenCa renal cell adenocarcinoma, and that local peritumoral injections of IL-12 can result in regression of established subcutaneous tumors. Based on results obtained using mice deficient in lymphocyte subsets and antibody depletion experiments, Brunda and colleagues concluded that the antitumor efficacy of IL-12 is mediated primarily through $CD8^+$ T cells (64,77).

Most anticancer therapeutic regimens involve systemic treatment with chemotherapy and/or local treatment with radiation therapy. In previous studies, treatment of animals bearing Lewis lung carcinoma with IL-12 in combination with fractionated radiation therapy was markedly dose-modifying, indicating that IL-12 was acting synergistically with radiation (78). A study was undertaken to understand the most effective scheduling of IL-12 administration with fractionated radiation therapy in the murine Lewis lung carcinoma known to be metastatic and responsive to IL-12.

Interleukin-12 (recombinant murine IL-12; rmIL-12) was found to be an active antitumor agent against the Lewis lung carcinoma. The antitumor activity was dependent upon rmIL-12 dose, the duration of treatment, and the tumor burden at the initiation of treatment. The effect of the schedule of rmIL-12 administration alone and along with a 1-week regimen of fractionated radiation therapy (Table 7; Fig. 8) or a 2-week regimen of fractionated radiation therapy (Table 8; Fig. 9) was examined. Beginning treatment with rmIL-12 on day 2 after tumor cell implantation and treating for 5 days resulted in about 5 days of tumor growth delay, while beginning treatment with rmIL-12 on day 2 and treating for 10 days and then for 5 days again resulted in about 7.7 days of tumor growth delay (Table 7). Delaying the initiation of rmIL-12 treatment to day 7 after tumor cell implantation and treating for 5 days resulted in a tumor growth delay of about 2.7 days, while extending that treatment to 10 injections increased the tumor growth delay to 5.4 days. Further delaying the initiation of rmIL-12 treatment until day 14 post–tumor cell implantation and treating for 10 injections resulted in about 4.3 days of tumor growth delay. Finally, treating bulky disease beginning on day 21 post–tumor cell implantation with rmIL-12 for 5 days did not alter tumor growth (79).

Fractionated radiation therapy in a 5-day regimen resulted in increasing tumor growth delay with increasing radiation dose (Table 7). Administering rmIL-12 for 5 days prior to radiation therapy resulted in an additive effect of the two treatments but did not increase the response of the tumor to the radiation therapy. Administration of rmIL-12 prior to, during, and after radiation therapy resulted in a highly effective therapy which included an additive effect of the two therapies and dose modification of the radiation therapy with a dose-modifying factor of 2. Administering rmIL-12 during and after fractionated radiation also resulted in a highly effective therapeutic regimen, including an additive effect of the two therapies and a radiation dose-modifying factor of 3. Delaying administration of rmIL-12 until 2 days or 1 week after completion of the radiation regimen resulted in less efficacious treatments than when the rmIL-12 was given concurrently and after the radiation therapy. Nevertheless, treatments where the rmIL-12 was administered

Table 7 Growth Delay of the Lewis Lung Carcinoma and Number and Percent of Large Lung Metastases on Day 20 After Treatment with IL-12 and Fractionated Radiation Therapy Delivered Locally to the Tumor-Bearing Limb

Treatment group	Tumor growth delay, days[a]	Lung metastases (% large)[b]
Control	—	25 (53)
IL-12 (45 µg/kg) IP[c]		
days 2–6	4.9 ± 0.4	15 (43)
days 7–11	2.7 ± 0.3	16 (47)
days 2–11; 14–18	7.7 ± 0.5	8.5 (29)
days 7–11; 14–18	5.4 ± 0.4	9 (31)
days 14–18; 21–25	4.3 ± 0.4	16 (50)
days 21–25	0.3 ± 0.3	
5×2 Gy, days 7–11[d]	3.1 ± 0.4	17.5 (62)
5×3 Gy, days 7–11	4.3 ± 0.4	17 (53)
5×4 Gy, days 7–11	6.2 ± 0.6	17 (55)
IL-12 (45 µg/kg) IP, days 2–6		
+ 5×2 Gy, d 7–11	6.8 ± 0.6	14 (27)
+ 5×3 Gy, d 7–11	7.8 ± 0.9	13 (35)
+ 5×4 Gy, d 7–11	10.0 ± 1.1	12 (39)
IL-12 (45 µg/kg) IP, days 2–11; 14–18		
+ 5×2 Gy, d 7–11	8.7 ± 0.8	8 (40)
+ 5×3 Gy, d 7–11	11.2 ± 1.3	7 (35)
+ 5×4 Gy, d 7–11	16.1 ± 1.9	6 (33)
IL-12 (45 µg/kg) IP, days 7–11; 14–18		
+ 5×2 Gy, d 7–11	6.9 ± 0.8	10 (24)
+ 5×3 Gy, d 7–11	12.5 ± 1.6	6 (30)
+ 5×4 Gy, d 7–11	19.8 ± 2.1	4 (27)
IL-12 (45 µg/kg) IP, days 14–18; 21–25		
+ 5×2 Gy, d 7–11	4.2 ± 0.3	17 (39)
+ 5×3 Gy, d 7–11	7.4 ± 0.5	15 (32)
+ 5×4 Gy, d 7–11	10.6 ± 1.2	14 (23)
IL-12 (45 µg/kg) IP, days 21–25		
+ 5×2 Gy, d 7–11	3.3 ± 0.3	19 (50)
+ 5×3 Gy, d 7–11	6.6 ± 0.4	18 (61)
+ 5×4 Gy, d 7–11	9.6 ± 1.0	16 (50)

[a]Tumor growth delay is the difference in days for treated tumors to reach 500 mm^3 compared with untreated control tumors. Untreated control tumors reach 500 mm^3 in 12.5 ± 0.3 days. Mean ± SE of 18 animals.

[b]The number of external lung metastases on day 20 post–tumor implant as counted manually and scored as ≥ 3 mm in diameter. Data are the means from 6–12 pairs of lungs. Numbers in parentheses, number of large (vascularized) metastases.

[c]IL-12 was administered by IP injection.

[d]Radiation therapy was delivered in fractions of 2, 3, or 4 Gy daily on days 7–11 locally to the tumor-bearing limb (100 rad/min; gamma cell 40).

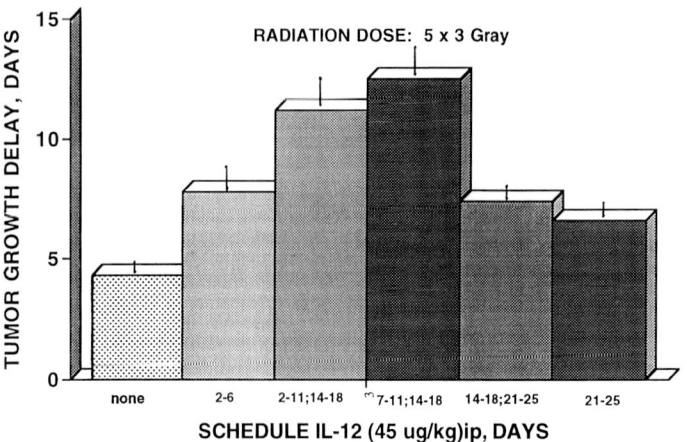

Figure 8   Growth delay of the Lewis lung carcinoma after treatment of the tumor-bearing animals with fractionated radiation therapy (2, 3, or 4 Gy) delivered locally to the tumor-bearing limb once per day on days 7–11 after tumor implantation alone or along with rmIL-12 (45 μg/kg, IP) on days 2–6; days 2–11 and 14–18; days 7–11 and 14–18; days-14–18 and 21–25; or days 21–25. Data are the means of three experiments ± SEM.

only after the radiation were as effective as or more effective than radiation alone. Using 3 Gy (×5) as a representative radiation dose, there was a maximal 2.8-fold increase in tumor growth delay when rmIL-12 was administered during and after fractionated radiation therapy (Fig. 8). The efficacy of these regimens against systemic disease, represented by lung metastases, paralleled the effects observed in the primary tumor (Table 7). When rmIL-12 was administered prior to, during, and after radiation therapy or during and after radiation therapy, the numbers of lung metastases was decreased to 20% to 40% of the controls. The percent of large (vascularized) metastases was also decreased by treatment with rmIL-12 (79).

When the fractionated radiation regimen was extended to 2 weeks, the results shown in Table 8 were obtained. Administration of rmIL-12 for 5 days prior to radiation therapy resulted in an additive effect of the two therapies but no dose modification of the radiation occurred. Concurrent administration of rmIL-12 just prior to each of the 10 radiation fractions formed a highly effective treatment regimen resulting in additivity of the two therapies and a radiation dose-modifying factor of 5. Administering rmIL-12 along with the second week of the fractionated radiation regimen and then for 5 days the week after radiation therapy also produced a highly effective treatment regimen with an additive effect of the two therapies and a radiation dose-modifying factor of 2.7. When rmIL-12 administration was delayed until the completion of the radiation therapy, only a modest increase

Table 8   Growth Delay of the Lewis Lung Carcinoma and Number and Percent of Large Lung Metastases on Day 20 After Treatment with IL-12 and 2 Weeks of Fractionated Radiation Therapy Delivered Locally to the Tumor-Bearing Limb

Treatment group	Tumor growth delay, days[a]	Lung metastases (% large)[b]
Control	—	25 (53)
10×2 Gy, days 7–11; 14–18[c]	4.1 ± 0.3	13 (32)
10×3 Gy, days 7–11; 14–18	5.1 ± 0.4	11 (38)
10×4 Gy, days 7–11; 14–18	8.9 ± 0.7	6 (27)
IL-12 (45 µg/kg) IP, days 2–6[d]		
$+ 10 \times 2$ Gy, d 7–11; 14–18	5.5 ± 0.4	7.5 (33)
$+ 10 \times 3$ Gy, d 7–11; 14–18	7.6 ± 0.7	6 (30)
$+ 10 \times 4$ Gy, d 7–11; 14–18	10.6 ± 0.9	5 (20)
IL-12 (45 µg/kg) IP, days 7–11; 14–18		
$+ 10 \times 2$ Gy, d 7–11; 14–18	7.2 ± 0.5	3.5 (43)
$+ 10 \times 3$ Gy, d 7–11; 14–18	16.6 ± 1.3	2.5 (40)
$+ 10 \times 4$ Gy, d 7–11; 14–18	28.9 ± 2.3	2 (50)
IL-12 (45 µg/kg) IP, days 14–18; 21–25		
$+ 10 \times 2$ Gy, d 7–11; 14–18	5.4 ± 0.5	10.5 (38)
$+ 10 \times 3$ Gy, d 7–11; 14–18	11.1 ± 0.9	6 (42)
$+ 10 \times 4$ Gy, d 7–11; 14–18	16.4 ± 1.1	5 (40)
IL-12 (45 µg/kg) IP, days 21–25		
$+ 10 \times 2$ Gy, d 7–11; 14–18	5.6 ± 0.4	15 (32)
$+ 10 \times 3$ Gy, d 7–11; 14–18	7.7 ± 0.6	14 (52)
$+ 10 \times 4$ Gy, d 7–11; 14–18	11.8 ± 1.1	6 (38)

[a]Tumor growth delay is the difference in days for treated tumors to reach 500 mm^3 compared with untreated control tumors. Untreated control tumors reach 500 mm^3 in 12.5 ± 0.3 days. Mean ± SE of 15 animals.

[b]The number of external lung metastases on day 20 post–tumor implant as counted manually and scored as ≥ 3 mm in diameter. Data are the means from 6–12 pairs of lungs. Numbers in parentheses, number of large (vascularized) metastases.

[c]Radiation therapy was delivered in fractions of 2, 3, or 4 Gy daily on days 7–11 locally to the tumor-bearing limb (100 rad/min; gamma cell 40).

[d]IL-12 was administered by IP injection.

in tumor growth delay compared with radiation therapy alone was observed. Using the fractionated radiation regimen of 3 Gy (×10) as a representative treatment, concurrent administration of rmIL-12 and radiation therapy resulted in a 3.3-fold increase in tumor growth delay compared with radiation therapy alone (Fig. 9). A reduction in the number of lung metastases on day 20 was observed

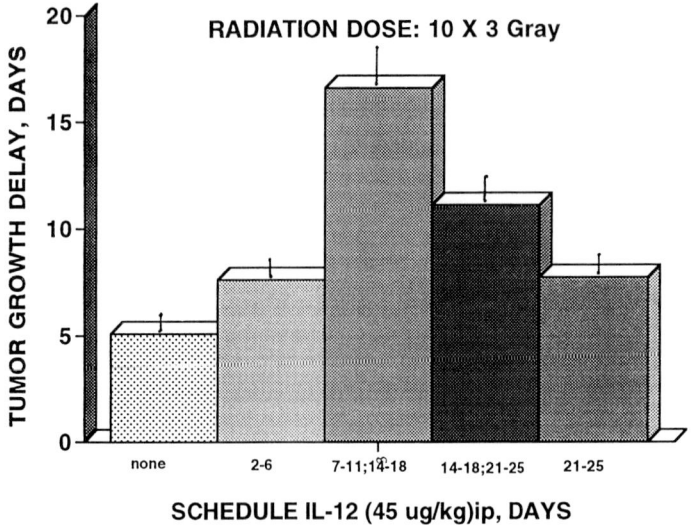

Figure 9   Growth delay of the Lewis lung carcinoma after treatment of the tumor-bearing animals with fractionated radiation therapy (2, 3, or 4 Gy) delivered locally to the tumor-bearing limb once per day on days 7–11 and 14–18 after tumor implantation alone or along with rmIL-12 (45 µg/kg, IP) on days 2 through 6; days 7–11 and 14–18; days 14–18 and 21–25; or days 21–25. Data are the means of three experiments ± SEM.

with each of the 2-week radiation therapy regimens (Table 7). However, the treatment regimen including concurrent administration of rmIL-12 and radiation therapy, which was most effective against the primary tumor, was also most effective in decreasing the number of lung metastases on day 20.

rmIL-12 (45 or 4.5 µg/kg) administered on days 7 through 11 and 14 through 18 was a highly effective radiosensitizer in the Lewis lung carcinoma (Fig. 10). GM-CSF is a growth factor for the granulocyte-macrophage lineage. rmGM-CSF (45 or 4.5 µg/kg) was administered on days 7 through 11 and 14 through 18 alone or along with fractionated radiation on days 7 through 11. rmGM-CSF was an active antitumor agent against the Lewis lung carcinoma and produced an increase in tumor growth delay in combination with radiation therapy that was parallel to the radiation effect alone, indicating additivity of the therapies. When the higher doses of rmIL-12 and rmGM-CSF were administered together with fractionated radiation therapy, a marked increase in tumor growth delay resulted. When lower doses of rmIL-12 and/or rmGM-CSF were administered

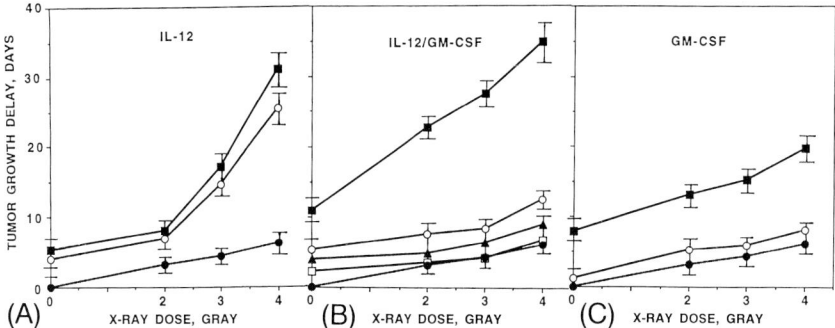

Figure 10 Growth delay of the Lewis lung carcinoma after treatment of the tumor-bearing animals with rmIL-12, GM-CSF, or rmIL-12 and GM-CSF along with fractionated radiation therapy. Symbols: (A) rmIL-12: radiation alone (●); rmIL-12 (4.5 µg/kg) days 7–11 and 14–18 along with radiation (○); rmIL-12 (45 µg/kg) days 7–11 and 14–18 along with radiation (■). (B) rmIL-12/GM-CSF: radiation alone (●); rmIL-12 (45 µg/kg)/GM-CSF (4.5 µg/kg) days 7–11 and 14–18 along with radiation (○); rmIL-12 (45 µg/kg)/GM-CSF (45 µg/kg) days 7–11 and 14–18 along with radiation (■); rmIL-12 (4.5 µg/kg)/GM-CSF (4.5 µg/kg) days 7–11 and 14–18 along with radiation (□); rmIL-12 (45 µg/kg) days 7–11 and 14–18 along with radiation (▲). (C) GM-CSF: radiation alone (●); GM-CSF (4.5 µg/kg) days 7–11 and 14–18 along with radiation (○); GM-CSF (45 µg/kg) days 7–11 and 14–18 along with radiation (■). Points are the means of three experiments; bars are the SEM.

along with fractionated radiation, the effects on tumor growth delay were less than those of rmIL-12 alone.

Like rmIL-12, treatment with rmGM-CSF decreased the number and size of Lewis lung metastases on day 20 (Table 9). In fact, administered at the same dose and on the same schedule, rmGM-CSF was a more effective agent against metastatic disease than rmIL-12. Coadministration of rmIL-12 (45 µg/kg) and rmGM-CSF (45 µg/kg) on days 7 through 11 and 14 through 18 was a highly effective therapy against metastatic Lewis lung carcinoma, nearly ablating lung metastases on day 20 even in the absence of radiation therapy (79).

Granulocyte-macrophage colony-stimulating factor (GM-CSF) is a cytokine acting on stimulates potent, specific, and long-lasting antitumor immunity in multiple murine model systems, including the Lewis lung carcinoma (84,88). Based on these results, a Phase I human clinical trial of vaccination with autologous lethally irradiated non-small-cell lung carcinoma cells engineered by

Table 9 Number and Size of Lung Metastases on Day 20 in Animals Bearing Subcutaneous Lewis Lung Carcinoma Treated with Fractionated Radiation Therapy Locally to the Tumor-Bearing Limb Alone or Along with rmIL-12 and/or rmGM-CSF[a]

	Number of lung metastases (% large) Radiation dose, Gy × 5			
Treatment group	0	2	3	4
X-rays	24.5 (56)	17.5 (62)	17 (53)	17 (55)
IL-12 (4.5 µg/kg)	17.5 (56)	14 (43)	10 (38)	8.5 (50)
IL-12 (45 µg/kg)	14 (36)	12 (38)	9 (36)	7 (40)
GM-CSF (4.5 µg/kg)	8.5 (46)	5.5 (27)	3 (0)	2.5 (0)
GM-CSF (45 µg/kg)	5 (11)	5 (10)	4.5 (0)	3.5 (0)
IL-12 (4.5 µg/kg) GM-CSF (4.5 µg/kg)	11 (36)	4 (25)	2 (0)	0 (0)
IL-12 (45 µg/kg) GM-CSF (0.45 µg/kg)	7 (50)	7 (50)	4.5 (0)	2 (0)
IL-12 (45 µg/kg) GM-CSF (4.5 µg/kg)	4.5 (22)	2.5 (0)	1.5 (0)	1 (0)
IL-12 (45 µg/kg) GM-CSF (45 µg/kg)	0.5 (0)	1 (0)	0.5 (0)	0 (0)

[a]The treatment regimens are described in the legend to Figure 2.

adenoviral-mediated gene transfer to secrete human GM-CSF is planned (Dr. Glenn Dranoff, personal communication).

The exact mechanism for the enhanced response to the triple combination of rmIL-12/rmGM-CSF/fractionated radiation therapy can be only speculative. rmIL-12, while directly activating NK and T cells, could also indirectly induce macrophage activation via induction of INF-γ. Macrophages could also be activated by release products resulting from cell damage induced by radiation. Local production of endogenous rmIL-12 by stimulated macrophages could act as a positive feedback mechanism on tumor-associated NK and T cells to promote additional tumor cell killing, which would be enhanced by the radiation-induced injury. The additional activation of granulocytes and macrophages by GM-CSF treatment would further augment the tumor-killing response.

III. Human Cell Lines and Xenografts

A. Human Cell Lines

With the development of reliable cell culture techniques, media, and serum, the possibility of establishing continuous lines of malignant cells in culture became real. Beginning around 1970 and continuing through the mid-1980s, a cohort of human lung cancer cell lines were developed. Table 10 presents the characteristics of 27 human lung cancer cell lines. The cell lines represent an important resource for testing potential new drugs and drug combinations and for elucidation of the molecular characteristics of human lung cancer. Several of the cell lines (NCI-H460, NCI-H520, NCI-H596, NCI-H661, NCI-H676B, NCI-H209, and NCI-H820) were established from tissues collected prior to any therapy. Others were from patients after known prior therapy (Calu-1, 5-fluorouracil, and adriamycin; Calu-3, cyclophosphamide, bleomycin, and adriamycin; Calu-6, radiation; ChaGo K-1, methotrexate, procarbazine, vincristine, and hydroxyurea) or unknown prior therapy (NCI-H441, NCI-H345, NCI-H69, NCI-H82, NCI-H128, NCI-H146, NCI-H446, and NCI-H510A). Some of these cell lines, such as A549 and Calu-3, are very widely used whereas others such as NCI-H441 (doubling time 58 hours), NCI-H520 (doubling time 32 hours) grow quite slowly, making them less favorable for many cell culture studies. The p53 status of several of the cell lines has been elucidated: NCI-H345, NCI-H460, NCI-H596, NCI-H661, and NCI-510A cell lines express easily detectable levels of p53 very similar to the levels found in normal lung; and NCI-H520 and NCI-H209 have greatly reduced levels of p53 much lower than the levels found in normal lung (89). The NCI-H676B cell line expresses an abnormally sized p53 mRNA (2.3 kb) as well as the normally sized p53 mRNA (2.8 kb). The NCI-H82 cell line expresses an abnormally sized p53 mRNA (3.7 kb) in greatly reduced amounts compared with normal lung (89). The NCI-H82 cell line also exhibits a 25-fold amplification of c-myc DNA and a 24-fold increase in c-myc mRNA compared with normal lung and other lines (90).

Even with the availability of these well-characterized cell lines, the application of single or combined drug sensitivity/resistance findings from cell culture experiments to improve clinical treatment regimens has not materialized. Recent advances in semiautomated cell culture techniques using dye-based assays of viability such as tetrazolium salt 3-(4,5-dimethylthiazol-2-yl)-2,5-diphenyltetrazolium bromide (MTT) or sulforhodamine B (SRB) along with improved methods of data analysis (isobologram methodology) to determine hematopoietic precursors and mature granulocytes and monocytes (80–82). GM-CSF may also play a role in the maturation and/or function of specialized antigen presenting cells (83). Dranoff et al. (84) showed that vaccination with irradiated tumor cells engineered to secrete GM-CSF stimulated potent, specific, and long-lasting antitumor immunity against B16 melanoma. Localized expression of GM-CSF by the irradiated vaccinating cells might enhance tumor-antigen presentation by host antigen presenting cells. Treatment with GM-CSF produced some antitumor activity against the Lewis lung carcinoma which appeared to be primarily additive with fractionated radiation therapy. Treatment with GM-CSF (45 µg/kg) on the same schedule as rmIL-12 augmented the radiosensitization by the rmIL-12 treatment of the tumor and formed a powerful treatment against the metastatic disease.

Table 10 Human Lung Cancer Cell Line Characteristics

Cell line	Age/gender	Tumor type and origin	Genetics	Growth	Reference
Non-small-cell lung cancer lines					
A549	58/M	Carcinomatous lung tissue; epithelial-like	Modal chromosome 65–67	Cell culture	105
A-427	52/M	Carcinomatous lung tissue; epithelial-like	Modal chromosome 70–72; N5 tetrasomic chromosomes N1 & N15 single; N10, N12, N21 triple	Cell culture	105
Calu-1	47/M	Epidermoid carcinoma; metastasis to pleura	Modal chromosome 62; hypotriploid; 13 marker chromosomes	Cell culture monolayer; forms tumors in nude mice	106
Calu-3	25/M	Adenocarcinoma; pleural effusion	Modal chromosome 62; hypotriploid; 7 marker chromosomes	Cell culture monolayer; forms tumors in nude mice	106
Calu-6	61/F	Anaplastic carcinoma proba bly lung	Modal chromosome 57–59; hypotriploid; 14 marker chromosomes	Cell culture monolayer; forms tumors in nude mice	106
SK-MES-1	65/M	Lung squamous carcinoma; pleural effusion	Modal chromosome 59; hypotriploid; 17–20 marker chromosomes	Cell culture monolayer	106
SK-LU-1	60/F	Primary lung adenocarcinoma	Modal chromosome 88; hypotetraploid; 7 marker chromosomes	Cell culture monolayer; forms tumors in immunodeficient rats	
SW900	53/M	Lung squamous carcinoma; epithelial-like	Modal chromosome 56; hypotriploid; >30 marker chromosomes	Cell culture monolayer; forms tumors in nude mice	107
SL-6		Large-cell carcinoma		Cell culture monolayer; forms tissues in nude mice	108
ChaGo K-1	45/M	Undifferentiated bronchogenic carcinoma; subcutaneous metastases	Modal chromosome 52; hyperdiploid	Cell culture monolayer	109
NCI-H292	32/F	Pulmonary mucoepidermoid carcinoma; cervical node metastasis	Modal chromosome 47; near-diploid; 12 marker chromosomes	Cell culture monolayer; forms tumors in nude mice	110
NCI-H441	—/M	Papillary adenocarcinoma; pericardial fluid	Modal chromosome 52; hyperdiploid; 14 marker chromosomes	Cell culture monolayer	111
NCI-H460	—/M	Large-cell carcinoma; pleural fluid; expresses p53	Modal chromosome 57–58; hypotriploid; 7 marker chromosomes	Cell culture monolayer; forms tumors in nude mice	89,110

Cell line	Age/Sex	Origin	Karyotype	Culture characteristics	Ref.
NCI-H520	—/M	Lung squamous cell carcinoma; lung mass; low p53	Modal chromosome 58; hypotriploid; 20 marker chromosomes	Cell culture monolayer; forms tumors in nude mice	89,111
NCI-H596	73/M	Lung adenosquamous carcinoma; chest wall mass	Modal chromosome 71; near-triploid; 20 marker chromosomes	Cell culture monolayer; forms tumors in nude mice	89,111
NCI-H661	43/M	Lung large-cell carcinoma; lymph node	Modal chromosome 142; hyperhexaploid; >70 marker chromosomes	Cell culture monolayer	89,111
NCI-H676B	63/M	Lung adenocarcinoma; pleural fluid	Modal chromosome 43; hypodiploid	Cell culture suspension	89,111
NCI-H820	53/M	Lung papillary adenocarcinoma; lymph node metastasis	Modal chromosome 69; near-triploid; 25–35 marker chromosomes	Cell culture suspension; forms tumors in nude mice	
Small-cell lung cancer lines					
SW-2		Small-cell lung carcinoma, pleural fluid		Cell culture suspension; forms tumors in nude mice	112,113
NCI-H69	55/M	Small-cell lung carcinoma; pleural fluid	Highly aneuploid; modal chromosome 72–78; subtetraploid	Cell culture suspension; forms tumors in nude mice	114
NCI-H82	40/M	Small-cell lung carcinoma; pleural fluid	Modal chromosome 68; near-triploid	Cell culture suspension; forms tumors in nude mice	114
NCI-H128	60/M	Small-cell lung carcinoma; pleural fluid	Modal chromosome 65–66; predominantly triploid	Cell culture suspension; forms tumors in nude mice	114
NCI-H146	59/M	Small-cell lung carcinoma; pleural fluid	Modal chromosome 68; near-triploid; 15 marker chromosomes	Cell culture suspension; forms tumors in nude mice	115
NCI-H209	—/M	Small-cell lung carcinoma; bone marrow	Modal chromosome 49; hyperdiploid; 11 marker chromosomes	Cell culture suspension; forms tumors in nude mice	115
NCI-H345	64/M	Small-cell lung carcinoma; bone marrow	Modal chromosome 63; hypotriploid; 16 marker chromosomes	Cell culture suspension; forms tumors in nude mice	115
NCI-H446	61/M	Small-cell lung carcinoma; pleural fluid	Modal chromosome 74; hypertriploid; >25 marker chromosomes	Cell culture mixed suspension and attached; forms tumors in nude mice	116
NCI-H510A	56/M	Small-cell lung carcinoma; adrenal metastasis		Cell culture mixed suspension and attached	115

Local radiation, like other tumor cell cytotoxic therapy, facilitates T-cell-mediated tumor regression. The exact mechanisms for this response are unknown, but they could involve reduced synthesis of immune suppressant factors from killed and/or damaged tumor cells, the exposure or expression of immunogenic epitopes by irradiated tumors, and/or the generation of rmIL-12-enhancing cytokines by the generation of an inflammatory response as a result of tumor cell killing. There is some evidence that patients may be able to recognize antigens on lung tumor cells (85). One study has suggested that the development of antibody responses to autologous lung cancer cells as measured by immunoblotting is associated with prolonged survival (86). Lung cancers express a variety of gene products which have been shown to be the targets of cellular and humoral responses in patients with various malignancies; these include mutant ras, mutant p53, her-2/neu, the epidermal growth factor receptor, and the MAGE, BAGE, and GAGE families (87). Among the approaches utilizing ex vivo modification of tumor cells, Dranoff et al. have shown that vaccination with irradiated tumor cells engineered to secrete GM-CSF additivity or synergy may broaden the utility of *in vitro* studies (91,92). Mogi et al. (93) have extended the isobologram methodology to three drug combinations in cell culture and found that the cisplatin/navelbine/CPT-11 combination was additive in cytotoxicity toward a non-small-cell lung cancer cell line.

Small-cell lung cancer has been a particularly frustrating disease because 80% or more of patients respond very well to primary chemotherapy but ultimately fail to respond upon recurrence of the disease. One hypothesis is that the recurrent disease represents the emergence of drug-resistant subpopulations of the tumor either present in the primary tumor or induced by the initial chemotherapy regimen. Several drug-resistant cell lines have been developed from the small-cell lung cancer cell line NCI-H69 including H69/DAU, H69/VP, and OC-NYH/VM selected for resistance to daunorubicin, VP-16, and VM-26, respectively (94). Other drug-resistant sublines of NCI-H69 are H69/BCNU, NYH/CIS, NYH/TPT, and NYH/CAM selected for resistance to BCNU, cisplatin, topotecan, and camptothecin. Jensen et al. (94) examined the response of this collection of small-cell lung cancer cell lines to topotecan, CPT-11, taxol, taxotere, and gemcitabine as representative new anticancer drugs. From data on collateral sensitivity and lack of cross resistance, they concluded that a platinum complex and a taxane or a topoisomerase I inhibitor along with a topoisomerase II inhibitor could be good drug combinations.

B. Human Tumor Xenografts

Just as the development of cell lines selects a subpopulation(s) of cells from the original tumor that can grow in cell culture, so the growth of human tumors in immunodeficient nude or SCID mice selects a subpopulation(s) of cells that can grow in the presence of murine vasculature and other normal cells (95,96). Most established human lung cancer cell lines can grow tumor nodules in immunodeficient mice, albeit some grow very slowly. Most human tumors are implanted subcutaneously in mice because this allows the growth and response of the tumor to therapy to be assessed readily over a time course of weeks or months (97,98). Subcutaneously implanted human tumor xenografts tend to grow locally as tumor nodules, but rarely metastasize (99,100). Tumor growth in lungs is most often achieved by intravenous injection of tumors cells, resulting in lung colony formation; however, orthotopic implantation of human lung cancer cells intrabronchially for growth in the lungs of nude mice or rats has been described (101,102), but is technically challenging. Corti et al. (103) grew the human large cell lung carcinoma NCI-H460 in nude mice, then selected a rare lung metastasis for implantation into fresh hosts. After three such serial transplantations, the H460M subline, which avidly metastasizes to the lungs from a subcutaneous implant, was developed. Yano et al. (104) found that by pretreating SCID mice implanted intravenously with human small cell lung cancer cells H69/VM with antimouse IL-2 receptor β chain antibody, numerous lymph node and liver metastases were observed.

Thus, refinement of human tumor xenograft models are leading to well-controlled experimental systems which increasingly mimic human disease and are proving to be better predictors of the response of human disease to therapy. The xenograft model is very useful for testing cytotoxic agents, and it may be useful for newer agents directed toward the vasculature, although in these tumors the vasculature is murine but it is, by definition, not useful for immunotherapy or vaccines.

IV. Conclusion

Preclinical models of a specific group of malignancies such as lung cancer can be particularly useful in elucidating single agents and drug combinations that may be active in those diseases. Investigators still make good use of the earliest established syngeneic models such as the Lewis lung carcinoma, and are still learning the most useful applications of human lung cancer cell lines grown in culture or in immunodeficient animals. Preclinical data from these models provide valuable scientific support for clinical trials of new drugs, drug combinations, and combined-modality regimens. Data from these models also allow the further molecular elucidation of the changes resulting in malignant transformation and the response of malignant cells to therapy.

References

1. Matthews M. Problems in morphology and behavior of bronchopulmonary malignant disease. In: Israel I, Chahanain P, eds. Lung Cancer: Natural History, Prognosis and Therapy. New York: Academic Press, 1976:23.

2. Sugiura K, Stock C. Studies in a tumor spectrum. III. The effect of phosphoramides on the growth of a variety of mouse and rat tumors. Cancer Res 1955; 15:38–51.

3. Sugiura K, Stock C. Studies in a tumor spectrum. I. Comparison of the action of methylbis(2-chloroethyl) amine and 3-bis (2-chlorethyl) aminomethyl-4-methoxymethyl-5-hydroxy-6-methlpyridine on the growth of a variety of mouse and rat tumors. Cancer 1952; 5:382–315.

4. Sugiura K, Stock C. Studies in a tumor spectrum. II. The effect of 2,4,6-triethylenimino-s-triazine on the growth of a variety of mouse and rat tumors. Cancer 1952; 5:979–991.

5. DeWys W. A quantitative model for the study of the growth and treatment of a tumor and its metastases with correlation between proliferative state and sensitivity to cyclophosphamide. Cancer Res 1972; 32:367–373.

6. DeWys W. Studies correlating the growth rate of a tumor and its metastases and providing evidence for tumor-related systemic growth-retarding factors. Cancer Res 1972; 32:374–379.

7. Steel G, Adams K. Stem-cell survival and tumor control in the Lewis lung carcinoma. Cancer Res 1975; 35:1530–1535.

8. Steel GG, Nill RP, Peckham MJ. Combined radiotherapy-chemotherapy of Lewis lung carcinoma. Int J Radiat Oncol Biol Phys 1978; 4:49–52.

9. Gemcitabine HCl (LY188011 HCl) Clinical Investigational Brochure. Indianapolis, IN: Eli Lilly Company, October 1993.

10. Huang P, Chubb S, Hertel L, Plunkett W. Mechanism of action of 2′,2′ difluorodeoxycytidine triphosphate on DNA synthesis (abstr 2530). Proc Am Assoc Cancer Res 1990; 31:426.

11. Hertel L, Boder G, Kroin J. Evaluation of the antitumor activity of gemcitabine 2′,2′-difluoro-2′-deoxycytidine. Cancer Res 1990; 50:4417–4422.

12. Bouffard D, Fomparler L, Momparler R. Comparison of the antineoplastic activity of 2′,2′ difluorodeoxycytidine and cytosine arabinoside against human myeloid and lymphoid leukemia cells. Anticancer Drugs 1991; 2:49–55.

13. Heinemann V, Hertel L, Grindey G, Plunkett W. Comparison of the cellular pharmacokinetics and toxicity of 2′,2′-difluorodeoxycytidine and 1-beta-D-arabinofuranosyl cytosine. Cancer Res 1988; 48:4024–4031.

14. Eckhardt I, VonHoff D. New drugs in clinical development in the United States. Hematol Oncol Clin North Am 1994; 8:300–332.

15. Anderson H, Lund B, Bach F. Single-agent activity of weekly gemcitabine in advanced non-small cell lung cancer: a Phase 2 study. J Clin Oncol 1994; 1821–1826.

16. Gatzemeier U, Shepard F, LeChevalier T, et al. Activity of gemcitabine in patients with non-small cell lung cancer: a multicentre, extended Phase II study. Eur J Cancer 1996; 32A:243–248.

17. Bertelli P, Mantica C, Farina G, et al. Cobelli S, LaVerde N, Gramegna G, Scanni A. Treatment of non-small cell lung cancer with vinorelbine. Proc Am Soc Clin Oncol 1994; 13:362.

18. Bore P, Rahmani R, VanCamtfort J. Pharmacokinetics of a new anticancer drug, navelbine, in patients. Cancer Chemother Pharmacol 1989; 23:247–251.

19. Cros S, Wright M, Morimoto M. Experimental antitumor activity of navelbine. Semin Oncol 1989; 16(suppl):15–20.
20. Cvitkovic E. The current and future place of vinorelbine in cancer therapy. Drugs 1992; 44(suppl 4):36–45.
21. Marquet P, Lachatre G, Debord J. Pharmacokinetics of vinorelbine in man. Eur J Clin Pharmacol 1992; 42:545–547.
22. Navelbine (vinorelbine tartrate) Clinical Investigational Brochure. Burroughs Wellcome Co., October 1995.
23. Fumoleau P, Delgado F, Delozier T, et al. Phase II trial of weekly intravenous vinorelbine in first line advanced breast cancer chemotherapy. J Clin Oncol 1993; 11:1245–1252.
24. Jehl F, Quoix E, Leveque D. Pharmacokinetics and preliminary metabolite fate of vinorelbine in humans as determined by high performance liquid chromatography. Cancer Res 1991; 51:2073–2076.
25. Lepierre A, Lemarie E, Dabouis G, Garnier G. A Phase 2 study of navelbine in the treatment of non-small cell lung cancer. Am J Clin Oncol 1991; 14:11519.
26. Teicher BA, Herman TS, Holden SA, Eder JP. Chemotherapeutic potentiation through interaction at the level of DNA. In: Chow T-C, Rideout DC, eds. Synergism and Antagonism in Chemotherapy. New York: Academic Press, 1991:541–584.
27. Teicher B. A systems approach to cancer therapy (antiangiogenics + standard cytotoxics' mechanism(s) of interaction). Cancer Metastasis Rev 1996; 15:247–272.
28. Alvarez Sotomayor E, Teicher BA, Schwartz GN, Holden SA, Menon K, Herman TS, Frei E III. Minocycline in combination with chemotherapy or radiation therapy in vitro and in vivo. Cancer Chemother Pharmacol 1992; 30:377–384.
29. Teicher BA, Alvarez Sotomayor E, Huang ZD. Antiangiogenic agents potentiate cytotoxic cancer therapies against primary and metastatic disease. Cancer Res 1992; 52:6702–6704.
30. Teicher BA, Alvarez Sotomayor E, Huang ZD, et al. β-Cyclodextrin tetradecasulfate/tetrahydrocortisol ± minocycline as modulators of cancer therapies in vitro and in vivo against primary and metastatic Lewis lung carcinoma. Cancer Chemother Pharmacol 1993; 33:229–238.
31. Teicher BA, Holden SA, Ara G, et al. Potentiation of cytotoxic cancer therapies by TNP-470 alone and with other antiangiogenic agents. Int J Cancer 1994; 57:920–925.
32. Teicher BA, Holden SA, Dupuis NP, et al. Potentiation of cytotoxic therapies by TNP-470 and minocycline in mice bearing EMT-6 mammary carcinoma. Breast Cancer Res Treat 1995; 36:227–236.
33. Teicher BA, Dupuis NP, Robinson M, Emi Y, Goff D. Antiangiogenic treatment (TNP-470/minocycline) increases tissue levels of anticancer drugs in mice bearing Lewis lung carcinoma. Oncol Res 1995; 7:237–243.
34. Teicher BA, Dupuis N, Kusumoto T, et al. Antiangiogenic agents can increase tumor oxygenation and response to radiation therapy. Radiat Oncol Invest 1995; 2:269–276.
35. Brem H, Ingber D, Blood CH, Bradley D, Urioste S, Folkman J. Suppression of tumor metastasis by angiogenesis inhibition. Surg Forum 1991; 42:439–441.

36. Ingber D, Fujita T, Kishimoto S, et al. Synthetic analogues of fumagillin that inhibit angiogenesis and suppress tumour growth. Nature 1990; 348:555–557.

37. Kusaka M, Sudo K, Matsutani E, et al. Cytostatic inhibition of endothelial cell growth by the angiogenesis inhibitor TNP-470 (AGM-1470). Br J Cancer 1994; 69:212–216.

38. Antoine N, Greimers R, De Roanne C, et al. AGM-1470, a potent angiogenesis inhibitor, prevents the entry of normal but not transformed endothelial cells into the G_1 phase of the cell cycle. Cancer Res 1994; 54:2073–2076.

39. Yamamoto T, Sudo K, Fujita T. Significant inhibition of endothelial cell growth in tumor vasculature by an angiogenesis inhibitor, TNP-470 (AGM-1470). Anticancer Res 1994; 14:1–4.

40. Kusaka M, Sudo K, Fujita T, et al. Potent anti-angiogenic action of AGM-1470: comparison to the fumagillin parent. Biochem Biophys Res Commun 1991; 174:1070–1076.

41. Brem H, Folkman J. Analysis of experimental antiangiogenic therapy, J Pediatr Surg 1993; 28:445–451.

42. Takayamiya Y, Friedlander RM, Brem H, Malick A, Martuza RL. Inhibition of angiogenesis and growth of human nerve sheath tumors by AGM-1470. J Neurosurg 1993; 78:470–476.

43. Brem H, Gresser I, Grossfeld J, Folkman J. The combination of antiangiogenic agents to inhibit primary tumor growth and metastasis. J Pediatr Surg 1993; 28:445–451.

44. Yanase T, Tamura M, Fujita K, Kodama S, Tanaka K. Inhibitory effect of angiogenesis inhibitor TNP-470 in rabbits bearing VX-2 carcinoma by arterial administration of microspheres and oil solution. Cancer Res 1993; 53:2566–2570.

45. Kamei S, Okada H, Inoue Y, Yoshioka T, Ogawa Y, Toguchi H. Antitumor effects of angiogenesis inhibitor TNP-470 in rabbits bearing VX-2 carcinoma by arterial administration of microspheres and oil solution. J Pharmacol Exp Ther 1993; 264:469–474.

46. Yamaoka M, Yamamoto T, Masaki T, Ikeyama S, Sudo K, Fujita T. Inhibition of tumor growth and metastasis of rodent tumors by the angiogenesis inhibitor O-(chloroacetyl-carbamoyl)fumagillin (TNP-470; AGM-1470). Cancer Res 1993; 53:4262–4267.

47. Toi M, Yamamoto Y, Imazawa T, Takayanagi T, Akutsu K, Tominaga T. Antitumor effect of the angiogenesis inhibitor AGM-1470 and its combination effect with tamoxifen in DMBA induced mammary tumors in rats. Int J Oncol 1993; 3:525–528.

48. Yamaoka M, Yamamoto T, Ikeyama S, Sudo K, Fujita T. Angiogenesis inhibitor TNP-470 (AGM-1470) potently inhibits the tumor growth of hormone-independent human breast and prostate carcinoma cell lines. Cancer Res 1993; 53:5233–5236.

49. Placidi L, Cretton-Scott E, de Sousa G, Rahmani R, Placidi M, Sommadossi J-P. Disposition and metabolism of the angiogenic moderator O-(chloroacetyl-carbamoyl) fumagillol (TNP-470; AGM-1470) in human hepatocytes and tissue microsomes. Cancer Res 1995; 55:3036–3042.

50. Tamargo RJ, Bok RA, Brem H. Angiogenesis inhibition by minocycline. Cancer Res 1991; 51:672–675.

51. Teicher BA, Holden SA, Ara G, et al. Influence of an anti-angiogenic treatment on 9L gliosarcoma: oxygenation and response to cytotoxic therapy. Int J Cancer 1995; 61:732–737.

52. Teicher BA, Holden SA, Ara G, Northey D. Response of the FSaII fibrosarcoma to antiangiogenic modulators plus cytotoxic agents. Anticancer Res 1993; 13:2101–2106.

53. Kakeji Y, Teicher B. Preclinical studies of the combination of angiogenic inhibitors with cytotoxic agnets. Invest Drugs 1997. In press.

54. Banks RE, Patel PM, Selby PJ. Interleukin 12: a new clinical player in cytokine therapy. Br J Cancer 1995; 71:655–659.

55. Gazzinelli RT, Hieny S, Wynn TA, Wolf S, Sher A. Interleukin 12 is required for the T-lymphocyte-independent induction of interferon γ by an intracellular parasite and induces resistance in T-cell-deficient hosts. Proc Natl Acad Sci USA 1993; 90:6115–6119.

56. Locksley RM. Interleukin 12 in host defense against microbial pathogens. Proc Natl Acad Sci USA 1993; 90:5879–5880.

57. Robertson M, Ritz J. Interleukin 12: basic biology and potential applications in cancer treatment. Oncologist 1996; 1:88–97.

58. Gately MK, Desai B, Wolitzky AG, et al. Regulation of human lymphocyte proliferation by a heterodimeric cytokine, IL-12 (cytotoxic lymphocyte maturation factor). J Immunol 1991; 147:874–882.

59. Perussia B, Chan SH, D'Andres A, et al. Natural killer (NK) cell stimulatory factor of IL-12 has differential effects on the proliferation of TCR-$\alpha\beta^+$, TCR-$\gamma\delta^+$ T lymphocytes, and NK cells. J Immunol 1992; 149:3495–3502.

60. Robertson MJ, Soiffer RJ, Wolf SF, et al. Responses of human natural killer (NK) cells to NK cell stimulatory factor (NKSF): cytolytic activity and proliferation of NK cells are differentially regulated by NKSF. J Exp Med 1992; 175:779–788.

61. Gately MK, Wolitzky AG, Quinn PM, Chizzonite R. Regulation of human cytolytic lymphocyte responses by interleukin-12. Cell Immunol 1992; 143:127.

62. Naume B, Gately M, Espevik T. A comparative study of IL-12 (cytotoxic lymphocyte maturation factor)-, IL-2-, and IL-7-induced effects on immunomagnetically purified CD56$^+$ NK cells. J Immunol 1992; 148:2429–2436.

63. Chan SH, Perussia B, Gupta JW, et al. Induction of interferon γ production by natural killer cell stimulatory factor: characterization of the responding cells and synergy with other inducers. J Exp Med 1991; 173:869–879.

64. Brunda MJ, Luistro L, Warrier RR, et al. Antitumor and antimetastatic activity of interleukin-12 against murine tumors. J Exp Med 1993; 178:1223–1230.

65. Nastala CL, Edington HD, McKinney TG, et al. Recombinant IL-12 administration induces tumor regression in association with IFN-γ production. J Immunol 1994; 153:1697–1706.

66. Noguchi Y, Richards EC, Chen Y-T, Old LJ. Influence of interleukin 12 on p53 peptide vaccination against established Meth A sarcoma. Proc Natl Acad Sci USA 1995; 92:2219–2223.

67. Brunda M, Luistro L, Rumennik L, et al. Antitumor activity of interleukin 12 in preclinical models. Cancer Chemother Pharmacol 1996; 38(suppl):S16–S21.

68. Fujiwara H, Hamaoka T. Antitumor and antimetastatic effects of interleukin 12. Cancer Chemother Pharmacol 1996; 38:S22–S26.

69. Voest EE, Kenyon BM, O'Reilly MS, Truitt G, D'Amato RJ, Folkman J. Inhibition of angiogenesis *in vivo* by interleukin 12. J Natl Cancer Inst 1995; 87:581–586.

70. Kedar E, Klein E. Cancer immunotherapy: are the results discouraging? Can they be improved? Adv Cancer Res 1992; 59:245.

71. Seder RA, Gazzinelli R, Sher A, Paul WE. Interleukin 12 acts directly on CD4+ T cells to enhance priming for interferon γ production and diminishes interleukin 4 inhibition of such priming. Proc Natl Acad Sci USA 1993; 90:10188–10192.

72. Yoshida A, Koide Y, Uchijima M, Yoshida TO. IFN-γ induces IL-12 mRNA expression by a murine macrophage cell line, J774. Biochem Biophys Res Commun 1994; 198:857–861.

73. Gately MK, Warrier RR, Honasoge S, et al. Administration of recombinant IL-12 to normal mice enhances cytolytic lymphocyte activity and induces production of IFN-γ *in vivo*. Int Immunol 1994; 6:157–167.

74. Zeh HJ III, Hurd S, Storkus WJ, Lotze MT. Interleukin-12 promotes the proliferation and cytolytic maturation of immune effectors: implications for the immunotherapy of cancer. J Immunother 1993; 14:155–161.

75. Caruso M, Pham-Nguyen K, Kwong Y, et al. Adenovirus-mediated interleukin-12 gene therapy for metastatic colon carcinoma. Proc Natl Acad Sci USA 1996; 93:11302–11306.

76. Nishimura T, Watanabe K, Yahata T, et al. Application of interleukin 12 to antitumor cytokine and gene therapy. 1996; 38:S27–S34.

77. Brunda MJ. Interleukin-12. J Leuk Biol 1994; 55:280–288.

78. Teicher BA, Ara G, Menon K, Schaub RG. *In vivo* studies with interleukin-12 alone and in combination with monocyte-colony stimulating factor and/or fractionated radiation therapy. Int J Cancer 1995; 65:80–84.

79. Teicher B, Ara G, Buxton D, Leonard J, Schaub B. Optimal scheduling of interleukin-12 and fractionated radiation therapy in the murine Lewis lung carcinoma. Clin Cancer Res 1997. Submitted.

80. Aglietta M, Monzeglio C, Pasquino P, Carnino F, Stern AC, Gavosto F. Short-term administration of granulocyte-macrophage colony stimulating factor decreases hematopoietic toxicity of cytostatic drugs. Cancer 1993; 72:2970–2973.

81. Miller AM. Hematopoietic growth factors in autologous bone marrow transplantation. Semin Oncol 1993; 20:88–95.

82. Naparstek E, Ohana M, Greenberger JS, Slavin S. Continuous intravenous administration of rmGM-CSF enhances immune as well as hematopoietic reconstitution following syngeneic bone marrow transplantation in mice. Exp Hematol 1993; 21:131–137.

83. Steinman RM. The dendritic cell system and its role in immunogenicity. Annu Rev Immunol 1991; 9:271–296.

84. Dranoff G, Jaffee E, Lazenby A, et al. Vaccination with irradiated tumor cells engineered to secrete murine granulocyte-macrophage colony-stimulating factor stimulates potent, specific, and long-lasting anti-tumor immunity. Proc Natl Acad Sci USA 1993; 90:3539–3543.

85. Perlin E. Carcinoma of the lung: immunotherpay with intradermal BCG and allogenic tumor cells. Int J Radiat Oncol Biol Phys 1980; 6:1033–1039.

86. Winter S. Antibodies against autologous tumor cell proteins in patients with small-cell lung cancer: association with improved survival. J Natl Cancer Inst 1993; 85:2012–2018.

87. Boon T, Cerottini J, VandenEynde B, vanderBruggen P, PelVan A. Tumor antigens recognized by T lymphocytes. Annu Rev Immunol 1994; 12:337–365.

88. Dranoff G, Mulligan R. Gene transfer as cancer therapy. Adv Immunol 1995; 58:417–454.

89. Takahashi T, Nau M, Chiba I, et al. p53: a frequent target for genetic abnormalities in lung cancer. Science 1989; 246:491–494.

90. Little C, Nau M, Carney D, Gazdar A, Minna J. Amplification and expression of the c-myc oncogene in human cancer cell lines. Nature 1983; 306:194–196.

91. Kratzke R, Kramer B. Evaluation of *in vitro* chemosensitivity using human lung cancer cell lines. J Cell Biochem Suppl 1996; 24:160–164.

92. Kratzke R, Shimizu E, Kaye F. Molecular genetics of lung cancer. In: Benz C, Yu E, eds. Tumor Suppressors and Oncogenes in Human Malignancies. Boston: Kluwer Academic Publishers, 1992.

93. Mogi H, Hasegawa Y, Watanabe A, Nomura F, Saka H, Shimokata K. Combination of effects of cisplatin, vinorelbine and irinotecan in non-small cell lung cancer cell lines *in vitro*. Cancer Chemother Pharmacol 1997; 39:199–204.

94. Jensen P, Holm B, Sorensen M, Christensen I, Sehested M. In vitro cross-resistance and collateral sensitivity in seven resistant small-cell lung cancer cell lines: preclinical identification of suitable drug partners to taxotere, taxol, topotecan and gemcitabin. J Cancer 1997; 75:869–877.

95. Houghton J, Houghton P. The suitability and use of human tumor xenografts. In: Kallman R, ed. Rodent Tumor Models in Experimental Cancer Therapy. New York: Pergamon, 1987.

96. Steel G. How well do tumor xenografts maintain the therapeutic response characteristics of the source tumor in the donor patient? In: Kallman R, ed. Rodent Tumor Models in Experimental Cancer Therapy. New York: Pergamon, 1987.

97. Sharkey F, Fogh J, Hajdu S, Fitzgerald P, Fogh J. Experience in surgical pathology with human tumor growth in the nude mouse. In: Fogh J, Giovanella B, eds. The Nude Mouse in Experimental and Clinical Research. New York: Academic Press, 1978:187–214.

98. Sharkey F, Fogh J. Considerations on the use of nude mice for cancer research. Cancer Met Rev 1984; 3:341–360.

99. Fidler I. Rationale and methods for use of nude mice to study the biology and therapy of human cancer metastasis. Cancer Met Rev 1986; 5:29–49.

100. Manzotti C, Audisio R, Pratesi G. Importance of orthotopic implantation for human tumors as model systems: relevance to metastasis and invasion. Clin Exp Met 1993; 11:5–14.

101. McLemore T, Blacker P, Gregg M, et al. Intrabronchial implanation. A method for the orthotopic propagation of human lung tumors in athymic nude mice. Chest 1987; 91:5S–8S.

102. Mulvin D, Howard R, Mitchell D, et al. Secondary screening system for preclinical testing of human lung cancer therapies. J Natl Cancer Inst 1992; 84:31–37.
103. Corti C, Pratesi G, DeCesare M, et al. Spontaneous lung metastases in human lung tumor xenograft: a new experimental model. J Cancer Res Clin Oncol 1996; 122:154–160.
104. Yano S, Nishioka Y, Izumi K, et al. Novel metastasis model of human lung cancer in scid mice depleted of NK cells. Int J Cancer 1996; 67:211–217.
105. Giard D, Aaronson S, Todaro G, et al. In vitro cultivation of human tumors: establishment of cell lines derived from a series of solid tumors. J Natl Cancer Inst 1973; 51:1417–1423.
106. Fogh J. Human tumor cells *in vitro*. In: Fogh J, ed. New York: Plenum Press, 1975:115–159.
107. Fogh J, Wright W, Loveless J. Absence of HeLa cell contamination in 169 cell lines derived from human tumors. J Natl Cancer Inst 1977; 58:209–214.
108. Teicher BA, Frei E III. Development of alkylating agent–resistant human tumor cell lines. Cancer Chemother Pharmacol 1988; 21:292–298.
109. Rabson A, Rosen S, Tashjian A. Production of human chorionic gonadotropin *in vitro* by a cell line derived from a carcinoma of the lung. J Natl Cancer Inst 1973; 50:669–674.
110. Banks-Schlegel S, Gazdar A, Harris C. Intermediate filament and cross-linked envelope expression in human lung tumor cell lines. Cancer Res 1985; 45:1187–1197.
111. Brower M, Carney D, Oie H, Gazdar A, Minna J. Growth of cell lines and clinical specimens of human non-small cell lung cancer in a serum-free defined medium. Cancer Res 1986; 46:798–806.
112. Francis J, Bernal S, Gazdar A, Thompson R, Baylin S. L-Dopa decarboxylasa activity (DDC): a distinguishing biomarker for the growth of small cell lung cancer (SCCL) in tissue culture. AACR Proc 1980; 21:52.
113. Francis K, Thompson R, Bernal S, Luk G, Baylin S. Effects of dibutyral cyclic adenosine 3′, 5′-monophosphate on the growth of cultured human small cell lung carcinoma and the specific cellular activity of L-dopa decarboxylase. Cancer Res 1983; 43:639.
114. Gazdar A, Carney D, Russell E, et al. Establishment of continuous, clonable cultures of small-cell carcinoma of the lung which have amine precursor uptake and decarboxylation cell properties. Cancer Res 1980; 40:3502–3507.
115. Carney D, Gazdar A, Bepler G, et al. Establishment and identification of small cell lung cancer cell lines having classic and variant features. Cancer Res 1985; 45:2913–2923.
116. Gazdar A, Carney D, Nau M, Minna J. Characterization of variant subclasses of cell lines derived from small cell lung cancer having distinctive biochemical, morphological, and growth properties. Cancer Res 1985; 45:2924–2929.

Part Three

SMALL-CELL LUNG CANCER

15

Surgery for Small-Cell Lung Cancer

DEAN M. DONAHUE

The MGH Cancer Center
Massachusetts General Hospital, and
Harvard Medical School
Boston, Massachusetts

DOUGLAS J. MATHISEN

Massachusetts General Hospital, and
Harvard Medical School
Boston, Massachusetts

I. Introduction

The biological behavior of small-cell lung cancer (SCLC) usually results in systemic spread in approximately 70% of patients at presentation. Up to an additional 20% will have regionally advanced disease with local lymph node metastases predicting unrecognized distant disease. This phenotypic trait explains the historically dismal outcome of surgery for SCLC in the prechemotherapy era.

The current standard therapy for limited-stage SCLC is chemotherapy with etoposide and cisplatin with concurrent thoracic radiotherapy (1). This still results in a 2-year local failure rate of 70% (2). The area of primary tumor or its regional lymph nodes is the most frequent site of relapse in SCLC. One way for surgery to play a role in therapy would be to show an improvement in local control. Whether this possible improvement in local control would translate into improved survival has been controversial. The results of two meta-analyses of patients with limited-stage SCLC treated with chemotherapy show a small but significant survival benefit for patients receiving thoracic radiation therapy (3,4). Whether the addition of surgery would further improve survival is unproven. What has been shown is that certain patients with small-cell lung cancer do well following resection. It has yet to be clearly elucidated what factors are important in selecting surgical patients.

337

II. Historical Background

Most early surgical series of SCLC reported 5-year survival of <3% (5,6). In 1973 Takata and colleagues reported 161 patients presenting with SCLC. Only 35 (21.7%) were felt to be resectable (5). Of these only two patients had a complete resection, surviving a total of 47 and 77 months. In 1978 Mountain reported 41 patients undergoing complete resection out of 368 patients with SCLC (11.1%) (6). The median survival following resection was 5 months. This was identical to the 146 patients with limited-stage disease who did not undergo a resection.

The disappointing results of primary surgical therapy led to a prospective randomized trial of surgery versus radiotherapy by the Medical Research Council of Great Britain (7,8). A total of 144 patients with limited-stage SCLC were included in this trial. The median survival in the surgical patients was 199 days, compared to 300 days in the radiation therapy group. At 10-year follow-up, only three patients remained alive, all treated with radiotherapy. The conclusion drawn was that radiotherapy was preferable to surgery. While the results had a dramatic impact on the treatment of this disease, there were several flaws in the study. The most glaring was that *one-half* of the surgical group did not undergo resection. These patients either had a thoracotomy and were found to be unresectable, or had no operation because they were thought to be medically unfit. More than 50% of these patients received local radiotherapy instead of resection. These unresected patients were included in the surgical survival data.

In response to the Medical Research Council report, Lennox and colleagues retrospectively reviewed 275 patients with SCLC (9). They reported a 58% resection rate and a 5-year survival of 10.6% among cases treated with surgery alone. It is difficult to explain the difference between the survival in this series compared to the 1% to 3% survival in others (5,6). One possibility is the selection of patients with "limited-stage" SCLC for surgery. This broadly defined stage could be narrowed down with the application of surgical staging procedures such as mediastinoscopy. This could help in selecting the subset of patients who could benefit from surgery.

III. Role of Surgery in Staging SCLC

The TNM classification universally applied to most solid tumors has been slower to gain acceptance in small-cell lung cancer. The Veterans Administration Lung Cancer Study Group classification of *limited disease* and *extensive disease* is still frequently used in today's literature. The TNM stage of limited disease would range from T1N0 to T3N3. This broad clinical spectrum is significant, as the likelihood of disease control in SCLC varies inversely with TNM stage (10). Shields and colleagues were early proponents of TNM staging in SCLC (11). They

Table 1 Survival of Completely Resected SCLC Patients by TNM Stage

TNM	Stage	Number of patients	5-Year survival (%)
T1 N0 M0	IA	26	59
T2 N0 M0	IB	23	27.9
T1 N1 M0	IIA	16	31.3
T2 N1 M0	IIB	39	9.0
T3 OR N2	III	28	3.6

Source: Ref. 11.

reported 148 cases of SCLC who underwent complete resection with negative microscopic margins. Survival for each TNM stage (Table 1) was more favorable than the next advanced stage, underscoring the significance of the TNM system.

Mediastinoscopy should be used to accurately stage the mediastinum in patients with SCLC, especially if surgical resection is an option. The use of CT scans to obtain a clinical stage is particularly deceptive in small-cell lung cancer. Shepherd and colleagues from the University of Toronto reported 63 patients with resectable SCLC (12). The preoperative TNM clinical stage correlated with the postoperative pathologic stage only 35% of the time. As many as one-third of patients had falsely negative mediastinal lymph nodes by CT scan. These patients would have clinically been stage I or II, but pathologically were stage III, carrying a worse prognosis. Wada and associates found that 47.4% of the clinically node-negative patients had nodal involvement (N1, 2, or 3) found at resection (13).

IV. Role of Surgery in Treatment of Early-Stage SCLC

It is unusual for SCLC to present as an early-stage lesion. Of 370 patients with peripheral lung nodules evaluated in a Veterans Administration Surgical Oncology Group trial, only 15 (4%) were found to have small-cell cancer (14). As discussed earlier, Shields and colleagues were early advocates for the use of TNM staging in SCLC (11). Following a complete resection with negative microscopic margins, 148 patients were randomized to receive single-agent chemotherapy with either nitrogen mustard or cyclophosphamide, or no additional treatment. There was no survival advantage to either of these mild chemotherapuctic regimens compared to surgery alone. Stage-related survival is reported in Table 1. Their survival results were similar to those of completely resected non-small-cell lung cancer of equivalent stage.

A study from McGill University identified 15 confirmed solitary tumors out of 375 patients presenting with SCLC (15). These 15 patients underwent a variety of treatment regimens. Their median survival of 24 months was significantly better than the 11-month survival in a group of limited-stage disease treated at the same institution. This improved prognosis may reflect an earlier stage of presentation; however, almost half of the solitary nodule patients did not have their hilar or mediastinal lymph nodes biopsied.

Meyer performed resection followed by combination chemotherapy in patients with stage I or II SCLC (16). Seventy percent of his patients were alive and disease-free 5 or more years following surgery, including two of the four patients with positive N1 nodes. Shah and colleagues reported that 35% of patients with SCLC referred to a single surgeon at the Royal Brompton Hospital for evaluation were found suitable for thoracotomy (17). Following a negative mediastinoscopy, 28 patients went on to resection. Fourteen patients had stage I SCLC, five had stage II, and 11 had stage III. Chemotherapy or radiation therapy was not used in this series. For the patients with negative lymph nodes, including eight patients with T3N0 lesions, the actual 5-year survival was 59.1%. There were no 5-year survivors in any of the N1- or N2-positive patients. Tumor location had little effect on survival, as the 5-year survival rates for central and peripheral lesions were 42.8% and 50%, respectively.

It is possible that these early-stage lesions are a pathologic subgroup of the more common perihilar small-cell tumors. It has been shown that some tumors characterized as small-cell by light microscopy show ultrastructural features of squamous cell or adenocarcinoma (18,19). Warren and associates postulated the existence of a lower-grade pulmonary neuroendocrine carcinoma with features similar to small cell cancer (20). They retrospectively reviewed pathologic specimens from 46 peripheral lung tumors thought to be small-cell carcinoma. Each patient had undergone a complete resection. The diagnosis of a small-cell neuroendocrine tumor was confirmed in 34 patients. Twelve patients (26%) were reclassified as well-differentiated neuroendocrine tumors based on the presence of detectable organoid architecture with scant or focal necrosis.

Clinically, these two groups behaved differently. In the small-cell tumors, the 2-year survival for stage I lesions was only 9%. This contrasts with the 2-year survival for all stages of well-differentiated neuroendocrine carcinomas of 82%. It seems possible that this entity represents a different phenotype, and may complicate the data analysis if a clinical series contains patients with this tumor subtype.

V. Role of Surgery Combined with Chemotherapy

Small-cell lung cancer is a highly chemosensitive tumor. Current chemotherapy with etoposide- and platinum-based regimens have an overall response rate as high as 95% (21). However, autopsy studies have identified SCLC at the primary site in 64% and in local lymph nodes in 53% of patients who had a complete clinical response (22). Several studies have evaluated the role of surgical resection combined with chemotherapy (Table 2).

Table 2 Survival by Stage in Resected SCLC Treated with Chemotherapy

Investigators	No. patients	Chemo	Survival	Stage survive (%)				
				I		II		
				A	B	A	B	III
Shields et al., 1982 (11)	148	None vs. N mustard or cyclophosphamide	5-year	59.5	27.9	31.3	9.0	3.6
Ichinose et al., 1992 (23)	37	Variable CAV or CAV II	5-year	67.7		34.3		15.6
Davis et al., 1993 (24)	37	CAV	5-year	50		35		21
Karrer and Ulsperger, 1995 (25)	183	Mostly CAV	4-year	56		29		N/A
Fujimori et al., 1997 (21)	21	CAV II	3-year	All stages = 63.6				

CAV: cyclophosphamide, doxorubicin, vincristine; CAV II: cisplatin, doxorubicin, etoposide (VP-16).

Ichinose and colleagues reported a series of 69 stage I to IIIA patients (23). This group underwent either surgical resection or radiation therapy (50 to 75 Gy). All but two patients had received chemotherapy. The patients were assigned to each group in a nonrandomized fashion. Surgical resection was not considered if the patient required a pneumonectomy for complete resection; however, overt N2 disease seen on CT scan was *not* a contraindication to resection. Comparison between these two groups should therefore be made cautiously.

The local failure rates for the patients treated surgically were 0%, 25%, and 25% for stage I, II, and IIIA, respectively. The overall local and distant failure rates in the surgical group were 16% and 37.8%, compared to 25% and 50% in the non-resected group (Table 3). Because the pathologic staging of the radiation therapy group is not known, the survival was reported based on preoperative clinical stage. The stage I, II, and IIIA 5-year survival rates in the surgical group were 67.7%, 34.3%, and 15.6% (Table 2). This compares to 50%, 14.3%, and 4.1% in the non-surgical group.

In 1993, Davis and colleagues reported 37 consecutive patients with clinical stage I and II SCLC treated with chemotherapy and surgery only (24). Patients with peripheral lesions were excluded from the study, eliminating a group shown to benefit from resection (11). Following a negative mediastinoscopy, patients underwent resection. Postoperatively, patients were treated with CAV chemotherapy and 20 Gy of cranial irradiation. There were no postoperative or chemotherapy-related deaths. Seven patients (19%) were upstaged when positive N2 nodes were found at thoracotomy. Stage I patients (n = 10) had a median survival of 162 weeks and a calculated 5-year survival of 50%. The median survival times for

Table 3 Sites of Failure in SCLC

Investigators	Patients	Surgery	Chemotherapy	Radiation therapy		Recurrence (%)	
				Chest	Brain	Local	Distant
Sheperd et al., 1991 (26)	119	Yes	Mostly CAV	68 pts. 25–35 Gy	20 GY	8.3	N/R
Ichinose et al., 1992 (23)	37	Yes	VCMC	None	None	16	37.8
	32	No	CAV EP	50.2–75 Gy	None	25	50
Davis et al., 1993 (24)	37	Yes	CAV	None	20 Gy	0	N/R
Lad et al., 1994 (28)	182	Yes	CAV	50 Gy	30 Gy	25	N/R
Fujimori et al., 1997 (21)	21	Yes	CAVII	None	None	4.7	23.8
Work et al., 1997 (2)	199	No	CAV plus EP	40–45 Gy	25–33 Gy	70	63

CAV: cyclophosphamide, doxorubicin, vincristine; VCMC: vincristine, cyclophosphamide, mitomycin C, chromomycin A3; CAV II: cisplatin, doxorubicin, etoposide; EP: etoposide (VP-16): cisplatin.

stage II (n = 14) and III (n = 8) patients were 86 and 63 weeks, respectively. The 5-year survival times for these two groups were 35% and 21%, respectively. With a minimum follow-up of 18 months, there were only two local recurrences (6%). Both patients had distant failures concurrently. No radiotherapy had been given to the tumor bed or mediastinum or hilum.

The Lung Cancer Study Group (LCSG) of the International Society of Chemotherapy reported in 1995 a prospective study of clinical stage I patients who were resected and then randomized to different chemotherapy protocols postoperatively (25). None of the chemotherapy regimens included combination etoposide and platinum. Prophylactic cranial irradiation was added if the patients were disease-free following their chemotherapy. Of the 183 patients enrolled in the study, 50 (27%) were found to have more advanced disease at thoracotomy. One hundred fifty-two patients were able to have a complete resection (83%). The 4-year survival rates for pathologic stage I and II patients were 56% and 29%, respectively. The 27 patients with N2 disease who could be completely resected had a 33% 4-year survival.

In 1997, Fujimori and associates reported a Phase II trial examining surgery following induction chemotherapy with cisplatin, adriamycin, and etoposide (CAV II) (21). Of the 150 patients seen with small-cell lung cancer, 22 (14.6%) had clinically resectable disease (N0, N1, or early N2) and were entered into the study. Mediastinoscopy was not done, which could have improved the pretreatment staging. The clinical response rate to preoperative chemotherapy was 95.5%. Twenty-one patients underwent resection including a radical lymph node dissection. The pathologic complete response rate to the CAV II chemotherapy was 25%. With a minimum follow-up of 41 months, there has only been one known local recurrence. Survival was reported for the preoperative clinical stage rather than the pathologic stage. The median survival for all stages was 61.9 months, with an actuarial 3-year survival of 66.7%. There were six relapses during a minimum follow-up of 41 months. This included one local failure and five distant failures (four brain, one liver). Of note, no prophylactic cranial irradiation was given during the study.

VI. Role of Surgery in Multimodality Therapy

Combination chemotherapy and radiotherapy remain the mainstay of therapy for limited-stage SCLC. In 1997, Work and colleagues reported a study of 199 patients with "limited-stage" SCLC treated with multidrug chemotherapy including etoposide and cisplatin, and randomized to early or late radiation therapy (2). The 2-year local recurrence rate was 70%, and the median survival was 11 months. There was no significant difference with the timing of radiation therapy. Comparing these data to several of the surgical series should be made cautiously, as patients with involved N3 nodes (contralateral mediastinal, ipsilateral supraclavicular)—typically excluded in surgical series—could be included in this study. Local failure rates from combined modality studies are reported in Table 3.

The University of Toronto Lung Oncology Group reported 119 patients with clinically resectable SCLC (26). Patients with bulky mediastinal adenopathy, supraclavicular lymph node involvement, or pleural effusions were excluded. Chemotherapy was given to 107 patients, with 40 patients treated preoperatively. Regimens containing etoposide and cisplatin were administered in only nine patients. Postoperative thoracic irradiation (25 to 35 Gy) was given to most stage II and III patients (n = 68). Cranial irradiation (20 Gy) was given to 85 patients. Four patients were unable to be resected. No patient treated with preoperative chemotherapy had gross residual disease following resection, but six patients had surgical margins positive for microscopic disease. All patients had a complete lymph node staging intraoperatively. The pathologic complete response rate was 10% for the 40 patients treated with preoperative chemotherapy. Ten patients (8.3%) had a relapse at the primary site alone, with seven others (5.9%) failing both locally and distantly. The projected 5-year survival rates for pathological stage I (n = 35), II (n = 36), and IIIa (n = 48) were 51%, 28%, and 19%, respectively (Table 4). The overall median survival was 111 weeks. There was no difference in survival between patients receiving preoperative or postoperative chemotherapy.

This same group reported a retrospective analysis of "salvage" surgery for patients who failed to improve or who progressed during their chemotherapy (27). A group of 28 patients without bulky mediastinal or N3 disease underwent resection. The median survival was 74 weeks from the time of operation, with a projected 5-year survival of 23%.

In 1994 the LCSG reported a prospective randomized series of 328 patients with limited, potentially resectable small-cell lung cancer (28). This study excluded patients with peripheral lesions or a normal bronchoscopy, thereby reducing the number of early-stage lesions that respond favorably to surgery. All patients were treated with CAV chemotherapy (cyclophosphamide, doxorubicin, and vincristine) for five cycles. Clinical responders to the chemotherapy were then randomized to either thoracotomy and resection, or no surgery. All patients were then treated with 50 Gy of thoracic irradiation and 30 Gy of cranial irradiation. There were no postoperative complications reported. There was a 40% clinical complete response in both groups and a 19% pathologic complete response to chemotherapy in the surgical group. The two groups demonstrated a similar pattern of failure, with 25% relapsing in the chest only and 12% in the brain. The median survival in the surgical group was 15.4 months, compared to 18.6 months in the nonsurgical group. This study concluded that resection did not influence the pattern of relapse or the survival. No subsets were identified that would benefit from multimodality therapy.

However, the statistical power of the study was not great, especially for indi-

Table 4 Survival by Stage in Resected SCLC Treated with Multimodality Therapy

Investigators	No. patients	Chemo	Radiation therapy		Survival	Stage survive (%)				
			Chest	Brain		I		II		III
						A	B	A	B	
Sheperd et al., 1991 (26)	119	Mostly CAV	79 pts. 25–35 Gy	85 pts. 20 Gy	5-year	51		28		19
Lad et al., 1994 (28)	70	CAV	50 Gy post op	30 Gy	Median (Months)	11.4	17.1	14.5		12.5
Xiaojia et al., 1995 (29)	199	Cyclophospha- mide based	For positive nodes	None	5-year	52.3		31		15.5

CAV: cyclophosphamide, doxorubicin, vincristine; CAV II: cisplatin, doxorubicin, etoposide (VP-16).

vidual TNM groups. Of note, even the pathologic complete responders (T0N0) had a median survival of only 17 months, and in stage IA, 11.4 months. This possibly reflects the ineffectiveness of CAV chemotherapy employed in this study compared with today's etoposide- and platinum-based regimens. The major drawback in this series is that in nearly one-quarter of the surgical patients (16/70) an incomplete resection was done. Some of the local failures would represent progression of this residual local disease. These patients would predictably lower the median survival in the surgical group.

In 1995, Xiaojia and colleagues reported 199 SCLC patients treated with surgery combined with different cyclophosphamide-based chemotherapy regimens (29). Those with hilar or mediastinal lymph node involvement were given postoperative radiation therapy. The 5-year survival rates for stage I, II, and III were 52.3%, 31%, and 15.5%, respectively. No significant difference in survival was found in patients receiving preoperative compared with postoperative chemotherapy.

Wada and associates reported a retrospective review of 46 patients who received either preoperative and/or postoperative chemotherapy in a nonrandomized fashion (13). All patients were completely resected, which included a mediastinal lymph node dissection. This series would therefore represent a very accurate postoperative pathologic staging. The 5-year survival rates for stages I, II, and III were 39%, 40%, and 29%. Of note, there were no long-term survivors in the subset of patients who refused chemotherapy. Nine of 19 patients (47.4%) with clinical N0 disease were found to have positive lymph nodes at surgery.

Coolen and colleagues reported two consecutive groups of 15 patients each who underwent resection for small-cell lung cancer (30). Adjuvant chemotherapy was added to the second group, and three patients received radiation therapy. The 5-year survival in the first group treated without chemotherapy was 13%. This increased to 27% in the second group with better preoperative staging and the addition of postoperative chemotherapy. The survival for pathologic stage I patients improved from 12% to 60% between the two groups. Survival was <2 years in all eight patients who had positive mediastinal lymph nodes. Two of these N2 patients who were treated with etoposide and carboplatin had a greater survival time (18.5 months) than the three CAV-treated patients (5 months).

Takei and associates retrospectively reviewed a series of 49 patients who underwent resection for small-cell lung cancer (31). Twenty-two patients underwent preoperative chemotherapy, with 10 of these receiving radiation therapy as well. Eighteen patients had surgery with postoperative chemotherapy, and nine patients were treated with resection alone. The 15 patients who presented with clinical stage I disease and underwent initial surgery had a 5-year survival of 79.4%. With current chemotherapy regimens, the neoadjuvant therapy patients with clinical stage IIIA disease had a 5-year survival of 23.1%. The combined clinical stage IIIB and IV patients had 3-year and 5-year survival of 40% and

26.2%. Again the CT scan proved to be limited in assessing lymph node involvement, as the accuracy was only 63.3%.

VII.   Conclusion

While small-cell lung cancer tends to present at a more clinically advanced stage, there is reasonable evidence to support approaching this disease in a similar manner to non-small-cell lung cancer. The broader application of the TNM staging system in SCLC, and the use of surgical staging techniques such as mediastinoscopy, may assist in the evolution of treatment strategies.

SCLC is a chemosensitive disease. Combination chemotherapy has shown impressive remission rates, yet long-term survivors are rare. The addition of radiation therapy to improve local treatment has been shown to improve survival (3,4). The question of a surgical role in addition to current chemoradiotherapy protocols has yet to be answered. It seems possible that surgical resection as a means of improving local disease control may further improve survival.

There is good evidence to support the role of surgery in early-stage SCLC. Shah and associates reported a 59.1% 5-year survival for T1–3N0 lesions treated by resection alone (17). The earlier series by Shields and colleagues showed similar survival between SCLC and non-small-cell early stage lesions (11). The addition of chemotherapy to surgery for stage I SCLC has resulted in 5-year survival ranging from 50% to 70% (16,23–25). Trimodality therapy results in similar survival rates for stage I tumors (26,29).

Unfortunately, only a small percentage of patients present with early-stage lesions. The presence of lymph node metastasis, predicting distant spread, negatively affects survival. With lymph node involvement confined to the lung parenchyma (stage II) the 5-year survival for combined modality series is as high as 28% to 50% (16,23–26,29).

Evaluating stage III disease can be difficult, as T3N0 lesions seem to exhibit a different biological behavior than patients with positive mediastinal lymph nodes (T1–3N2). Long-term survivors have been reported for T3N0 tumors (17,25). While the survival for N2-positive patients has generally been poor (11,30,32), it remains to be seen if current chemotherapy agents will improve in the systemic control of SCLC enough to warrant surgery for locally advanced SCLC.

References

1. Turrisi AT III. Concurrent chemoradiotherapy for limited small-cell lung cancer. Oncology 1997; 11 (suppl 9):31–37.
2. Work E, Nielsen OS, Bentzen SM, Fode K, Palshof T. Randomized study of initial

versus late chest irradiation combined with chemotherapy in limited-stage small-cell lung cancer. J Clin Oncol 1997; 15:3030–3037.

3. Pingnon J-P, Arriagada R, Ihde D, et al. A meta-analysis of thoracic radiotherapy for small cell lung cancer. N Engl J Med 1992; 327:1618–1624.

4. Warde P, Payne D. Does thoracic irradiation improve survival and local control in limited-stage small-cell carcinoma of the lung? A meta-analysis. J Clin Oncol 1992; 10:890–895.

5. Takita H, Brugarolas A, Marabella P, Vincent RG. Small cell carcinoma of the lung. J Thorac Cardiovasc Surg 1973; 66:472–477.

6. Mountain C. Clinical biology of small cell carcinoma: relationship to surgical therapy. Semin Oncol 1978; 5:272–279.

7. Working Party on the Evaluation of Different Methods of Therapy in Carcinoma of the Bronchus. Comparative trial of surgery and radiotherapy for the primary treatment of small-celled or oat-celled carcinoma of the bronchus. Lancet 1966; 2:979–986.

8. Miller AB, Fox W, Tall R. Five year follow-up of the medical research council comparative trial of surgery and radiotherapy for the primary treatment of small-celled or oat-celled carcinoma of the bronchus. Lancet 1969; 2:501–505.

9. Lennox SC, Flavell G, Pollock DJ, Thompson VC, Wilkins JL. Results of resection for oat-cell carcinoma of the lung. Lancet 1968; 2:925–927.

10. Meyer, JA. Effect of histologically verified TNM stage on disease control in treated small cell carcinoma of the lung. Cancer 1985; 55:1747–1752.

11. Shields TW, Higgins GA, Matthews MJ, Keehn RJ. Surgical resection in the management of small cell carcinoma of the lung. J Thorac Cardiovasc Surg 1982; 84:481–488.

12. Shepherd FA, Evans WK, Feld R, et al. Adjuvant chemotherapy following surgical resection for small-cell carcinoma of the lung. J Clin Oncol 1988; 6:832–838.

13. Wada H, Yokomise H. Teneka F, et al. Surgical treatment of small cell carcinoma of the lung: advantage of preoperative chemotherapy. Lung Cancer 1995; 13:45–46.

14. Higgins GA, Shields TW, Keehn RJ. The solitary pulmonary nodule. Arch Surg 1975; 110:570–575.

15. Quoix E, Fraser R, Wolkove N, Finkelstein H, Kreisman H. Small cell lung cancer presenting as a solitary pulmonary nodule. Cancer 1990; 66:577–582.

16. Meyer JA. Five-year survival in treated stage I and II small cell carcinoma of the lung. Ann Thorac Surg 1986; 42:668–669.

17. Shah SS, Thompson J, Goldstraw P. Results of operation without adjuvant therapy in the treatment of small cell lung cancer. Ann Thorac Surg 1992; 54:498–501.

18. Nomori H, Shimogato Y, Kodama T, Morinaga S, Nakajima T, Watanabe S. Subtypes of small cell carcinoma of the lung: morphometric, ultrastructural, and immunohistochemical analysis. Hum Pathol 1986; 17:604–613.

19. Churg A, Johnston WH, Stulbarg M. Small cell squamous and mixed small cell squamous-small cell anaplastic carcinomas of the lung. Am J Surg Pathol 1980; 4:255–263.

20. Warren WH, Memoli VA, Jordan AG, Gould VE. Reevaluation of pulmonary neoplasms resected as small cell carcinomas. Cancer 1990; 65:1003–1010.

21. Fujimori K, Yokoyama A, Kurita Y, Terashima M. A pilot Phase 2 study of surgical

treatment after induction chemotherapy for resectable stage I to IIIA small cell lung cancer. Chest 1997; 111:1089–1093.

22. Elliot JA, Osterlind K, Hirsch FR, Hansen HH. Metastatic patterns in small cell lung cancer: correlation of autopsy findings with clinical parameters in 537 patients. J Clin Oncol 1987; 5:246–254.

23. Ichinose Y, Hara N, Ohta M, Takamori S, Kawasaki M, Hata K. Comparison between resected and irradiated small cell lung cancer in patients stages I through IIIa. Ann Thorac Surg 1992; 53:95–100.

24. Davis S, Crono L, Tonato M, Darwish S, Pelicci PG, Grignani F. A prospective analysis of chemotherapy following resection of clinical stage I–II small-cell lung cancer. Am J Clin Oncol (CCT) 1993; 16:93–95.

25. Karrer K, Ulsperger E. Surgery for cure followed by chemotherapy in small cell carcinoma of the lung. Acta Oncol 1995; 34:899–906.

26. Shepherd FA, Ginsberg RJ, Feld R, Evans WK, Johansen E. Surgical treatment for limited small-cell lung cancer. J Thorac Cardiovasc Surg 1991; 101:385–393.

27. Shepherd FA, Ginsberg R, Patterson GA, et al. Is there ever a role for salvage operations in limited small-cell lung cancer? J Thorac Cardiovasc Surg 1991; 101:196–200.

28. Lad T, Piantadosi S, Thomas P, Payne D, Ruckdeschel J, Giaccone G. A prospective randomized trial to determine the benefit of surgical resection of residual disease following response of small cell lung cancer to combination chemotherapy. Chest 1994; 601 (suppl 6):320S–323S.

29. Xiaojia C, Shiyei L, Dongling Z, et al. Multimodality therapy including surgical resection for limited small cell lung cancer. Chin Med J 1995; 109:689–691.

30. Coolen L, Van den Eckhout A, Deneffe G, Demedts M, Vansteenkiste J. Surgical treatment of small cell lung cancer. Eur J Cardiothorac Surg 1995; 9:59–64.

31. Takei H, Ohe Y, Tamura T, et al. Indication of surgery for small cell lung cancer based on clinical stage (abstr). Proc Am Soc Clin Oncol 1997; 16:485a.

32. Meyer JA, Gullo JJ, Ikins PM, et al. Adverse prognostic effect of N2 disease in treated small cell carcinoma of the lung. J Thorac Cardiovasc Surg 1984; 88:495–501.

16

Role of Thoracic Radiation Therapy and Prophylactic Cranial Irradiation in the Management of Small-Cell Lung Cancer

PARVESH KUMAR

Robert Wood Johnson Medical School/UMDNJ
Cancer Institute of New Jersey
New Brunswick, New Jersey

I. Introduction

Almost 180,000 new cases of lung cancer will be diagnosed and approximately 160,000 people will die of this disease in 1999 (1). Small-cell lung cancer (SCLC) will represent 20% to 25% of all newly diagnosed cases of lung cancer. In contrast to non-small-cell lung cancer (NSCLC), which is a locoregional disease amenable to surgical therapy, small-cell lung cancer is a systemic disease characterized by rapid proliferation and early distant dissemination for which surgery usually plays a minimal therapeutic role. As shown by Matthews et al. (2) in a series of autopsies performed on a group of SCLC patients who had died within 1 month of an attempted curative surgical resection, the cause of death in most cases was systemic metastases despite a rigorous preoperative evaluation which had demonstrated only locoregional disease. These differences in the "biologic behavior" of SCLC as compared to NSCLC eventually led the World Health Organization in 1967 to recognize "oat cell carcinoma" as a distinct histological and clinical entity.

Given the systemic nature of SCLC, it is not surprising that chemotherapy has become the cornerstone of therapeutic management of this disease. Despite being extremely responsive to both chemotherapy and radiotherapy, improving survival outcome for SCLC has been changing. However, modern-era treatments which have combined cisplatin-based chemotherapy with thoracic radiation therapy (TRT) provide optimism for improving survival outcome, especially for limited-stage (LS) SCLC. The role of radiation therapy in the management of SCLC can be either curative (i.e., TRT for LS SCLC), prophylactic (i.e., prophylactic cranial irradiation), or palliative. This chapter will focus on the curative and prophylactic role of radiation therapy, especially for the treatment of LS SCLC, although its potential use in extensive-stage disease will be also discussed.

II. Staging System

The primary role of staging investigations is to assess anatomical extent of disease so that only the most appropriate therapies may be optimally used. Given that the majority of the patients diagnosed with SCLC present with "metastatic" disease, the TNM staging system offers little prognostic value except possibly to identify a few early local tumors which may be amenable to surgical resection. Hence, the simple two-stage system of "limited" and "extensive" stage disease as proposed by the Veterans Administration Lung Cancer Study Group (3) almost two decades ago continues to be widely used. This two-tier staging system provides prognostic significance as well as guidance in directing the most appropriate therapies. Limited-stage SCLC is defined as disease encompassable by a single continuous, usually hemithoracic, normal tissue tolerable, "therapeutic" radiation port; extensive-stage (ES) disease is defined as tumor extension beyond these bounds. Hence, both anatomic and physiologic criteria define LS disease. At presentation, LS SCLC represents about one-third of all cases of SCLC while ES disease accounts for the remaining two-thirds.

III. Thoracic Radiation Therapy
A. Limited-Stage Disease

The role of thoracic radiation therapy (TRT) in the treatment of LS SCLC has evolved with a better understanding of the natural history of this disease and of the patterns of failure. Given that SCLC is a systemic disease, modern-era treatment philosophy of LS disease integrates chemotherapy (CT) for the treatment of undetectable micrometastases usually present at diagnosis while TRT is used to improve locoregional tumor control.

Although survival is the major endpoint used to judge the success of chemoradiation therapy, local control within the radiation port is the most direct measure of the efficacy of TRT. Long-term survival cannot be achieved or maintained without local control of disease! However, determination of local control is not an exact science, and it can be affected by many factors as follows:

1. Definition of local failure (relapse at primary site or other additional areas within the chest such as mediastinum, contralateral hilum, supraclavicular fossae).
2. Differentiating recurrence from fibrosis.
3. Duration of control of systemic disease by chemotherapy (i.e., "competing risk" phenomenon).
4. Length of follow-up interval.
5. Statistical methods (e.g., overall crude failure or first failure)

All of these factors may under- or overestimate local control and thus the measured efficacy of TRT.

1. Historical Perspective: Where Have We Been?

Although TRT has been used to treat SCLC for over three decades, its role in the "standard" management of LS disease was not well established until the mid- to late 1980s. A series of treatment paradigms ranging initially from surgery followed by mainly TRT, and then mostly CT, to now combined chemoradiation therapy best represents the evolution of treatment for SCLC (Fig. 1).

The radiosensitivity of SCLC was discovered during the 1960s; this eventually led to a shift in the treatment of SCLC from surgical management to TRT. In a randomized trial of 144 patients comparing TRT alone (n = 73) to surgery only (n = 71) in "limited-stage" SCLC conducted by the Medical Research Council (4), both the median survival (43 weeks vs. 28.5 weeks; $P = .04$) and overall survival (4% vs. 1%) were superior in the radiotherapy arm. In fact, the sole survivor on the surgery arm refused thoracotomy after randomization and instead underwent TRT. During the same time period, the systemic nature of SCLC was clinically recognized, which led to the use of chemotherapy.

In 1969, the VA Lung Cancer Study Group randomized almost 2000 patients with "extensive-stage" SCLC to several alkylating agents at various dose schedules or placebo therapy. This trial showed that the median survival could be more than doubled by using cyclophosphamide versus placebo treatment (4 months vs. 1.5 months, respectively; $P = .0005$) (5). Hence this landmark study began the era of CT in the treatment of SCLC. As first suggested by Watson and Berg (6), chemotherapy was then combined with TRT as the "new model" for the treatment of SCLC by several investigators. In the first randomized trial comparing TRT to cyclophosphamide and TRT conducted by Bergsagel et al. (7), both progression-free survival (16 weeks vs. 29 weeks) and overall survival (21 weeks vs. 42 weeks) were significantly superior in the combined-modality arm.

Other randomized trials also subsequently confirmed the survival benefit of using combined chemoradiation therapy over TRT alone (8,9). Eventually, trials (10) were conducted using combination CT alone which yielded survival outcomes similar to combined chemoradiation therapy studies. Given the higher tox-

Where Have We Been?

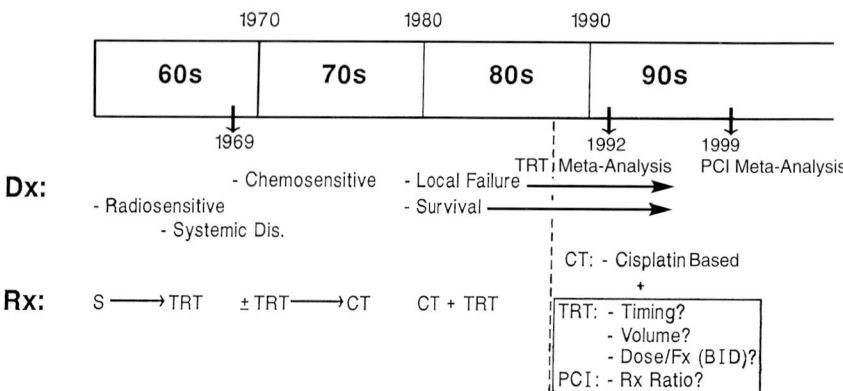

Figure 1 The historical evolution of the management of SCLC can be best described as a series of treatment paradigms ranging initially from surgery to TRT during the 1960s, then shifting from TRT to CT during the 1970s, followed by integration of TRT into the overall therapy regimen during the late 1980s to the early 1990s. Dx: diagnostic issues or discoveries relating to a specific era; Rx: therapy; S: surgery; TRT: thoracic radiation therapy; CT: chemotherapy; PCI: prophylactic cranial irradiation.

icities associated with combined chemoradiation therapy, and the high chemoresponsiveness of SCLC, many investigators began to either relegate TRT to an adjuvant role (11) or omit it altogether from the treatment regiment (12). Hence, during the late 1960s and the early 1970s, multiagent chemotherapy became the primary treatment for SCLC, reflecting a "philosophical" change in the management of this disease. However, the high frequency of local recurrence and poor survival led to a reassessment of the role of TRT in the treatment of SCLC (13).

2. "Standard of Therapy": Where Are We Now?

Beginning in the late 1970s and continuing throughout the 1980s, multiple cooperative group randomized trials were initiated in the United States to test the role of TRT in the treatment of LS SCLC (14–18). Major trials initiated by the Southeastern Cancer Study Group (SECSG) (14), National Cancer Institute (NCI) (15), Cancer and Leukemia Group B (CALGB) (16), Eastern Cooperative Oncology Group (ECOG) (17), and Southwest Oncology Group (SWOG) (18) randomized patients with LS SCLC to chemotherapy with or without TRT (Table 1). The schedule of TRT (i.e., concurrent, sequential, or alternating) and the dose/fractionation schemes varied among the cooperative groups, although prophylactic cranial irradiation (PCI) was included as part of the radiation regiment in all of the trials. All of the trials showed a decrease in local failure (LF) rates in the combined modality arm(s), and all but the SWOG study reported a statistically significant

Table 1 Major U.S. Randomized Trials of Chemotherapy (CT) Alone Versus Chemoradiation Therapy (CRT) in LS SCLC[a]

Cooperative group trial (investigators)	CRT sequence	Thoracic radiotherapy	Local failure (%) CT	Local failure (%) CRT	2-Year survival (%) CT	2-Year survival (%) CRT
CALGB, 1981–84	CON	50 Gy/25 fxs	67		8	
(Perry et al., 16),		wk 1		40		15[b]
n = 399		wk 9		41		25[b]
			(LF only)			
ECOG, 1981–95	SEQ	50 Gy/25 fxs	—	—	13	19[b]
(Creech et al., 17),		wk 8				
n = 310						
SECSG I, 1978–82	ALT	40 Gy/14 fxs	52	36	16	24[b]
(Birch et al., 14),		wk 5, 8, 11				
n = 291		(split course)				
NCI, 1977–86	CON	40 Gy/15 fxs	67	30	12	28[b]
(Bunn et al., 15),		day 1				
n = 96						
SWOG, 1980–83	SEQ	48 Gy/22 fxs	72	50	25	35
(Kies et al., 19),		wk 12				
n = 93 (CR)						

[a]Survival and local control results of major U.S. prospective randomized trials comparing chemotherapy alone to chemoradiation therapy in LS SCLC. All of the trials showed a significant improvement in local control, and all but the SWOG study showed a statistically significant improvement in survival with chemoradiation therapy vs. CT alone. CR: complete response; LF: local failure; CRT: chemoradiation therapy; CON: concurrent; SEQ: sequential, ALT: alternating.
[b]$P < .05$

improvement in survival with the addition of TRT. Generally, LF rates are reduced by half, from about 60% with CT alone to 30% with the addition of TRT.

In the early 1990s, two meta-analyses (19,20) confirmed the results of the previous prospective randomized trials by showing that TRT improves survival in LS SCLC (Fig. 2). Pignon et al. (19) reported an *absolute* survival advantage of at least 5% at 3 years with the addition of TRT to chemotherapy (~15%) versus chemotherapy alone (~10%; $P = .001$). In relative terms, the combination of TRT and CT improved survival by 50% as compared to CT alone! Additionally, since the review by Pignon et al. (19) was an intent-to-treat analysis, it may have actually underestimated the impact of TRT in improving survival. The impact of an *absolute* 5% survival advantage with the addition of TRT to chemotherapy for the treatment of LS SCLC should not be underestimated. Within the United States, this survival improvement translates annually into almost 2000 more living patients who would otherwise have succumbed to SCLC. Thus, the "positive" results obtained from these randomized cooperative group trials and the meta-analyses reestablished TRT as an integral part of the "standard of therapy" for LS SCLC.

Efficacy of Conventional TRT

- Reduces Local Failure Rates
  - CT Only ≈ 60%
  - CT + TRT ≈ 30%

- Survival Benefit at 3 years*
  - Absolute ≈ 5%
  - Relative ≈ 50% (CT = 10% vs. CT/TRT = 15%)

Figure 2   The efficacy of conventional TRT in reducing local failure rates and in improving survival for limited-stage SCLC. (*Ref. 19.)

Although these prospective randomized studies (14–18) and the meta-analyses demonstrated that radiation therapy reduces LF rates and improves survival in the treatment of LS SCLC, several issues regarding the role of TRT still remain unresolved:

Timing of TRT with chemotherapy (i.e., concurrent vs. sequential vs. alternating)

Volume of radiation port (i.e., pre-CT vs. post-CT disease extent)

Optimal total dose/fractionation scheme

As these radiation therapy–related issues are explored below, one must always "place" them within the context of chemotherapy agents, doses, schedules, and their interaction with TRT.

3. Timing of TRT

Thoracic radiation therapy can be integrated with chemotherapy in three major ways: concurrently, sequentially, or alternatingly (Fig. 3). The optimal time to combine TRT with chemotherapy remains unknown. In the meta-analysis by Pignon et al. (19), no significant difference in survival outcome was observed between "early" (i.e., radiation given within 60 days of start of therapy) and "late" TRT. Furthermore, this analysis also found no significant difference in survival between sequential and nonsequential (i.e., concurrent or alternating) TRT. Each approach offers its unique therapeutic advantages and disadvantages.

a. Concurrent TRT

In the concurrent approach, TRT is delivered simultaneously with chemotherapy. With this approach, TRT can be given either "up-front" (early) or "delayed" (late) during the chemotherapy. The mathematical model of Goldie and Coldman suggests that the most effective regimens should be given "early" in the treatment course to prevent the emergence of resistant tumor clonogens. Additionally, tumor clonogens resistant to chemotherapy may be sensitive to ionizing radiation (21).

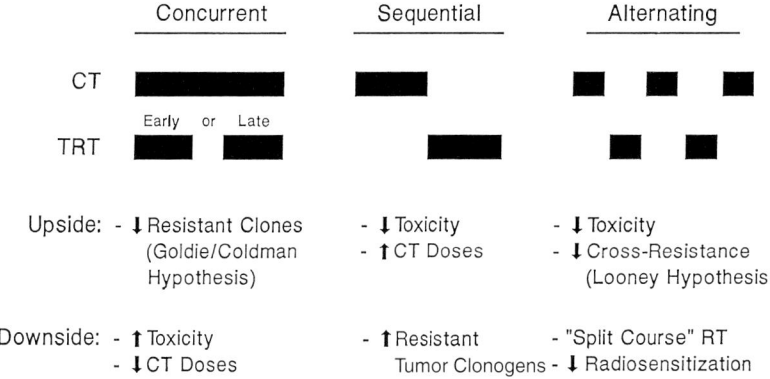

	Concurrent	Sequential	Alternating
CT			
TRT	Early or Late		

Upside: - ↓ Resistant Clones (Goldie/Coldman Hypothesis) - ↓ Toxicity - ↑ CT Doses - ↓ Toxicity - ↓ Cross-Resistance (Looney Hypothesis)

Downside: - ↑ Toxicity - ↓ CT Doses - ↑ Resistant Tumor Clonogens - "Split Course" RT - ↓ Radiosensitization

Figure 3 TRT can be integrated with CT either concurrently, sequentially, or alternatingly. Upside (advantages); downside (disadvantages); ↑ = increased; ↓ = decreased.

However, the disadvantages of the concurrent approach include increased toxicity from the simultaneous combining of the two therapies, and the decreased ability to deliver the full dose of chemotherapy.

Generally, some of the better survival outcomes in the treatment of LS SCLC have been achieved with the use of concurrent TRT and CT. For example, both the CALGB trial (protocol 8083) (16) and the National Cancer Institute of Canada (NCIC) study (22) compared concurrent TRT and CT to CT alone. In both of these trials, survival outcome was significantly improved with the addition of concurrent TRT to the CT regiment. In the NCIC study, 2-year survival was improved from 12% with CT alone to 28% with chemoradiation therapy. Local failure was also significantly reduced, from 67% in the CT-only arm to 30% in the combined modality arm. This same pattern of improvement in survival and reduction in LF rates was also evident with chemoradiation therapy versus CT alone in the CALGB trial. However, "negative" randomized trials such as the SWOG (18), Copenhagen (23), and GETCB (24) studies, which showed no significant survival advantage of adding TRT to the CT regimen, used either alternating or sequential TRT.

In a recently completed large Phase III study by the Japanese Clinical Oncology Group (JCOG) (25), 228 eligible patients were randomized to concurrent (day 2, cycle 1) or sequential (after cycle 4) BID TRT (45 Gy at 1.5 Gy/fraction twice a day) in conjunction with cisplatin-based chemotherapy. Preliminary results were very encouraging in both arms of this trial, though both median and 2-year survival favored concurrent over sequential TRT (29 months and 50% vs. 19 months and 40%, respectively). The use of both cisplatin-based CT and twice-a-day TRT accounts for the initial good results obtained in both arms of this trial.

i. "Early" Versus "Late" Concurrent TRT. Two large randomized studies have evaluated the role of "early" versus "delayed" concurrent TRT: CALGB protocol 8083 (16) and the NCIC trial (22) (Table 2), which showed opposite results. The CALGB protocol was a three-arm trial, two of which used either early (day 1 with cycle 1) or delayed (day 64 with cycle 4) TRT. Although local control was the same for the two TRT arms, 2-year failure-free survival favored delayed radiotherapy (25%) over the early radiotherapy (15%) arm ($P = .078$). Updated results of this study continue to confirm the earlier reported findings; 5-year overall survival still favors the delayed TRT (12%) over the early TRT (6%) arm or no TRT at all (3%) (26). On the other hand, the NCIC trial showed just the opposite results of the CALGB study. The NCIC study randomized patients with LS SCLC to either "early" (day 21 with cycle 2 of 6) or "late" (day 106 with cycle 6 of 6) TRT in conjunction with CT. As in the CALGB study, local control in the NCIC trial was virtually identical on the "early" versus the "late" TRT arms, though both 3-year progression-free survival (26% vs. 19%, $P = .036$, respectively) and 5-year overall survival (20% vs. 11%, $P = .008$, respectively) were superior in the "early" arm.

So why are there conflicting results between these two studies assessing the optimal concurrent timing of TRT with CT, especially given relatively the same intrathoracic local chest control rates between the early and late arms on both trials? Direct comparisons between these two trials are hampered by differences in the dose/fractionation and timing of TRT (i.e., "early" and "late" are not the same for both studies), and in the chemotherapy agents and duration (Table 3). Despite these dissimilarities, three possible reasons may explain the outcome differences between the two trials. First, the decreased ability to deliver the full dose of chemotherapy in the "early" (day 1) relative to the "late" TRT arm in the CALGB trial (verbal communication with Michael C. Perry) may have compromised survival in the early TRT arm. Additionally, the earlier administration of TRT in the NCIC trial allowed for "earlier" control of local disease, which may have reduced the incidence of brain metastases from 28.1% in the late arm to 18.1% ($P = .042$) in the early arm, partially contributing to the survival advantage observed in the early TRT arm. Finally, the design of late TRT arm (i.e., day 106 with cycle 6/6) in

Table 2 Limited-Stage SCLC Concurrent TRT: Early Versus Late[a]

Trial	Local control (%)	5-Year survival (%)
Early TRT		
CALGB 8083 (d 1, c 1)	54	6.6
NCIC (d 22, c 2)	59	20.0
Late TRT		
CALGB 8083 (d 64, c 4)	54	12.8
NCIC (d 106, c 6)	61	11.0

[a]Comparison of local control and survival outcome between CALGB protocol 8083 and NCIC study using "early" versus "late" *concurrent* thoracic radiation therapy. Note the similarities in local control rates between the early and the late TRT arms in *both* trials, and similar survival results in both late TRT arms.

Table 3 Limited-Stage SCLC Concurrent TRT: Early Versus Late Protocol Therapy Differences[a]

Therapy differences	CALGB 8083	NCIC Study
CT agents/cycles	CEV × 6/CAV × 7–18	CAV/EP × 6
TRT	50 Gy/25 fxs	40 Gy/15 fxs
Timing		
Early	day 1, cycle 1	day 22, cycle 2
Late	day 64, cycle 4/18	day 106, cycle 6/6

[a]Comparison between CALGB protocol 80–83 and the NCIC study revealed differences in the chemotherapeutic agents and duration, the TRT dose/fractionation scheme, and the timing of TRT. Although the total TRT dose may have been "radiobiologically equivalent," the timing of "early" (day 1, cycle 1 for CALGB protocol 80–83, and day 22, cycle 2 for NCIC study) and "late" (day 64, cycle 4/18 for CALGB study versus day 106, cycle 6/6 for NCIC study) were different. The "late" timing for the NCIC study was more a sequential TRT than a "true" concurrent approach. CT, chemotherapy; CEV, cyclophosphamide, etoposide, vincristine; CAV, cyclophosphamide, adriamycine, vincristine; EP, etoposide, cisplatin.

the NCIC trial was more like "sequential" chemotherapy followed by TRT than a "true" concurrent approach. Generally, survival outcome using sequential TRT is inferior to concurrent TRT; thus the NCIC trial design for the late TRT arm may have inadvertently advantaged the early TRT arm.

Although the question of early versus late concurrent TRT remains unresolved, each approach still offers its unique therapeutic advantages. Early concurrent TRT may reduce the incidence of brain metastases possibly due to "earlier" control of intrathoracic disease before development of chemoresistant micrometastases. On the other hand, "late" concurrent TRT does not appear to compromise local control though it potentially offers the opportunity to decrease lung toxicity by treating only the residual post-CT thoracic disease through a smaller-volume radiation portal.

b. Sequential TRT

In the sequential approach, the chemotherapy treatment is completed first and then TRT is delivered. The advantages of sequential therapy include overall decreased toxicity and potentially improved ability to deliver the full dose of chemotherapy. The downside includes an increased probability of developing therapy-resistant tumor clonogens. One large (18) and two small (27,28) randomized trials using non-cisplatin-based CT followed by sequential TRT in complete responders have been conducted. In the large SWOG study (18), complete responders (CRs) (n = 153) following induction CT were randomized to either split-course TRT (48 Gy in 22 fractions) or more additional CT. No difference in survival was observed between those patients undergoing TRT or CT only. However, local control was significantly improved with the addition of TRT (44% vs. 10%).

In the Northern California Oncology Group study (27), complete responders were randomized to either sequential involved-field TRT (n = 24) or observation or more additional CT (n = 24). Although no significant difference in survival between those patients receiving TRT or CT/observation was observed, intrathoracic local control was again significantly better on the radiation therapy arm (71% vs. 42%; P = .042). In the Petites Cellules Group trial (28), complete responders with both LS and ES disease were randomized to sequential TRT (n = 27) or observation (n = 25). No difference in survival was observed between the TRT and the observation group. In all three of the above studies, survival was unaffected by the addition of sequential TRT, although local control was significantly improved. The development of CT-resistant tumor clonogens resulting in a failure pattern dominated by systemic relapse may have contributed to this lack of survival improvement. Additionally, overall survival results seen in all three of these studies were relatively inferior to modern-day trials using cisplatin-based chemotherapy.

c. Alternating TRT

In the alternating approach, split-course TRT is interdigitated between cycles of chemotherapy. Besides potentially reducing toxicity and increasing the ability to deliver the full dose of chemotherapy, alternating TRT may also decrease the probability of developing cross-therapy-resistant tumor clonogens (i.e., Looney hypothesis). However, the disadvantages of this approach include split-course TRT and the loss of concomitant chemotherapy radiosentization. Multiple Phase II studies have confirmed the feasibility and efficacy of using alternating CT with either conventional (29) or hyperfractionated (HFX) TRT (30,31). Two large Phase III trials have evaluated the role of alternating CT and TRT (14,32). In the SECSG trial (14), 291 patients received either CAV chemotherapy alone or alternatingly with TRT. Both local control (64% vs. 48%; P = .06) and 2-year survival (28% vs. 19%; P = .03) outcomes were significantly improved with the addition to TRT. In a recently completed trial by the Petites Cellules Group (32), alternating TRT (55 Gy in 22 fractions tri-split course) was compared to concurrent TRT (50 Gy in 20 fractions) using non-cisplatin-based CT regimen. In this study, the 3-year survival rate was not statistically different between the concurrent arm (4%) and the alternating arm (7%). Survival was poor in both arms of this study, probably due to the use of non-cisplatin-based CT.

Generally, the addition of alternating TRT when compared to CT alone improves survival in LS SCLS, although this survival advantage is inferior to the results obtained with concurrent TRT.

4. The Best Timing!

Although the optimal temporal integration of TRT (i.e., concurrent vs. sequential vs. alternating) has not been conclusively resolved, most "positive" trials comparing chemoradiation therapy to CT alone have used "early," usually concurrent radiotherapy versus "late," usually sequential or alternating TRT. Additionally, some of the best survival results achieved in the treatment of LS SCLC have occurred using early concurrent TRT along with cisplatin-based CT. The current data highly support the use of concurrent over either sequential or alternating TRT in LS SCLC.

5. Volume of TRT

In the delivery of TRT for LS SCLC, the achievement of an optimal therapeutic ratio which minimizes toxicity while maximizing local control requires a careful balance between the dose/fractionation scheme and the radiated volume. This therapeutic ratio is also influenced by the combination of CT and TRT, which is usually more toxic than CT alone. For example, in the NCI trial (15), treatment-related mortality in the combined modality arm (11%) was almost three times as high as in the CT-alone arm (4%). Radiation therapy–related factors which may contribute to increased toxicity include the dose/fractionation scheme and the volume of the radiation portal. From a toxicity standpoint, radiation dose and volume encompassed within the radiation port are inversely related. Radiation dose escalation requires a reduction in volume so that toxicity can be kept at acceptable levels. However, within the context of standard radiation doses of 45 to 50 Gy level currently used in LS SCLC, there is considerable room for variation of the portal volume.

Historically, large radiation portals have been used to treat SCLC for multiple reasons. One of the tenets of radiation therapy mandates the coverage of next-echelon-uninvolved lymph nodes along with the primary tumor and involved lymphatic nodal stations. Confirmation of this tenet in LS SCLC came from an analysis of the patterns of failure in the SECSG trial (14). In this trial, exclusion of the contralateral hilum or the entire mediastinum increased the intrathoracic failure rate from 33% with adequate portals to 69% ($P = .026$) in portals with compromised "margins." Though SCLC invariably responds to CT, total clearance of local disease at the peripheral edges of the primary tumor by systemic therapy is not always certain. In a study reported by Mira and Livingston (33), radiation ports encompassing only the post-CT residual local chest disease were used. In this study, five of seven *intrathoracic* failures occurred outside of the radiation port at the lung periphery or with a malignant pleural effusion. The authors postulated that microscopic disease at the edges of the primary tumor had not been totally eradicated by initial CT alone, resulting in local recurrence. The authors concluded that perhaps larger radiation ports encompassing the pre-CT disease extent may have avoided these intrathoracic failures. Hence, the rationale for coverage of pre-CT disease extent within the radiation portal is to address both anatomical and chemoresponsive uncertainties.

However, this above rationale was recently challenged by a retrospective analysis from the Mayo Clinic (34). In this study, radiation ports encompassing either pre-CT (n = 31) or post-CT (n = 28) disease extent were correlated to patterns of locoregional failure. The rates of locoregional failure were similar for pre-CT (n = 10/31) and post-CT (n = 9/28) radiation portals. Additionally, no marginal local failures were observed in the post-CT radiation ports. In fact, all of the local failures occurred in the epicenter of the primary tumor, suggesting intrinsic tumor resistance rather than peripheral "geographic misses" as the cause of relapse. Furthermore, in a study conducted by the SWOG (18), partial responders to initial CT were randomized to either wide-field (pre-CT) or involved-field (post-CT) radiation treatment volume; no difference in local chest control rates was observed between these two groups of patients.

The retrospective analysis from the Mayo Clinic and the results from the SWOG trial challenge the historical rationale for prophylacticly covering uninvolved lymphatic nodal regions and pre-CT disease extent. Given the pulmonary toxicity associated with large portals with questionable benefit, the inclusion of only residual post-CT thoracic disease into a smaller radiation volume appears reasonable and should be prospectively evaluated.

6. Dose and Fractionation Scheme

Although TRT significantly reduces local failure rates in LS SCLC, there is still considerable room for improvement in local control. Recognizing the limitation that the volume of the radiation port places upon dose escalation, there are two potential ways of improving local control: increasing the total conventional radiation dose, or using alternative fractionation schemes (i.e., accelerated fractionation), hyperfractionated radiation, or a combination of both [i.e., CHART (continuous hyperfractionated accelerated radiation therapy)].

In order to improve local control with increasing doses of radiation, a dose-response relationship must first exist. Choi and Carey (35) showed a dose-response relationship between the total doses of radiation delivered and locoregional tumor control rates (Fig. 4). In this report, local control was only 20% to 25% in the radiation dose range of 30 to 35 Gy level, though it improved exponentially to 60% to 70% with doses in the 45 to 50 Gy range. However, whether a dose-response relationship exists beyond the conventional 50 Gy level is unclear. Arriagada et al. (29) increased the total thoracic tumor dose from 45 to 65 Gy level, albeit using split radiation courses, and found no significant improvement in local control. In a recently completed Phase I/II CALGB study (36), the maximum tolerated radiation dose given with cycle 4 of cisplatin/etoposide CT was determined to be 70 Gy in 35 fractions for conventional once-a-day TRT as compared to 45 Gy for twice-a-day irradiation at 1.5 Gy/fx. Acute esophageal toxicity was the dose-limiting factor for both arms of the study. Local control data were not reported in the abstract.

Another strategy to potentially improve local control involves the use of accelerated radiotherapy (AR). The aim of this strategy is to reduce repopulation

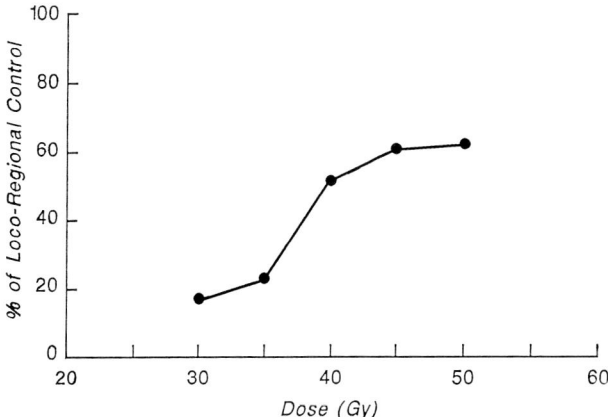

Figure 4 Dose-response relationship of thoracic radiotherapy in LS SCLC. Locoregional tumor control is improved with increasing TRT doses reaching a plateau at the 45 to 50 Gy level. From Ref. 35.

of malignant clonogens in rapidly proliferating tumors by delivering twice-a-day radiation therapy to shorten the overall treatment interval. Generally, overall total dose in this strategy is maintained at levels similar to conventional once-a-day radiotherapy. Several completed Phase II studies have already confirmed the efficacy of using AR in conjunction with CT (37–39). The results of a phase III intergroup trial (protocol 0096) were recently updated. In this trial, patients were randomized to either twice-a-day (45 Gy in 3 weeks) or conventional single daily fraction (SDF) (45 Gy in 5 weeks) concurrent (day 1, cycle 1) TRT along with four cycles of cisplatin and etoposide CT (40). At a median follow-up of almost 8 years, significant difference in 5-year survival outcome was found between BID and SDF TRT (126% vs. 16%, respectively; $P = .04$). Median survival was also improved from 19 months in those patients receiving once-daily TRT versus 23 months for those receiving BID TRT. Local control was better in the BID arm (64%) than the SDF arm (48%; $P = .06$). However, the improvement in local control came at a significantly higher rate of grade ≥ 3 esophageal toxicity (BID = 27% vs. SDF = 11%, $P < .001$, respectively).

 Given the conflicting results in improving local control with conventionally fractionated TRT beyond the 50 Gy level and the significant improvement in survival outcome using BID versus. SDF TRT, the use of BID TRT should be considered in LS SCLC for those patients who are likely to tolerate such aggressive therapy. However, among patients with a marginal or poor performance status or older age, the use of SDF of 1.8 or 2.0 Gy to total thoracic dose levels of 45–50 Gy is still reasonable (Fig. 5).

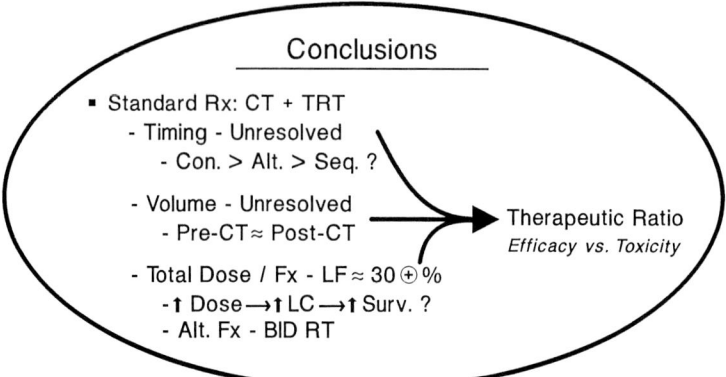

Figure 5 The current "standard" of therapy for the treatment of LS SCLC consists of combining chemotherapy with thoracic radiation therapy. Although not yet completely resolved, the most optimal time to combine TRT with CT appears to be concurrently rather than sequentially or alternatingly. Issues relating to the most optimal volume (i.e., pre-CT vs. post-CT) and the total dose and fractionation scheme remain unresolved. Whether alternative fractionation schemes such as accelerated radiotherapy or an increase in the total conventional radiation dose will lead to improvement in local control and subsequentially survival remains unclear. LF, local failure; LC, local control.

B. Extensive-Stage Disease

The efficacy of thoracic radiation therapy in the treatment of ES disease is limited by the inefficacy of systemic chemotherapy! As was the case in LS SCLC, TRT significantly reduces local failure rates in ES disease, from generally 70% with CT alone to usually <40% with the addition of chest irradiation. In two consecutive studies conducted by SWOG in ES SCLC, LF at the primary site was only 20% when TRT (30 Gy/10 fx) was used (41), compared to 67% when chest irradiation was omitted for patients in CR (42). However, the local efficacy of TRT has failed to improve survival in ES SCLC (43,45).

In a Phase III randomized trial conducted by the NCIC and SWOG (45) following completion of a phase II study (44), CODE chemotherapy and TRT were compared to an alternating regimen of CAV (cisplatin, adriamycin, vincristine)/ PE (cisplatin and etoposide) chemotherapy only. The response rates were significantly higher on the CODE/TRT arm (66.4%) than the CAV/EP arm (52.3%; $P =$ .039). However, in comparing CODE/TRT arm to the CAV/EP arm, no significant difference in either median progression-free survival (34.3 weeks for both arms) or median survival (51 weeks vs. 46.3 weeks, respectively) was observed between the two treatment groups.

Generally, overall response rates in ES SCLC with cisplatin-based chemotherapy vary from 50% to 70%, although the CR rate is much lower, at 15% to 20%. Unless chemotherapy dramatically improves control of systemic disease in ES SCLC, the addition of TRT to the overall treatment regimen is not likely to improve survival despite significantly improving local tumor control rates, a paradigm that has already been observed in LS SCLC.

IV. Prophylactic Cranial Irradiation

Rarely has the use of radiation therapy in the management of a malignant disease created so much controversy as the use of prophylactic cranial irradiation (PCI) in the treatment of SCLC. On the surface, SCLC and PCI seem to be "made for each other." Small-cell lung cancer is a systemic disease which has a high propensity for distant metastases including involvement of the central nervous system (CNS). The CNS, which is protected by the blood-brain barrier, is a "pharmacologic sanctuary" site only "partially" permeable to systemic chemotherapy. Prophylactic cranial irradiation is highly efficacious in reducing the incidence of brain metastases. Yet, despite these made-for-each-other indications, opponents of PCI argue that the lack of survival benefit and the neurocognitive morbidity associated with PCI outweigh its potential benefits.

A. CNS Involvement in SCLC

In 1973, Hanson (46) reported a 40% crude incidence of cerebral metastases in 20 patients following treatment with chemotherapy and thoracic irradiation, and thus suggested the addition of PCI to the overall therapeutic regimen for SCLC. Yet almost three decades later, after PCI was first tested in a clinical trial by CALGB (47), its role remains controversial. Why is there a controversy surrounding PCI? First, it is important to recognize that various treatment factors can influence the probability of developing cerebral metastases in patients with SCLC. These factors include the duration of survival, the efficacy of chemotherapy, statistical methods used to calculate the frequency of CNS involvement, and the timing of TRT (Fig. 6).

The crude frequency of CNS metastases increases with longer duration of survival until the cumulative actuarial incidence reaches a plateau. In a review of 10 randomized trials comparing PCI to no PCI, Kristjansen and Kristensen (48) reported an overall crude CNS relapse rate of 22% among patients not receiving PCI. However, among the studies reporting actuarial risks of CNS involvement, such as by Nugent et al. (49), the overall frequency of CNS metastases was 49% but increased to a cumulative probability of 80% for patients surviving beyond 2 years. Similarly, Arriagada et al. (50) reported an overall and isolated brain relapse rate of 67% and 45%, respectively, at 2 years for patients not undergoing PCI using a "competing risk" approach. Hence, as systemic chemotherapy for SCLC improves, CNS relapse will be an increasing cause of treatment failure. This hypothesis was recently confirmed by an NCI Phase II trial using accelerated hyperfractionated TRT and alternating cisplatin-based chemotherapy. In this study reported by Johnson et al. (51) the 2- and 5-year actuarial survival rates were 43% and 19%, respectively, but fully *one-third* of all patients experienced an *isolated* brain relapse.

Statistical methods used to calculate CNS involvement in SCLC can vary widely. Crude failure rates tend to underestimate the effect of CNS metastases on the natural history of SCLC, whereas actuarial and "competing risk model" approaches tend to more accurately reflect the true impact of brain metastases in terminating event-free survival.

Systemic chemotherapy can also affect the incidence of CNS metastases in two different ways. First, the more efficacious the systemic chemotherapy, the greater the likelihood of achieving a complete response, and therefore the higher the probability of longer survival. Longer duration of survival usually leads to an increasing incidence of brain metastases. Secondly, recent clinical observations also suggest that the hydrophobic blood-brain barrier is not completely impervious to the effects of systemic chemotherapy, as had been suggested earlier. Treatment of cerebral metastases by systemic chemotherapy *only* without cranial irra-

---

Non-PCI Factors

- Duration of Survival: ↑ Surv → ↑ CNS Met

     ↑ ↓

- Systemic CT
  - Efficacy → RR (CR vs. PR), Survival
  - CNS: "Partial" Pharmacologic Sanctuary Site
- Timing of TRT: ↑ Earlier → CNS Met
- Statistical Methods
  - Overall vs. First Failure vs. Competing Risk
  - Crude vs. Acturial

Figure 6 The incidence of CNS involvement in SCLC is dependent upon multiple factors including duration of survival, efficacy of systemic chemotherapy, timing of thoracic radiation therapy, and the statistical methods used to calculate the risk of brain metastases. Generally, the higher the efficacy of chemotherapy, the longer the duration of survival and the greater the likelihood of brain metastases. Statistical methods such as overall or crude brain metastatic rates tend to less optimally reflect the impact of CNS upon terminating event-free survival as compared to the "competing risk model" and actuarial approaches. ↑ = increased or improved, ↓ = decreased.

diation has recently been reported to induce responses, albeit mostly partial responses (PRs), suggesting at least a partial penetration of the blood-brain barrier by cytotoxic chemotherapy (52,53). Additionally, the therapeutic evidence that only moderate doses of PCI (i.e., 24 to 36 Gy) are necessary to effectively eradicate subclinical disease in the brain also suggests at least a "partial, synergistic" cytotoxic effect of systemic chemotherapy upon the CNS.

The timing of TRT may also affect the subsequent development of brain metastases. In a Canadian trial reported by Murray et al. (22), patients with LS SCLC were randomized to receive either early (week 3, cycle 2) or late (week 15, cycle 5) TRT. Complete responders were then given PCI following completion of all chemotherapy. Brain metastases were more common among patients who were randomized to late (28.1%) than early (18.1%; $P = .042$) TRT. Since the timing of the PCI was the same for both randomized groups, the authors postulated that early thoracic radiotherapy may have eradicated chemoresistant clones at the primary site before the development of metastatic disease. In comparison, the use of delayed TRT may have allowed chemoresistant clones to proliferate outside of the radiotherapy portal unaffected by chemotherapy. Hence, it is important to recognize the influence of all these factors upon the efficacy and toxicity of PCI.

B. Therapeutic Ratio of PCI: Efficacy vs. Toxicity

Prophylactic cranial irradiation significantly reduces the incidence of brain metastases!

Ever since the first clinical trial by CALGB to some of the more recent randomized studies (50,54,55) testing the value of PCI, the efficacy of PCI to significantly reduce brain metastases remains undisputed. In a review of 10 randomized trials which included patients with LS and ES SCLC, in complete remission (CR) and PR, using early or delayed cranial irradiation and various TRT dose fractionation schemes, Kristjansen and Kristensen (48) reported a CNS relapse rate of 6% for patients undergoing PCI, compared to 22% for patients not receiving PCI. Hence, patients who did not receive PCI were almost four times more likely to experience a relapse in the brain as than patients who underwent PCI.

Recent randomized trials which have included only patients in complete remission continue to confirm the efficacy of PCI in significantly reducing the brain metastatic rate. The French at the Institut Gustave-Roussy (IGR) (50) randomized 505 patients in complete remission to PCI or observation on two consecutive protocols (i.e., PCI-85 and PCI-88). The majority of the patients enrolled to these two protocols had LS disease (83%), and a majority had also received TRT (80%). Using a competing risk model to compare the efficacy of observation-only to PCI, the 2-year overall brain metastatic rate (59% vs. 40%, respectively; $P = .00001$), and the isolated brain relapse rate (57% vs. 39%, respectively; $P = .00001$) were significantly reduced by cranial irradiation. The overall 2-year survival reached borderline statistical significance in favor of patients receiving PCI (31% vs. 27%; P = .10). Similarly, the United Kingdom Coordinating Council for Cancer Research (UKCCCR)/European Organization for Research and Treatment of Cancer (EORTC) trial (55) randomized 314 patients in complete remission to PCI or observation-only. This trial also showed a statistically significant benefit in favor of PCI to reduce the brain metastatic rate as compared to observation-only (P = .0001), but no survival advantage (P = .15).

The design of these three recent randomized trials comparing PCI to observation-only was fundamentally different from past randomized studies in one significant aspect: Only those patients who had achieved a complete response to initial chemotherapy, and mostly those with LS disease, and thus the subset of patients most likely to benefit from PCI, were eligible for protocol entry. Results from these three trials confirmed, not all that surprisingly, the efficacy of PCI to significantly reduce the brain metastatic rate. However, the high incidence of the overall and the isolated brain metastatic rate observed in these recent trials was far greater than previously reported results. Previous studies (48,56–58) have reported overall brain relapse rates of 20% to 25% without PCI, which is generally reduced to less than 10% with PCI. Similarly, these studies have also reported a very low *isolated* CNS relapse rate of generally <5%. These "historical" brain relapse rates reflect the inclusion of patients with partial response to initial chemotherapy (usually non-cisplatin-based), ES disease, and "crude" (vs. actuarial) statistical methods used to calculate the CNS metastatic rate. Furthermore, the inclusion of only patients in complete remission with mostly LS disease also explains the observed high incidence of brain metastases in these recent trials (50,55). Despite a significant reduction in the incidence of brain metastases, none of these recent individual randomized trials have confirmed a significant survival benefit for the use of PCI.

1. Why No Survival Benefit?

Why has PCI failed to significantly improve survival outcome in SCLC? Of course, that is the $64,000 question! In order for PCI to show a survival benefit, it should be delivered to the most favorable subset of patients who are at greatest risk of developing an *isolated* brain relapse. Ideally, this subset includes patients with LS disease who have achieved a complete response to initial chemoradiation therapy and who are therefore the most likely to be long-term survivors. As noted earlier, this hypothesis was recently confirmed by an NCI Phase II trial (51) using accelerated hyperfractionated TRT and aggressive alternating chemotherapy for patients with LS SCLC. In this NCI study, among the 37 of 54 patients who experienced a treatment failure, 19 relapsed in the brain, of which 13 were isolated events. Twelve of these 13 patients who relapsed only in the brain had no evidence of metastatic disease outside the CNS during the rest of their lives or at autopsy. The cumulative actuarial risk of developing an *isolated* brain relapse was nearly 40% in this trial.

There are multiple reasons for which the use of PCI in SCLC has failed to demonstrate a significant survival advantage, including selection of "unfavorable" subgroups of patients and small trials which have lacked adequate statistical power. Historically, randomized trials of PCI have included a heterogeneous group of patients not likely to benefit from PCI, such as those with only a partial response to initial therapy and/or those with ES disease. This unfavorable subset of patients are just as likely to relapse in non-CNS sites as in the brain, a pattern of relapse which is not likely to best assess the impact of PCI upon survival. For example, in a review of 10 randomized PCI trials by Kristjansen and Kristensen (48), none showed a statistically significant survival advantage to using PCI. However, only four of these 10 trials included patients with LS disease; the remaining six studies also included patients with ES disease. Additionally, these trials also included patients who had *not* achieved a CR to initial therapy. Moreover, various dose/fractionation and timing schemes were used for both PCI and TRT. Hence, all of these factors may have negated or underestimated the impact of PCI upon survival.

Virtually all of the *historical* randomized trials have lacked the statistical power to detect a moderate survival benefit for the use of PCI. The majority of these PCI trials have randomized <50 patients (59–64), and only one trial (56) enrolled >200 patients. Hence, a recent meta-analysis of seven modern-day randomized trials comparing PCI to observation-only in patients with SCLC in *complete remission* (Table 4) was undertaken and completed (78). Six of these seven trials included patients with ES disease who had achieved a CR. The meta-analysis covered an accrual period from 1977 to 1995 involving almost 1000 patients. The meta-analysis showed what had been suspected for a long time: PCI improves survival for those SCLC patients in complete remission. The survival rate was improved from 15.3% in the control group to 20.7% in the PCI group at 3 years, which corresponds to an *absolute* increase in survival of 5.4% and a *relative* improvement of 35%. As expected, PCI also significantly decreased the cumulative incidence of brain metastases from 58.6% in the control group of 33.3% in the PCI group ($P < .001$), a $54 \pm 7\%$ reduction in the brain metastatic rate (Table 4). This meta-analysis overcame two previous hurdles that had prevented the assessment of PCI upon survival: unfavorable patient selection bias (i.e., inclusion of those patients *not* in CR who are unlikely to benefit from PCI) and not having enough statistical power to detect a modest but significant survival difference.

2. *Neurotoxicity: Separating Myth from Truth*

Opponents of PCI argue that the neurotoxicity associated with cranial irradiation outweighs its potential benefits. Reported neurotoxicities from PCI have included confusion, ataxia, psychomotor retardation, aphonia, cerebellar dysfunction, optic neuropathy, inability to take care of oneself, "intellectual deficits," dementia, and leukoencephalopathy. In fact, opponents of PCI also argue that neurotoxicity following PCI could be avoided for patients who would not develop brain metastases anyway.

Table 4 Randomized Trials Comparing PCI Versus No PCI in Patients with SCLC in Complete Remission[a]

Trial (ref.)	Accrual period	Stage	PCI dose (Gy/fractions)	No. patients	Median Follow-up (yrs)
UMCC (63)	1977–80	All	30/10	29	18.5
Danish/NCI (48)	1985–91	All	24/8	55	8.8
Okayama (75)	1981–86	All	40/20	46	11.7
ECOG 3589/ RTOG 9201 (76)	1991–94	All	25/10	32	3.9
PCI 85 (54)	1985–1993	All	24/8	300	8.4
PCI 88 (77)	1988–1994	All	24/8	211	5.1
UKCCCR/EORTC (55)	1987–1995	Limited disease	8–36/1–18	314	3.5

Abbreviations: UMMC, University of Maryland Cancer Center NCI, National Cancer Institute; ECOG, Eastern Cooperative Oncology Group; RTOG, Radiation Therapy Oncology Group; UKCCR, United Kingdom Co-ordinating Committee on Cancer Research; EORTC, European Organization for Research and Treatment of Cancer.

[a]Meta-analysis of seven randomized trials by Dr. R. Arriagada involving almost 1000 patients in CR to assess the impact of PCI on survival

Historically, the neurotoxicities associated with PCI have been diagnosed by a process of exclusion rather than a true search for all potential etiologies, such as preexisting neurocognitive deficits or the impact of SCLC and systemic chemotherapy on higher brain function. The article published by Fleck et al. (58) demonstrates the inherent pitfalls of most studies examining neurotoxicities in SCLC. In this study of 114 patients with LS SCLC treated at Indiana University, complete remission was documented in 58 (51%) patients after initial chemoradiation therapy. Thirty-eight of the 58 patients underwent PCI while the remaining 20 did not. Only one (3%) of 38 patients undergoing PCI experienced a brain relapse; four (20%) of the 20 patients not receiving PCI experienced a CNS failure ($P = .04$). Among the 11 of 38 long-term survivors, significant neurotoxicity was documented in seven of these 11 patients. The authors were left with the "inescapable conclusion" that if PCI had not been used, these patients would not have experienced such major neurotoxicity.

This article by Fleck et al. (58) classically highlights what is "wrong" in assessing neurotoxicity in SCLC: retrospective analysis, shrinking denominator of evaluable patients, no initial pre-PCI neurocognitive evaluation, and a "toxic" dose/fractionation/timing scheme chosen for PCI. This analysis from Indiana University was a retrospective study not designed to assess the various etiologies which could adversely effect neurocognitive function. In this analysis, the "shrinking denominator phenomenon" penalized patients who had lived long enough to develop neurotoxicity after PCI without comparing neurocognitive function among the remaining patients who either relapsed in the brain with its attendant morbidity or those not undergoing PCI! Additionally, no pretherapy neurocognitive evaluations were conducted among patients to explore preexisting cognitive deficits prior to PCI. Furthermore, the dose/fractionation/timing schemes used for PCI (i.e., 36 Gy at 2.4 Gy/fx tri-split or 30 Gy at 3.0 Gy/fx) at Indiana University were "begging" for neurotoxicity. PCI was delivered using high doses per fraction and during concurrent CT, factors both known to adversely affect neurocognitive function. Also, the authors failed to appreciate that the neurotoxicity associated with brain metastases (i.e., ultimate complete loss of neurocognitive abilities and death) is far worse than most of the sequelae following PCI.

Recent prospective studies evaluating neurocognitive function in SCLC now confirm what had been suspected earlier: the preexistence of neurocognitive deficits prior to the delivery of PCI. In a prospective study conducted by Komaki et al. (65), 30 patients (29 with CR) with LS SCLC underwent neuropsychological examination prior to PCI and following PCI. Neurocognitive deficits were evident in 29 (97%) of 30 patients *prior* to PCI. Eleven patients subsequently underwent further neuropsychological testing 6 to 20 months after PCI, and no significant deterioration in their neurocognitive function was observed. Similar lack of deterioration in neurocognitive function following PCI was documented in another prospective study, by Van Oosterhout et al. (66). Two large prospective studies (46,47) also found preponderance of neurocognitive deficits prior to PCI, but no deterioration in neurocognitive function after PCI. In the Institut Gustave-Roussy (IGR) PCI-85 trial by Arriagada et al. (54), almost 60% of the 229 tested patients were found to have an abnormal neuropsychological exam at time of randomization. Follow-up neurocognitive testing after PCI revealed no significant deterioration in neurocognitive function. In the UKCCCR/EORTC trial (55), which randomized 314 patients to PCI or observation, cognitive function impairment was demonstrated in 17% to 42% of 136 tested patients prior to PCI. In paired follow-up assessments, the majority of the patients remained stable without neurocognitive deterioration. In a follow-up of this trial reported at the 8th International Association for the Study of Lung Cancer in Dublin (Ireland) (67), no significant neurocognitive differences were detected between the PCI group and the controls at 6 months following cranial irradiation. In fact, neurocognitive impairment was not related to age, gender, or previous therapy, and was distributed evenly between the PCI and the control arms. Similar observations have also been made in the treatment of pediatric acute lymphoblastic leukemia (ALL). In a prospective study evaluating *long-term* neurocognitive function among children will ALL who had experienced an *isolated* CNS relapse (68), the authors found no deterioration in group full-scale intelligence quotient (FSIQ) scores between pre-craniospinal irradiation (CSI) and post-CSI measurements at a median follow-up interval of 4.6 years. Factors which significantly correlated with final individual FSIQ scores in this pediatric study included initial pre-CSI FSIQ score (P = .00005), age at diagnosis (P = .009), and age at CSI (P = .011).

As highlighted by the study from Indiana University (58), other factors, such as the timing of systemic chemotherapy and the dose/fractionation scheme used for PCI, can also influence neurotoxicity. The recognition of preexisting neurocognitive deficits prior to PCI possibly due to systemic chemotherapy should come as no surprise given that the CNS is at least partially permeable to the cytotoxic effects of chemotherapy. In particular, chemotherapy regimens containing such drugs as methotrexate, procarbazine, or nitrosoureas can cross the blood-brain barrier, and therefore induce neurotoxicity. This neurotoxic effect of certain cytotoxic agents may be further exacerbated when PCI is delivered simultaneously with chemotherapy, as was the case in the Indiana University study.

Radiobiologically, fractionation of radiation therapy spares normal tissue by allowing for repair of sublethal damage between treatments. Late-responding tissues such as the CNS are particularly sensitive to the dose/fraction size compared to early-responding tissues, such as the skin, which are more affected by overall treatment time. The majority of the PCI regimens in the past have used high-dose/fraction size (i.e., >2.5 to 3.0 Gy/fx) to relatively high radiobiological doses (i.e., ≥30 Gy). Given the "sensitivity" of the brain to the radiation dose/fraction size, PCI regimens which use a high-dose/fraction size (i.e., >2.5 Gy/fx) should be avoided, to potentially further limit neurotoxicity from PCI.

Another etiologic factor that may contribute toward the neurotoxicity is the disease itself. In a study by Meyers et al. (69), neurocognitive function between two groups of patients with SCLC treated with or without CT was compared. No difference in cognitive function was found between the two groups. The authors concluded that the detectable neurocognitive deficits were possibly due to subclinical CNS disease rather than to any therapy-related factors. Hence, many factors other than PCI contribute to neurotoxicity often observed in patients with SCLC (Fig. 7).

C. PCI: The Bottom Line

In evaluating a SCLC patient for PCI, consideration should be given to several factors including the following: the high incidence of brain metastases with its attendant morbidity and mortality; the efficacy of PCI to significantly reduce brain metastases and to improve survival for those patients in complete remission, and the multifactorial etiologies which contribute to the development of neurotoxicity (i.e., "baseline" cognitive deficits, the disease process, CT, PCI timing, and dose/fx scheme) (70). Hence, PCI should be considered for SCLC patients in complete remission (generally in the United States, this option is also limited to patients with LS disease).

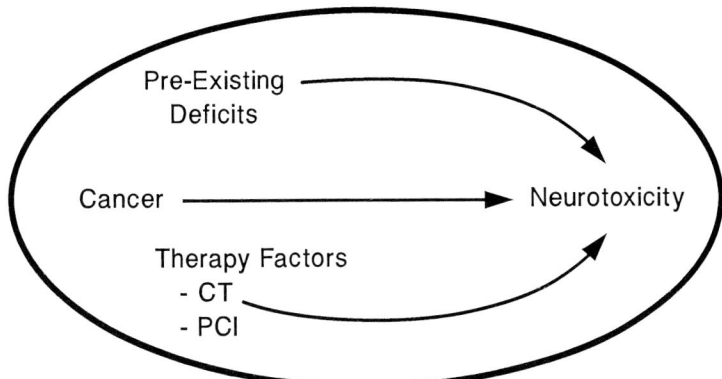

Figure 7 Many factors other than PCI impact upon neurotoxicity and neurocognitive functioning of patients following brain irradiation. These factors include pre-existing neurocognitive deficits, the disease itself, and systemic chemotherapy. CT; chemotherapy; PCI; prophylactic cranial irradiation.

D. The Future

Given that almost one-third of patients with LS SCLC treated with chemoradiation therapy continue to fail locally, strategies that attempt to improve local control will certainly dominate the "theme" of future clinical trials. Factors that affect local control of chest disease include timing of TRT with chemotherapy, volume encompassed within the radiation portal, and of course the total dose and fractionation scheme (Fig. 8).

As already discussed, TRT may be combined with CT either concurrently, sequentially, or alternatingly. Although toxicity may be somewhat increased in the concurrent approach, better local control and survival outcome appear to justify its use over either sequential or alternating TRT. However, whether to use "early" versus "late" concurrent TRT remains largely unresolved.

Given that both volume encompassed within the radiation portal and the total dose of TRT impact upon local control and toxicity, both issues will be addressed jointly. The necessity to encompass pre-CT disease extent and uninvolved lymphatic drainage areas within the radiation port has been recently challenged. Additionally, escalation of total conventional dose of TRT beyond the current standard of 45 to 50 Gy levels may be necessary to potentially improve local control of disease. Within CALGB, current "standard policy" is to deliver concurrent but "late" conventional TRT to 40 Gy with cycle 4 (day 64) to the pre-CT disease extent, followed by a boost of 10 Gy to the residual disease still uneradicated by three cycles of induction chemotherapy for a total radiation dose of 50 Gy. This approach of late concurrent TRT may be exploited by including only the remaining residual disease following induction CT within the radiation port to escalate total doses to much higher levels (e.g., 65 to 70 Gy). This strategy requires a careful balance between volume encompassed within the radiation port and total dose of TRT. Significant improvement in both local control and survival has been shown with the use of accelerated BID radiotherapy. However, this improvement in survival and local control should be weighed against the acute and chronic toxicities of using AR.

As combined chemotherapy and TRT becomes more effective in prolonging survival of patients with SCLC, especially those with LS disease, CNS prophylaxis will need to be systematically incorporated into the therapeutic regimen. Isolated CNS relapses that terminated initial complete remission were first observed in childhood ALL. Effective induction combination CT prolonged the survival of children from a few months to 1 to 2 years during the first treatment era (i.e., Total Protocol I-IV) at St. Jude Children's Research Hospital (SJCRH). However, CNS leukemia terminated complete remission in up to 75% of children (71). During the second treatment era (Total Protocols V-IX), the use of effective CNS prophylaxis (i.e., craniospinal irradiation to 24 Gy or cranial irradiation to 24 Gy and intrathecal methotrexate) significantly reduced the CNS failure rate and also improved 5-year event-free survival by fourfold (i.e., from 9% to 36%) (72). Are we at this threshold of a "CNS prophylaxis" treatment era for the management of SCLC? Yes! (Fig. 8.) The selection of the appropriate patient population most likely to achieve a survival benefit from CNS prophylaxis is crucial to properly integrating PCI into the overall curative regiment for SCLC.

Is there hope for the future? Yes! In an analysis from the National Cancer Institute (73) evaluating outcome in SCLC over the past two decades, patients with LS SCLC treated most recently with cisplatin/etoposide CT and TRT experienced a significant improvement in median survival when compared to those patients treated with cyclophosphamide-based CT (median survival = 21.3 months vs. 11.1–14.2 months, respectively, P = .011). So, it appears that the recent therapeutic advances have improved median and short-term survival for patients with LS SCLC. However, no improvement in overall survival was observed in this analysis over the past two decades (i.e., first decade = 1973–1982; second decade = 1983–1992) for all patients with LS or ES SCLC. In a similar report from the Dartmouth-Hitchcock Medical Center (74) detailing their survival outcome in SCLC during the past 25 years, patients treated on investigational protocols achieved better survival results than nonprotocol patients. Interestingly enough, survival for the patients of LS and ES SCLC did not change until the 1990s, when the median survival for the entire population increased from 8 months to 11.3 months (P = .0001). Hence, a lot more work needs yet to be done.

Though this review has focused upon the role of thoracic radiation therapy and prophylactic cranial irradiation in the management of small-cell lung cancer, one must always remember that the efficacy of radiation therapy is intimately interconnected to the efficacy of systemic chemotherapy in all issues relating to this dis-

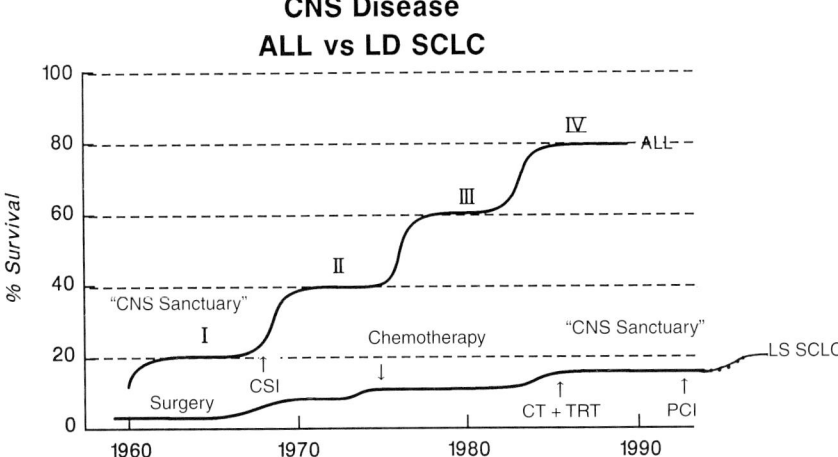

Figure 8 There are many parallels between ALL and LS SCLC in the treatment of CNS disease, although on a far less dramatic scale. Cranio-spinal irradiation significantly improved survival by a factor of 4 in ALL for selected pediatric patients. Later, the use of lower doses cranial irradiation with intrathecal chemotherapy also reduced neurotoxicity. Similarily, the use of PCI has significantly improved survival for approximately selected patients with SCLC. ALL; acute lymphoblastic leukemia; CT; chemotherapy; CSI; cranio-spinal irradiation.

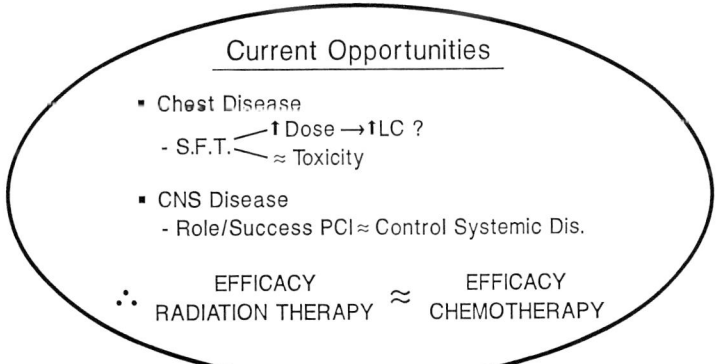

Figure 9 Current opportunities to improve survival in SCLC include escalation doses of conventional once-a-day thoracic radiation therapy (using a SFT), or twice-a-day accelerated irradiation to further reduce local failure rates. For CNS disease, the efficacy of PCI is intricately tied to the control of systemic disease by chemotherapy. Overall, the efficacy of radiation therapy in the management of SCLC is inherently tied to the efficacy of systemic therapy and, hence, a close collaboration between the radiation oncologist and medical oncologist will always be necessary in order to improve therapeutic ratio for this disease. SFT; shrinking field technique; LC local control; PCI; prophylactic cranial irradiation.

ease, including toxicity, local and CNS control, and survival. Hence, a close collaboration among the radiation oncologist, the medical oncologist, and the thoracic surgeon will be necessary if we are to succeed in improving survival of patients diagnosed with SCLC by better defining the role of PCI and by optimizing the timing, volume, and dose/fractionation of TRT through investigative clinical protocols. (Fig. 9.)

References

1. Landis SH, Murray T, Bolden S, Wingo PA. Cancer Statistics, 1999. CA Cancer J Clin 1999; 49:8–31.
2. Matthews MJ, Kanhouwa S, Pickren J, Robinette D. Frequency of residual and metastatic tumor in patients undergoing curative resection for lung cancer. Cancer Chemother Rep 1973; 4:63.
3. Petrovich Z, Ohanian M, Cox J. Clinical research on the treatment of locally advanced lung cancer. Cancer 1978; 42:1129–1134.
4. Scadding J, Bignall J, Blair L, et al. Comparative trial of surgery and radiotherapy for the primary treatment of small celled or oat-celled carcinoma of the bronchus. Lancet 1966; 2:979–986.
5. Green RA, Humphrey E, Close H, et al. Alkylating agents in bronchogenic carcinoma. Am J Med 1969; 46:516–525.
6. Watson WL, Berg JW. Oat cell lung cancer. Cancer 1962; 15:759.
7. Bergsagel DE, Jenkin RDT, Pringle JF, et al. Lung cancer: clinical trial of radiotherapy alone vs. radiotherapy plus cyclophosphamide. Cancer 1972; 30:621.
8. Eagan RT, Maurer LH, Forcier RJ, Tulloh M. Combination chemotherapy and radiation therapy in small cell carcinoma of the lung. Cancer 1973; 32:371.
9. Medical Research Council Lung Cancer Working Party. Radiotherapy alone or with chemotherapy in the treatment of small cell carcinoma of the lung. Br J Cancer 1979; 40:1.
10. Cohen MH, Ihde DC, Bunn PA Jr, et al. Cyclic alternating combination chemotherapy for small cell bronchogenic carcinoma. Cancer Treat Rep 1979; 63:163.
11. Byhardt RW, Cox JD, Holoye PY, et al. The role of consolidation irradiation in combined modality therapy of small cell carcinoma of the lung. Int J Radiat Oncol Biol Phys 1982; 8:1271.
12. Cohen MH. Is thoracic radiation necessary for patients with limited-stage cell lung cancer? No. Cancer Treat Rep 1983; 67:217.
13. Byhardt RW, Cox JD. Is chest radiotherapy necessary in any or all patients with small cell carcinoma of the lung? Yes. Cancer Treat Rep 1983; 67:290.
14. Birch R. Omura G, Greco FM, et al. Patterns of failure in combined chemotherapy and radiotherapy for limited small cell lung cancer: South Eastern Cancer Study Group experience. Monogr Natl Cancer Inst 1988; 6:265–270.
15. Bunn PA Jr, Lichter AS, Makuch RW, et al. Chemotherapy alone or chemotherapy with chest radiation therapy in limited stage small cell lung cancer: a prospective randomized trial. Ann Intern Med 1987; 106:655–662.
16. Perry MC, Eaton WL, Propert KJ, et al. Chemotherapy with or without radiation

therapy in limited small-cell carcinoma of the lung. N Engl J Med 1987; 316:912–918.

17. Creech R, Richter M, Finkelstein D. Combination chemotherapy with or without consolidation radiation therapy for regional small cell carcinoma of the lung. Proc Am Soc Clin Oncol 1988; 7:196 (#756).

18. Kies MS, Mira JG, Crowley JJ, et al. Multimodality therapy for limited small-cell lung cancer: a randomized study of induction combination chemotherapy with or without thoracic radiation in complete responders; and with wide-field versus involved field radiotherapy in partial responders: a Southwest Oncology Group study. J Clin Oncol 1987; 5:592–600.

19. Pignon JP, Arriagada R, Ihde DC, et al. A meta-analysis of thoracic radiotherapy for small-cell lung cancer. N Engl J Med 1992; 327:1618–1624.

20. Warde P, Payne D. Does thoracic irradiation improve survival and local control in limited stage small cell carcinoma of the lung? A meta-analysis. J Clin Oncol 1992; 10:890–895.

21. Ochs JJ, Tester WJ, Cohen MH. Salvage radiation therapy for intrathoracic small cell carcinoma of the lung progressing on combination chemotherapy. Cancer Treat Rep 1983; 67:1123–1126.

22. Murray N, Coy P, Pater JL, et al. Importance of timing for thoracic irradiation in the combined modality treatment of limited stage small cell lung cancer. J Clin Oncol 1993; 11:336–344.

23. Osterlind K, Hansen HH, Hansen HS, Dombernowsky P, Hansen M, Rorth M. Chemotherapy versus chemotherapy plus irradiation in limited small cell lung cancer: results of a controlled trial with 5 years follow-up. Br J Cancer 1986; 54:7–17.

24. LeBeau B, Chastang C, Bréchot JM. Small cell lung cancer (SCLC): negative results of a randomized clinical trial on delayed thoracic radiotherapy administered to complete responders (CR) patients (abstr). Lung Cancer 1991; 7(S94).

25. Takada M, Fukuoka M, Furuse K, et al. A Phase III study of concurrent versus sequential thoracic radiotherapy in combination with cisplatin and etoposide for limited stage small cell lung cancer: preliminary results of the Japan Clinical Oncology Group. Proc Am Soc Clin Oncol 1996; 15:372 (#1103).

26. Perry MC, Herndon JE II, Eaton WL, et al. Thoracic radiation therapy added to chemotherapy in limited small cell lung cancer: an update of cancer and leukemia group b (CALGB) study 8083. Proc ASCO 1996; 15:384 (#1150).

27. Carlson RW, Sikic BI, Gandara DR, et al. Late consolidative radiation therapy in the treatment of limited stage small cell lung cancer. Cancer 1991; 68:948–958.

28. Lebeau B, Chastang C, Brechot JM, Capron F, for the Petites Cellules Group. A randomized trial of delayed thoracic radiotherapy in complete responder patients with small cell lung cancer. Chest 1993; 104:726–733.

29. Arriagada R, LeChevalier T, Ruffie P, et al. Alternating radiotherapy and chemotherapy in 173 consecutive patients with limited stage small cell lung carcinoma. Int J Radiat Oncol Biol Phys 1990; 19:1135–1138.

30. Mornex F, Trillet V, Chauvin F, et al. Hyperfractionated radiotherapy alternating with multidrug chemotherapy in the treatment of limited small cell lung cancer. Int J Radiat Oncol Biol Phys 1990; 19:23–30.

31. Johnson DH, Turrisi AT, Chang AY, et al. Alternating chemotherapy and twice-daily

thoracic radiotherapy in limited stage small cell lung cancer: a pilot study of the Eastern Cooperative Oncology Group. J Clin Oncol 1993; 11:879–884.

32. LeBeau B, Chastaf CL, Urban T, et al. A randomized clinical trial comparing concurrent and alternating thoracic irradiation in limited small cell lung cancer (SCLC). Proc Am Soc Clin Oncol 1996; 15:383 (#1148).

33. Mira J, Livingston R. Evaluation and radiotherapy implications of chest relapse in small cell lung carcinoma treated with radiotherapy-chemotherapy: study of 34 cases and reviews of the literature. Cancer 1980; 46:2557–2565.

34. Liengswangwong V, Bonner J, Shaw E, et al. Limited stage small cell lung cancer: patterns of intrathoracic recurrence and the implications for thoracic radiotherapy. J Clin Oncol 1994; 12:496–502.

35. Choi N, Carey R. Importance of radiation dose in achieving improved loco-regional tumor control in limited stage small cell lung carcinoma: an update. Int J Radiat Oncol Biol Phys 1989; 17:307–310.

36. Choi N, Herndon J, Rosenman J, et al. Phase I study to determine the maximum tolerated dose (MTD) radiation in standard daily (QD) and accelerated twice daily (BID) radiation schedules with concurrent chemotherapy (CT) for limited stage small cell lung cancer (SCLC). Proc Am Soc Clin Oncol 1995; 14:363 (#1113).

37. Turrisi A, Glover DJ, Mason B, et al. Long term results of platinum etoposide (PE) + twice daily thoracic radiotherapy (TRT) for limited small cell lung cancer. Proc Am Soc Clin Oncol 1992; 11:292 (#975).

38. Armstrong JG, Rosenstein MM, Kris MG, et al. Twice daily thoracic irradiation for limited small cell lung cancer. Int J Radiat Oncol Biol Phys 1991; 21:1269–1274.

39. Johnson BE, Salem C, Nesbit J, et al. Limited (Ltd) stage small cell lung cancer (SCLC) treated with concurrent BID chest radiotherapy (RT) and etoposide, cisplatin (VP/PT) followed by chemotherapy (CT) selected by in vitro drug sensitivity testing (DST). Lung Cancer 1991; 7:152.

40. Turrisi III, AT, Kim K, Blum R, et al. Twice-daily compared c̄ once daily thoracic radiotherapy in limited small cell lung cancer treated concurrently with cisplatin and etoposide. New England J Med 1999; 340:265–71.

41. Livingston RM, Moore TN, Heilbrun L, et al. Small-cell carcinoma of the lung: combined chemotherapy and radiation. A Southwest Oncology Group study. Ann Intern Med 1978; 88:194–199.

42. Livingston RB, Mira JG, Chen TT, et al. Combined modality treatment of extensive small cell lung cancer: a Southwest Oncology Group study. J Clin Oncol 1984; 2(6): 585–590.

43. Livingston R, Schulman S, Mira J, et al. Combined alkylators and multiple-site irradiation for extensive small cell lung cancer: a Southwest Oncology Group study. Cancer Treat Rep 1986; 70:1395–1401.

44. Murray N, Gelmon K, Shah A, et al. Potential for long-term survival in extensive small cell lung cancer (ESCLC) with CODE chemotherapy and radiotherapy. Proc Am Soc Clin Oncol 1994; 13:338 (#1124).

45. Murray N, Livingston R, Shepherd F, et al. A randomized study of CODE plus thoracic irradiation versus alternating CAV/EP for extensive stage small cell lung cancer (ESCLC). Proc Am Soc Clin Oncol 1997; 16:456a (#1638).

46. Hanson HH. Should initial treatment of small cell lung carcinoma include systemic chemotherapy and brain irradiation. Cancer Chem Rep 197; 4:239–241.

47. Maurer LH, Tulloh M, Weiss RB, et al. A randomized combined modality trial in small cell carcinoma of the lung. Cancer 1980; 45:30–39.

48. Kristjansen PEG, Kristensen CA. The role of prophylactic cranial irradiation in the management of small cell lung cancer. Cancer Treat Rep 1993; 19:3.

49. Nugent JL, Bunn PA, Matthews MJ, et al. CNS metastases in small cell bronchogenic carcinoma: increasing frequency and changing pattern with lengthening survival. Cancer 1979; 44:1885–1893.

50. Arriagada R, Monnet I, Riviere A, et al. Prophylactic cranial irradiation for patients with small cell lung cancer in complete remission. Eur J Cancer 1995; 31A(suppl 5)S19.

51. Johnson BE, Bridges JD, Sobczeck M, et al. Patients with limited-stage small cell lung cancer treated with concurrent twice-daily chest radiotherapy and etoposide cisplatin followed by cyclophosphamide, doxorubicin, and vincristine. J Clin Oncol 1996; 14:806–813.

52. Postmus PE, Smit EF, Haaxma-Reiche H. Treatment of central nervous system metasases from small cell lung cancer with chemotherapy. Lung Cancer 1993; 9:281.

53. Twelves CJ, Souhami RL, Harper PG, et al. The response of cerebral metastases in small cell lung cancer to systemic chemotherapy. Br J Cancer 1990; 61:147.

54. Arriagada R, LeChevalier T, Borie F, et al. Prophylactic cranial irradiation for patients with small cell lung cancer in complete remission. J Natl Cancer Inst 1995; 87:183–190.

55. Gregor A, Cull A, Stephens RJ, Macbeth FR, Thatcher N. Effects of prophylactic cranial irradiation (PCI) in small cell lung cancer (SCLC): results of UKCCCR/EORTC randomised trial. Proc Am Soc Clin Oncol 1996; 15:381 (#1139).

56. Lucas CF, Robinson B, Hoskin PJ, et al. Morbidity of cranial relapse in small cell lung cancer and the impact of radiation therapy. Cancer Treat Rep 1986; 70:565–570.

57. Feld R, Clamon GH, Blunn R, et al. Short course prophylactic cranial irradiation for small cell lung cancer. Am J Clin Oncol 1985; 8:371–376.

58. Fleck JF, Einhorn LH, Lauren RC, et al. Is prophylactic cranial irradiation indicated in small cell lung cancer? J Clin Oncol 1990; 8:209–214.

59. Jackson DV, Richards F, Cooper MR, et al. Prophylactic cranial irradiation in small cell carcinoma of the lung. A randomized study. JAMA 1983; 237(25):2730–2733.

60. Cox JD, Petrovish Z, Paig C, Stanley K. Prophylactic cranial irradiation in patients with inoperable carcinoma of the lung. Cancer 1978; 42:1135–1140.

61. Eagan RT, Frytak S, Lee RE, et al. A case for preplanned thoracic and prophylactic whole brain radiation therapy in limited small cell lung cancer. Cancer Clin Trials 1981; 4:261–266.

62. Katsensis AT, Karpasitis N, Giannakakis D, et al. Elective brain irradiation in patients with small cell carcinoma of the lung: preliminary report. Lung Cancer International Congress Series 558, Excerpta Medica 1982; 277–284.

63. Aroney RS, Aisner J, Wesley MN, et al. Value of prophylactic cranial irradiation given at complete remission in small cell lung carcinoma. Cancer Treat Rep 1983; 67:675–682.

64. Seydel HG, Creech R, Pagano M, et al. Prophylactic versus no brain irradiation in regional small cell lung carcinoma. Am J Clin Oncol 1985; 8:218–223.
65. Komaki R, Meyers C, Shin D, et al. Evaluation of cognitive function in patients with limited small cell lung cancer prior to and shortly following prophylactic cranial irradiation. Int J Radiat Oncol Biol Phys 1995; 33:179–182.
66. Van Oosterhout AGM, Boon P, Houx P, et al. Follow-up of cognitive functioning in patients with small cell lung cancer. Int J Radiat Oncol Biol Phys 1995; 31:911–914.
67. Cull A, Gregor A, Stephens RJ. Neuropsychometric impairment in patients with small cell lung cancer (SCLC): evidence from a randomised trial of prophylactic cranial irradiation (PCI). Lung Cancer 1997; 18(1):125 (#488).
68. Kumar P, Mulhern RK, Regine WF, et al. A prospective neurocognitive evaluation of children treated with additional chemotherapy and craniospinal irradiation following isolated central nervous system relapse in acute lymphoblastic leukemia. Int J Radiat Oncol Biol Phys 1995; 31(3):561–566.
69. Meyers CA, Byrne, KS, Komaki R. Cognitive deficits in patients with small cell lung cancer before and after chemotherapy. Lung Cancer 1995; 12:231–235.
70. Pedersen AG, Bishop JF, Bleehen NM, et al. Management of CNS metastases in small cell lung cancer—a consensus report. In: Hansen HH, Kristjansen PEG, eds. Third IASLC Workshop on Small Cell Lung Cancer. Elsinore, Denmark. Lung Cancer 1989; 5:140–142.
71. Aur RJA, Hustu HO, Verzosa MS, Wood A, Simone JV. Comparison of two methods of preventing central nervous system leukemia. Blood 1973; 42:349.
72. Rivera GK, Pinkel D, Simone JV, et al. Treatment of acute lymphoblastic leukemia—30 years experience at St. Jude Children's Research Hospital. N Engl J Med 1993; 329:1289–1295. Lung Cancer 1997; 18(1):14 (#44).
73. Chute JP, Venzon DJ, Hankins L, Ihde DC, Johnson BE. Twenty years of clinical research on patients (PTS) with small cell lung cancer (SCLC) shows modest prolongation of survival (SUR) in recently treated limited stage pts. Proc ASCO 1995; 14:354 (#1074).
74. Mauer LH, West P, Eaton W, Rigas K, et al. Small cell lung cancer: 25 year experience from the Dartmouth Hitchcock medical center (DHMC): how much has changed? Lung Cancer 1997; 18(1):14 (#44).
75. Ohnoshi T, Ueoka H, Kawahara S, et al. Comparative study of prophylactic cranial irradiation in patients with small cell lung cancer achieving a complete response: a long-term follow-up result. Lung Cancer 1994; 10:47–54.
76. Wagner HJ, Kim K, Turrusi A, et al. A randomized Phase III study of prophylactic cranial irradiation vs observation in patients with small cell lung cancer achieving a complete response: final report of an incomplete trial by the ECOG and RTOG. Proc Am Soc Clin Oncol 1996; 15:376.
77. Arriagada R, Pignon JP, Laplanche A, et al. Prophylactic cranial irradiation for small cell lung cancer. Lancet 1997; 349:138.
78. Auperin A, Arriagada R, Pignon JP, et al. Prophylactic cranial irradiation for patients with small-cell lung cancer in complete remission. New Engl J Med 1999; 341:476–484.

17

Chemotherapy of Small-Cell Lung Cancer

ANTHONY L. BORAL and THOMAS J. LYNCH, JR.

The MGH Cancer Center
Massachusetts General Hospital
Boston, Massachusetts

I. Introduction

Small-cell lung cancer (SCLC) is one of the most chemotherapy-sensitive epithelial malignancies. As in acute leukemia, response rates to combination chemotherapy range from 60% to 80%. However, unlike the hematological malignancies, very few patients are cured.

There are many reasons for our failure to cure SCLC with chemotherapy. Important host factors include comorbid disease, impaired performance status, and the presence of pharmacological sanctuaries, such as bulky mediastinal tumors and CNS disease. Disease factors include a combination of poorly understood mechanisms that allow for the rapid emergence of drug-resistant clones.

Traditionally the World Health Organization has divided SCLC into three histological subtypes: oat cell or lymphocytelike; intermediate type; and a combined subtype, in which elements of squamous and/or adenocarcinoma are also seen. However, there is little evidence that prognosis or response to treatment is dependent upon histology. In practice, the diagnosis is made on the basis of histopathology complemented with staining for neuroendocrine markers that include neuron-specific enolase, synaptophysin, chromogranin A, and bombesin

(1). This allows the distinction to be made between small-cell and the more common non-small-cell lung cancers.

In the National Cancer Institute's Surveillance, Epidemiology, and End Results Program (SEER) SCLC represented 18% of cases of lung cancer (2). This amounts to 31,000 new cases of SCLC expected to be diagnosed in 1998 (3). The epidemiology of SCLC is closely tied to tobacco use, as <2% of SCLC patients do not have a history of cigarette smoking (4). The association with smoking accounts for the high incidence of coexisting cardiopulmonary disease in these patients, and is a major challenge in their treatment.

Clinically, SCLC typically presents as a central lung mass with associated mediastinal adenopathy. It generally grows as a submucosal, endobronchial lesion, which frequently causes cough, dyspnea, wheezing, postobstructive pneumonitis, and, less frequently, hemoptysis. Due to its central location and mediastinal involvement it can be associated with superior vena cava (SVC) syndrome and hoarseness due to injury to the recurrent laryngeal nerve. In 60% to 70% of cases SCLC is metastatic at diagnosis, and in more than 90% of cases there is mediastinal lymph node involvement (5–7).

SCLC is the most common cause of paraneoplastic syndromes. Often, these symptoms are a patient's presenting complaint. Cushing's syndrome due to ectopic production of ACTH, and the syndrome of inappropriate ADH secretion (SIADH) associated with increased ADH (and, less commonly, increased atrial natriuretic peptide) are both most commonly associated with SCLC. About 50% of SCLC patients have elevated serum ACTH and/or ADH levels, but only 5% of patients have symptoms of Cushing's syndrome and <5% have symptomatic hyponatremia (8,9). Hypercalcemia is most commonly seen in squamous-cell lung cancer, but in a series of 55 patients with hypercalcemia and lung cancer five (12.5%) had SCLC (9,10). An assortment of paraneoplastic neuropathies associated with specific autoantibodies have been described in patients with SCLC. Three-fourths of patients with paraneoplastic neuropathies associated with the anti-Hu antibody have SCLC. In most of these patients the predominant symptoms are of a diffuse sensory neuropathy, but in a minority, limbic, brainstem, or cerebellar degeneration are seen. More typically paraneoplastic cerebellar degeneration is associated with the anti-Yo antibody, but this is most often seen in patients with ovarian or breast cancers, and only rarely in SCLC (8,11). SCLC is the most common malignant cause of the Lambert-Eaton myasthenic syndrome, a symmetric, proximal muscle weakness. It is found in up to 3% of SCLC patients, and is associated with an antibody that inhibits acetylcholine release from the presynaptic neuron by disabling voltage-gated calcium channels (8,12,13). Other paraneoplastic neuropathies seen in SCLC include small-bowel dysmotility and pseudoobstruction, and photoreceptor degeneration with binocular visual loss. Digital clubbing and hypertrophic pulmonary osteoarthropathy are occasionally seen in SCLC, though they are much more common in non-small-cell lung cancer (8).

SCLC is usually a systemic disease at diagnosis; therefore, chemotherapy is an important part of the treatment plan for any stage of disease. Staging is important in determining which patients might benefit from local therapy, such as radiation, or surgery in rare cases. The most commonly used staging system is the two-stage system devised by the Veterans Administration Lung Group. By this scheme there are two stages: limited disease (LD), and extensive disease (ED) disease. LD is limited to a single hemithorax as defined by a "tolerable" radiation port. In the eyes of most radiation oncologists this includes ipsilateral supraclavicular and contralateral mediastinal lymph nodes. Originally ipsilateral malignant effusions were included in LD, but due to the poor prognosis of these patients ipsilateral effusions are now usually staged as ED (6,14). The outcome of patients with SCLC and pleural effusions is intermediate between that of patients with limited stage disease and extensive stage disease. Outside of a clinical trial, staging is directed at documentation of ED. This includes history and physical exam, complete blood counts, serum chemistries and liver function tests, chest radiograph and chest CT through the upper abdomen (including liver and adrenals), bone scan and head CT with intravenous contrast. If blood counts are normal, bone marrow biopsy is only necessary in the setting of a clinical trial of limited disease (15). Head CT reveals brain metastases in about 15% of patients at diagnosis, and about one-third of these are not symptomatic. Since early treatment of brain metastases may result in less neurological morbidity, patients should have head a CT even if ED has been documented (16).

A small minority of patients with SCLC present with isolated pulmonary nodules without evidence of lymph node involvement. In this subgroup surgical resection is associated with 5-year survival rates of 30% to 60% (7,17,18). These results are likely biased by the inadvertent inclusion of patients with well-differentiated neuroendocrine tumors, such as atypical carcinoid; nevertheless, patients with isolated pulmonary nodules should be surgically staged to identify lymph node–negative patients even if biopsy results demonstrate SCLC.

Stage at presentation with SCLC is the single most important predictor of response. Other indicators of poor prognosis include decreased performance status, increased tumor stage, male sex, elevated LDH, elevated alkaline phosphatase, hyponatremia, and lack of response to therapy, or early recurrence (19). In interpreting clinical trials of chemotherapeutic agents in SCLC it is important to consider the relative mix of stage of patients and other relevant prognostic factors of the given group of patients.

SCLC is a rapidly progressive, epithelial malignancy. While it accounts for a minority of patients with lung cancer, SCLC is among the 10 most commonly diagnosed cancers in the United States (2). Without treatment median survival is about 3 months in limited disease and 5 weeks in extensive disease (14), and with standard therapy only about 4% of all patients diagnosed with SCLC will live 5 or more years (20). However, SCLC is very responsive to both chemotherapy and radiotherapy, and modern treatment results in a substantial survival benefit.

The benefit of chemotherapy was first demonstrated in trials with single agents. Subsequently, combination regimens were shown to be superior to single agents, and in the 1990s a variety of exciting new agents have entered the clinic. Most recently, strides in understanding some of the molecular genetic processes underlying malignant transformation have given rise to trials of novel, biologically targeted treatments.

II. Single-Agent Chemotherapy in SCLC

SCLC is remarkably sensitive to both chemotherapy and radiotherapy, and treatment significantly improves survival. This was first demonstrated by the Veterans Administration Lung Cancer Study Group trial in 1969, which demonstrated that patients with extensive SCLC randomized to treatment with three cycles of cyclophosphamide had a median survival twice that of patients randomized to best supportive care (21). This finding was in marked contrast to results with chemotherapy in non-small-cell lung cancer and most other solid tumors, and it sparked interest in trials of chemotherapy in SCLC.

In the 1970s and 1980s at least 57 cytotoxic chemotherapeutic agents were evaluated for SCLC in Phase II trials. Active drugs were found among most classes of compounds evaluated (22). As described above, the alkylating agent cyclophosphamide was one of the first drugs shown to be active in SCLC. Other drugs found to have important single-agent activity during the 1970s and 1980s included the vinca alkaloids vincristine and vindesine; the anthracyclines doxorubicin and epirubicin; the platinum compounds cisplatin and carboplatin; the epipodophyllotoxins etoposide and teniposide; and the alkylating agent ifosfamide. Of these, etoposide and teniposide achieved the highest single-agent response rates (up to 80% to 90%) (23,24).

Since 1990 a number of new active agents, some with novel mechanisms of action, have been identified. These include the taxanes (paclitaxel and docetaxel), which stabilize microtubules; the camptothecins (topotecan and irinotecan), which inhibit topoisomerase I; gemcitabine, an antimetabolite closely related to cytarabine; and vinorelbine, a vinca alkaloid inhibitor of microtubule assembly. A listing of the drugs active against SCLC appears in Table 1.

Due to selection biases and other differences between patient populations it is not valid to compare the results among Phase II studies, but when studied as single agents, the active drugs have typically produced response rates of 25% to 50% in previously untreated patients (Table 1). Five of the newest agents—topotecan (25–27), irinotecan (28,29), docetaxel (30), paclitaxel (31), and vinorelbine (32,33)—have generated particular interest by demonstrating high single-agent activity in previously treated patients. Preliminary results of a randomized trial by Schiller et al. indicate that single-agent topotecan is as effective as the combination of cyclophosphamide, doxorubicin, and vincristine (34). Unfortunately,

Table 1 Single-Agent Chemotherapy in SCLC

Class	Compound[a]	Response rates	Selected refs.
Alkylating agents (covalently bind DNA)	CCNU	0–27%	39, 101
	methyl-CCNU	0–25%	102
	Cyclophosphamide	12–70%	38, 39
	Hexamethylmelamine	0–42%	103
	Ifosfamide	4–33%	104
	Prednimustine	11%	105
Platinum compounds (covalently bind DNA)	Cisplatin	0–31%	106–108
	Carboplatin	6–41%	109, 110
	Iproplatin	0–6%	111
Epipodophyllotoxins (inhibit topoisomerase II)	Etoposide	0–81%	23, 112–114
	Teniposide	0–90%	24, 115, 116
Anthracyclines (inhibit topoisomerase II)	Doxorubicin	21–50%	117, 118
	Epirubicin	33–50%	119, 120
	Idarubicin	0–14%	121
	Mitoxantrone	0–7%	122
Vinca alkaloids (inhibit microtubule assembly)	Vincristine	0–42%	
	Vindesine	0–33%	123
	Vinorelbine	12–26% (12–16% in previously treated)	124, 125 32, 33, 126–128
Antimetabolites	Fluorouracil	0–38%	129
	Mitoguazone	0–5%	130
	Cytarabine	0–7%	131
	Gemcitabine	27%	132
Taxanes (stabilize microtubules)	Docetaxel	8–25% (25% in previously treated)	30, 133
	Paclitaxel	34–50% (29% in previously treated)	31, 134, 135
Camptothecins (inhibit topoisomerase I)	Topotecan	6–39% (6–27% in previously treated)	25, 26, 136–139 28, 29, 140
	Irinotecan	16–47% (previously treated)	

[a]CCNU, lomustine.

regardless of the potent activity of these cytotoxic drugs, no single agent has provided cures or long-term survivals in patients with SCLC.

III. Combination Chemotherapy in SCLC
A.   Combination Therapy Is Superior to Single-Agent Therapy

The experience with hematological malignancies and models of the kinetics of
tumor cell killing in murine systems suggested that initial treatment with combinations of drugs would be more effective than single agents (35–37). In practice
this approach has only led to significant cure rates in a few solid tumors, such as
testicular cancer, choriocarcinoma, and high-grade lymphomas, but combination
chemotherapy has markedly increased the median survival of patients with SCLC,
and cured a minority of patients with limited disease. Landmark trials to document
the superiority of combination over single-agent therapy compared cyclophosphamide to cyclophosphamide and CCNU, and to cyclophosphamide, adriamycin,
and DTIC. In both trials the combination led to significant improvements in
response and survival (38,39). (See Table 2.)

The advantage of combination chemotherapy has been reconfirmed in
recent studies comparing single-agent oral etoposide to "modern" multidrug regimens in elderly or poor-performance status patients (40–42). The trial by the Medical Research Council Lung Cancer Working Party (Cambridge, U.K.) (40)
enrolled 339 previously untreated patients with poor performance status (WHO
performance status 2 to 4), and randomized them to four 21-day cycles of oral
etoposide (50 mg twice daily for 10 days) or "standard," intravenous therapy (four
21-day cycles of cycles of cyclophosphamide, doxorubicin, and vincristine
(CAV), or etoposide and vincristine). The trial by Souhami et al. (41) randomized
155 patients with extensive disease and a WHO performance status of 2 to 3 or
aged 75 years or older. Patients were assigned to either six 21-day cycles of oral
etoposide (100 mg twice daily for 5 days) or cisplatin and oral etoposide alternating with CAV. Both of these studies were terminated early due to excess mortality
in the groups treated with single-agent etoposide. furthermore, treatment with single-agent etoposide resulted in inferior control of lung cancer symptoms and overall quality of life. These results came as a surprise to many in the oncology community. They emphasize that many patients who are elderly or have advanced
disease will benefit from intensive chemotherapy, and that intensive treatment
may improve quality of life by decreasing cancer-related symptoms.

A large number of multidrug regimens have demonstrated activity in SCLC.
A summary of some of the important randomized trials comparing the most commonly used regimens is shown in Table 3. Due to its tolerability and high activity
(response rates of 80% to 90% in Phase II trials of patients with LD and/or ED),
CAV became a "standard" regimen in the late 1970s (43). The recognition of the
impressive single-agent activity of etoposide and cisplatin in the 1980s spawned a

Table 2 Randomized Trials of Combinations vs. Single Agents in SCLC

Regimens[a]	Pts[b]	Stage[c]	Response rate (PR + CR)[d]	Median survival	Summary	Ref.
Cy + CCNU	110	Incp	43%	4.6 mo	Increased response and survival in combination arm	39
Cy	118		22%	3.9 mo		
Cy + Dox + DTIC	217	Mixed	57%	7.1 mo	Increased response and survival in combination arm	38
Cy	34		12%	4.1 mo		
VP (oral for 10 days)	171	Mixed	45%	4.3 mo	Less toxicity and significant increased survival in combination arm. Stopped early	40
(Cy + Dox) or (Cy + Dox + Vcr)	66, 102		51%	6.0 mo		
VP (oral for 5 days)	75	ED	33%	4.8 mo	Less toxicity and increased response in combination arm. Stopped early	41
Cy + Dox + Vcr	80	ED	46%	5.6 mo		
VP (oral, 50 mg/d for 14 days)	32	ED	25%	5.1 mo	Less toxicity and increased response in combination arm. Stopped early	42
Cbo + VP (oral 240 mg/m², 3 days)	33		49%	6.9 mo		

[a]Cy, cyclophosphamide; CCNU, lomustine; Dox, doxorubicin; DTIC, dacarbazine; VP, etoposide; Vcr, vincristine; Cbo, carboplatin.

[b]Pts, number of patients.

[c]Inop, inoperable; LD, limited disease; ED, extensive disease; Mixed, LD and ED.

[d]CR, complete response; PR, partial response.

Table 3 Randomized Trials of Combination Chemotherapy in SCLC

Regimens[a]	Pts[b]	Stage[c]	Response rate (PR + CR)[d]	Median survival	Summary	Ref.
Cy + Dox + Vcr	49	Mixed	50%	8.3 mo	Increased response with VP16, no increased survival. More myelotoxicity with VP16	44
Cy + Dox + Vcr + VP	43		65%	10.3 mo		
Cy + Dox + Vcr	66	ED	46%	7.8 mo	Increased response with VP16, no increased survival. More myelotoxicity with VP16	45
Cy + Dox + Vcr + VP	70		70%	9.4 mo		
Cy + Dox + Vcr + XRT	113	LD	65%	12.4 mo	No difference in response or survival with VP16, Increased toxicity with VP16	46
Cy + Dox + Vcr + VP + XRT	118		70%	15.1 mo		
Mtx + Cy + CCNU + Vcr	89	ED	71%	5.3 mo	Increased survival and CR rate in early VP16 arm compared to Mtx. More myelotoxicity with VP16.	47
VP (late) + Cy + CCNU + Vcr	92		72%	6.2 mo		
VP (early) + Cy + CCNU + Vcr	88		84%	7.6 mo		
Cy-1200 + Dox-70 + Vcr	106	ED	72%	9.7 mo	No difference in response or survival. Similar myelotoxicity.	56
Cy-1000 + Dox-40 + Vcr + VP	108		74%	9.7 mo		
Cy-1000 + Dox-40 + Vcr	146	ED	53%	8.0 mo	No difference in response or survival. More myelotoxicity with high dose.	55
Cy-1200 + Dox-70 + Vcr	101		63%	6.7 mo		
Cis-80 + Cy-900 + Dox + VP	50	LD	54% CR	26% 2 yr	High dose only given at cycle 1. Increased 2 yr survival with high dose. No difference in CR rate.	58
Cis-100 + Cy-1200 + Dox + VP	55		67% CR	43% 2 yr		
Cis-80 day 1 + VP-80 days 1–3	46	ED	83%	11.4 mo	No difference in response or survival. More toxicity with high dose.	57
Cis-27 days 1–5 + VP-80 days 1–5	44		86%	10.7 mo		

Regimen	Pts	Disease	%	Months	Comment	Ref
Cy + Dox + Vcr	97	Mixed	55%	9.9 mo	Increased survival with alternating regimen. Increased response and less toxicity with Cis/VP compared to Cy/Dox/Vcr.	52
Cis + VP	97		78%	9.9 mo		
Alternating the two regimens	94		76%	11.8 mo		
Cy + Dox + Vcr	146	ED	51%	8.3 mo	No difference in response or survival. Less myelotoxicity with Cis/VP.	53
Cis + VP	148		61%	8.6 mo		
Alternating the two regimens	143		59%	8.1 mo		
Cis + Vcr + Dox + VP (with XRT)	110	ED	66%	11.7 mo	Increased response and toxic death with Cis/Vcr/Dox/VP. No difference in survival.	64
Cy + Dox + Vcr alt with Cis + VP	109		52%	10.6 mo		
Cis + VP (XRT in responders)	71	Mixed	69%	12.5 mo	No difference in CR rate or survival. Less non-heme toxicity with Cbo.	54
Cbo + VP (XRT in responders)	72		78%	11.8 mo		
Cis + VP (intravenous, days 1,2,3)	156	ED	57%	9.5	No difference in response or survival. More myelotoxicity with 21 day oral VP.	66
Cis + VP (oral, days 1–21)	150		61%	9.9		
Cis + VP (with XRT for LD)	73	Mixed	65%	11.6 mo	No difference in response or survival. In subgroup analysis Cis better than Ifos in LD.	70
Ifos + VP (with XRT for LD)	68		68%	9.4 mo		
Cis + VP (with XRT for LD)	42	Mixed	78%	12.6 mo	No difference in response or survival. More myelotoxicity with Ifos.	69
Cis + VP + Ifos (with XRT for LD)	47		74%	12.9 mo		
Cis + VP	84	ED	67%	7.3 mo	Increased time to relapse and survival with Ifos. No difference in response.	67
Cis + VP + Ifos	87		73%	9.0 mo		

[a]Cy, cyclophosphamide; CCNU, lomustine; Dox, doxorubicin; DTIC, dacarbazine; VP, etoposide; Vcr, vincristine; Cbo, carboplatin.
[b]Pts, number of patients.
[c]Inop, inoperable; LD, limited disease; ED, extensive disease; Mixed, LD and ED.
[d]CR, complete response; PR, partial response.

flurry of Phase II trials of combination regimens incorporating these agents. Three randomized studies have compared CAV to CAVE (CAV with etoposide). Two of the three found increased response with the addition of etoposide, but no significant increase in survival. In all three the addition of etoposide was associated with more myelotoxicity (44–46). The trial that did not show a difference in response (46) was confined to stage LD patients, and included thoracic radiotherapy; so, it is not directly comparable to the other two. Etoposide was also compared to methotrexate in a randomized fashion in combination with cyclophosphamide, CCNU, and vincristine (47). In this three-arm study there was a small but significant survival advantage (2 months) in the group that received etoposide early (days 3 to 6) in the 21-day treatment cycle in comparison to those who received methotrexate on days 14 and 17. Etoposide given days 14 to 17 was not significantly better than methotrexate. These results, in aggregate, do suggest an advantage to etoposide-containing combinations.

Simultaneous with these randomized studies the combinations of etoposide and cisplatin (EP), and etoposide and carboplatin (EC) produced response rates of 80% to 90% and complete response rates of 40% to 45% in Phase II trials (48,49). Furthermore, prospective and retrospective analyses indicated that up to 55% of patients who relapsed after CAV or had CAV-resistant disease responded to EP (50,51). Randomized trials in the early 1990s comparing CAV to EP in extensive disease had mixed results (52,53). The trial by Fukuoka et al. (52) found a higher response rate with EP, but no difference in survival. The trial by Roth et al. (53) found no difference in response or survival. Both trials allowed patients with progressive disease to cross over to the alternate regimen; so, survival is difficult to evaluate. However, in both trials EP was significantly less toxic than CAV. Subsequently a randomized comparison of cisplatin and carboplatin in combination with etoposide by the Hellenic Co-operative Oncology Group found no difference in complete response or survival rates, but EC was associated with significantly less nonhematological toxicity (54). Thus, a platinum compound in combination with etoposide has become the most commonly used regimen in SCLC.

Unfortunately, the outlook for patients with SCLC remains dismal. Among patients with extensive disease treated with a platinum and etoposide only 15% to 20% will achieve a complete response, half will die within 7 to 11 months, and only rare patients will live more than 2 years. Among patients with limited disease treated with a platinum, etoposide, and radiotherapy, 50% to 60% will achieve a complete response; nonetheless half will die within 12 to 20 months, and only 15% to 40% of patients will live >2 years (Tables 2, 3) (19).

B. Dose Intensification Without Stem Cell Support

Due to the remarkable sensitivity of SCLC to cytotoxic agents both in vivo and in vitro, many groups have attempted to improve on the successes of combination chemotherapy by escalating drug doses and/or increasing the number of drugs. "High-dose" CAV (cyclophosphamide 1200 mg/m^2, doxorubicin 70 mg/m^2, vincristine 1 mg/m^2) was found to be more toxic but no more efficacious than "standard dose" CAV (cyclophosphamide 1000 mg/m^2, doxorubicin 40 mg/m^2, vincristine 1 mg/m^2) (55). Using the same CAV regimens, high-dose CAV was found to be no more efficacious than standard CAV with etoposide (CAVE), and toxicity was similar (56). Higher (nontransplant) doses of EP have also been compared to standard doses with greater toxicity but no improvement in survival or response rate (57). Conversely, Arriagada et al. found that higher-dose cisplatin (100 mg/m^2) and cyclophosphamide (1200 mg/m^2) given during the first treatment cycle in combination with doxorubicin and etoposide resulted in superior 2-year survival compared to standard doses (cisplatin 80 mg/m^2 and cyclophosphamide 900 mg/m^2) in patients with limited disease. All treatment subsequent to cycle 1 was with standard doses, and patients received thoracic radiotherapy after completing chemotherapy (58).

Based on the model of drug resistance developed by Goldie and Coldman (35,36), rapid alternation of "non-cross-resistant" cytotoxic regimens will increase the likelihood of killing all of the malignant cells before a drug-resistant clone proliferates. Based on these concepts, various regimens of alternating drug combinations have been evaluated. Roth et al. (53) and Fukuoka et al. (52) have compared CAV, EP, and alternating cycles of CAV and EP (Table 3). In the Roth study all patients had ED, while in the Fukuoka study half had ED and half had LD. Both allowed crossover of patients with unresponsive or progressive disease between the CAV and EP arms. Fukuoka et al. (52) found a small (1.9 month) but significant increase in survival in CAV/EP versus CAV or EP, and a higher response rate with EP or CAV/EP as compared to CAV. In contrast, Roth et al. (53) found no differences in survival or response among the regimens. In both studies CAV and CAV/EP were more toxic than EP. Other groups have evaluated other alternating combinations with conflicting results (59–62). Therefore, there is no convincing evidence that alternating regimens are superior to repeating cycles of one combination regimen, as long as nonresponding patients are changed to a second combination.

An important limitation of all of these studies is that none used truly non-cross-resistant regimens, and it is unlikely that such regimens exist. Both Roth and Fukuoka found that after failing CAV or EP, only a minority of patients (8% to 23%) responded to the other regimen; thus, the regimens displayed a great deal of cross-resistance. As we learn more about the molecular genetics of malignant cells and the mechanisms of action of cytotoxic drugs, it is apparent that most if not all of the cytotoxic drugs in use today act through a limited number of common final pathways that depend upon disruption of cell cycle regulation and induction of apoptosis.

An alternative method of increasing treatment intensity is to select agents with different primary toxicities in order to increase the number of drugs and decrease the interval between treatments. The CODE regimen is a paradigm of this approach. In this regimen all four drugs are given the first day; then cisplatin/vincristine and cisplatin/doxorubicin/etoposide are given weekly, on alternate weeks for 8 weeks. This alternates weeks of milder myelosuppression with weeks of more intense myelosuppression. CODE results in very high response rates and CR rates of up to 40% in extensive disease (63), but a recent randomized trial comparing CODE to CAV/EP in patients with extensive disease found no difference in survival (64). Needless to say, CODE was substantially more toxic than CAV/EP. The logical extension of these approaches is the use of very high dose therapy and autologous stem cell support. Early reports suggest that high-dose chemotherapy supported by peripheral blood stem cells in selected patients can lead to a very promising outcome. Unfortunately, most patients with small-cell lung cancer do not have the performance status required to undergo high-dose chemotherapy. This continues to be an active area of research in the treatment of SCLC (65).

C. Combinations with New Cytotoxic Agents

At this time in the United States the combination of etoposide with a platinating agent, either cisplatin or carboplatin, is the most commonly used regimen in the treatment of SCLC. The specific drug schedules have varied among studies. In particular the etoposide has been delivered both on extended oral and 3-day intravenous schedules. In 1995 a large randomized study by the Cancer and Leukemia Group B found that an EP regimen given every 21 days with the cisplatin and etoposide delivered intravenously on days 1, 2, and 3 was equally efficacious to and less toxic than EP with the etoposide delivered by mouth, daily for 21 days (66). Thus, the 3-day EP regimen has become the "standard" regimen for initial treatment of SCLC in North America, against which new treatments should be compared (Table 3).

EP has been intensified by the addition of ifosfamide, and a randomized trial reported by Loehrer et al. showed an improved response rate and survival with EP plus ifosfamide compared to EP in patients with extensive disease (67,68). A similar comparison in a mixed population of patients with extensive and limited disease found no difference in response or survival (69). A German study compared etoposide/cisplatin with etoposide/ifosfamide, and the two combinations were shown to have similar efficacy (70). The advantage of ifosfamide added to etoposide/cisplatin in the Loehrer study many be explained by either superiority of the VIP combination or increased treatment intensity (Table 3).

The newer cytotoxic agents that have demonstrated important single-agent activity include the topoisomerase I inhibitors topotecan and irinotecan, the taxanes paclitaxel and docetaxel, the new vinca alkaloid vinorelbine, and the novel antimetabolite gemcitabine (Table 1). All of these agents are currently being tested in combination regimens in Phase II clinical trials. (See Table 4.)

Table 4 Combinations with New Drugs

Regimens[a]	Pts[b]	Stage[c]	Response rate	Median survival	Ref.
Txl + Cbo + VP	38	Mixed	76% (CR + PR)	17 mo in LD	76
(with XRT for LD)			40% CR in LD	7 mo in ED	
(Txl 135 mg/m^2, Cbo AUC = 5)			17% CR in ED		
Txl + Cbo + VP	98	Mixed	91% (CR + PR)	>16 mo in LD	73
(with XRT for LD)					
(Txl 200 mg/m^2, Cbo AUC = 6)			71% CR in LD	10 mo in ED	
			21% CR in ED		
Txl + Cbo + VP	35	LD	88% (CR + PR)		74
			37% CR	—	
Txl + Cbo + VP	35	Mixed	83% (CR + CR)	17 mo in LD	75
(with XRT for LD)			29% CR	7 mo in ED	
			40% CR in LD		
Txl + Cis + VP	26	ED	96% (CR + PR)		78
			19% CR	—	
Vnl + Cbo	33	ED	70% (CR + PR)		81
			25% CR	—	
Vnl + Dox	16	Relapsed	19% PR		84
(Stopped early for excess toxicity)			0% CR	—	
Top + Txl	12	ED	92% (CR + PR)	12 mo	71
			17% CR		
Irin + Cis	75	Mixed	84% (CR + PR)	13 mo	83
			29% CR	14 mo in LD	
			30% CR in LD		

[a]Txl, paclitaxel; Cbo, carboplatin; VP, etoposide; XRT, thoracic radiotherapy; Vnl, vinorelbine; Dox, doxorubicin; Top, topotecan; Irin, irinotecan.
[b]Pts, number of patients.
[c]LD, limited disease; ED, extensive disease; Mixed, LD and ED.

Topotecan is one of the most active single agents in the treatment of small-cell lung cancer. Efforts to combine this drug with existing agents have been challenging due to myelosuppression, notably neutropenia. Preliminary results from the trial by Jett et al. using the combination of topotecan and paclitaxel (topotecan 1 mg/m^2 on days 1 to 5 and paclitaxel 135 mg/m^2 over 24 hours, on day 5) in extensive disease demonstrated an overall response rate of 92%, a CR rate of 17%, and a median survival of 12 months. However, only 12 evaluable patients have been enrolled to date, and the regimen produces substantial toxicity. The original topotecan dose of 1.25 mg/m^2 was reduced due to grade 4 toxicity in two and fatal infection in the third of first three patients enrolled (not included in the results described above). Among the 12 patients treated at the lower dose, grade 3 or more severe leukopenia occurred in more than half of treatment cycles, despite the use of G-CSF (Table 4) (71). In a randomized Phase II trial conducted by the Cancer and Leukemia Group B that evaluated three two-drug combinations—topotecan/paclitaxel, topotecan/cisplatin, and paclitaxel/cisplatin—both topotecan arms were closed early due to excessive toxicity (72). The activity of the combination of topotecan and paclitaxel is very exciting, but bone marrow toxicity may limit its usefulness. Many groups are working at efforts to incorporate topotecan into the upfront therapy of SCLC.

The combination of paclitaxel with a platinum (carboplatin or cisplatin) and etoposide has also demonstrated very high activity with overall and complete response rates of 81% to 98% and 37% to 71% respectively in limited disease, and 65% to 84% and 17% to 21% respectively in extensive disease (patients with limited disease also received concurrent thoracic radiotherapy). Still, the median survival was only 7 to 10 months in extensive disease, and remained under 18 months in limited disease (73–78). Limited experience also indicates that paclitaxel can be added to the combination of carboplatin/etoposide/ifosfamide with acceptable toxicity and high response rates (79). Randomized studies comparing carboplatin and etoposide with and without paclitaxel are under way (80).

Preliminary data suggest that vinorelbine and carboplatin, vinorelbine and paclitaxel, and irinotecan and cisplatin are active combinations that deserve further study (81–83). Vinorelbine and doxorubicin was evaluated in patients with relapsed disease, but myelotoxicity was excessive and the trial was halted early (84). Tolerable combinations of cisplatin, etoposide, and gemcitabine, and of etoposide and gemcitabine have been devised in Phase I settings and will be tested in Phase II trials (85,86). A multitude of other combinations employing these newer cytotoxic drugs are being tested, and it is likely that some will demonstrate impressive response rates; however, past experience must make us skeptical of claims that higher complete response rates will be associated with improvements in survival. In the long term, novel therapeutic approaches are required.

IV. Novel Therapeutic Approaches

Tremendous strides have been made in understanding some of the fundamental biological processes that contribute to the malignant state. This knowledge is leading to the application of novel therapeutic approaches in the clinic that may be more effective than traditional cytotoxic chemotherapy at inhibiting the proliferation and metastasis of cancer cells.

Since the large majority of patients with limited-stage SCLC who achieve a complete response to initial therapy will die of metastatic disease, it is important to develop compounds that prevent the growth and invasion of microscopic metastatic deposits that evidently survive intensive cytotoxic chemotherapy.

Inhibitors of the matrix metalloproteinases (MMPI) are a group of antimetastatic agents that have recently entered Phase III clinical trials. The matrix metalloproteinases (MMP) are a family of Zn^{2+}-dependent enzymes that hydrolyze the protein components of the extracellular matrix. Increased MMP expression is associated with increased metastatic potential in a variety of tumors, and it is thought that MMP activity is important for metastatic tumor cells to invade and grow at distant sites (87). A number of MMPIs are in clinical development, including Phase III trials in patients with limited SCLC who have achieved a complete response to chemoradiotherapy.

SCLC cells express a number of surface marker molecules that are considered to be relatively specific to cells of neuroendocrine origin; these include GD2, GD3, and CD56 (88–92). These surface markers provide the opportunity to develop potent antibody-conjugated toxins that are directed at SCLC cells, and may be useful for eradicating minimal residual disease following debulking with traditional chemotherapy. N901-blocked ricin (N901-bR) is an immunoconjugate between a murine monoclonal antibody (N901) raised against CD56 and a form of the potent protein synthesis inhibitor, ricin, that has been modified to block the galactose binding sites and prevent nonselective cytotoxicity. In preclinical trials N901-bR cytotoxicity was highly specific for CD56-positive cells (93,94). In a Phase I trial in patients with relapsed or primary-refractory SCLC one partial response was observed in 21 patients, but systemic toxicities including capillary leak syndrome, cardiac toxicity, and peripheral nerve toxicity were noted and might have reflected cytotoxicity to normal tissues that express CD56 (95).

Another promising approach is the use of antisense oligonucleotides to inhibit the expression of specific oncogenes that are known to be mutated or overexpressed in SCLC cells. Two genes of interest are the C-*raf* gene, which encodes a critical intermediate in the Ras signal transduction pathway from tyrosine kinase growth factor receptors to the nucleus (96), and the *bcl2* gene, which encodes a potent inhibitor of apoptosis (97).

The antiapoptotic gene *bcl2* is overexpressed in most SCLC tumor samples and cell lines (98), and an antisense oligonucleotide directed against the *bcl2* gene has been shown to inhibit the growth of SCLC cell lines (99). An antisense oligonucleotide directed against *bcl2* is currently being evaluated in patients with lymphomas (100), and in the near future it will be tested in patients with other solid tumors, including SCLC. Phase I and II trials using an antisense inhibitor of the C-*raf* gene are in progress.

V. Conclusions

In contrast to most solid tumors and to non-small-cell lung cancer in particular, SCLC is usually highly responsive to treatment with cytotoxic chemotherapy and radiotherapy. This property has made SCLC of particular interest to medical oncologists. However, unlike many of the hematological malignancies, this responsiveness to treatment has not translated into a high cure rate. With current therapy long-term survival is only seen in about 4% of "all-comers" with SCLC. Further dose escalation of existing drugs with stem cell support, and combinations including the newer agents such as the camptothecins and taxanes will likely provide small improvements in response rates and survival, but novel approaches are necessary to cure a substantial fraction of SCLC patients. Biologically targeted approaches evolving from the astounding volume of molecular genetic knowledge that has accumulated over the past two decades are currently entering clinical trials. These approaches have the potential to alter the malignant phenotype at the cellular level, and may provide the means to eradicate residual disease that persists despite current cytotoxic therapies. Perhaps over the coming decade we will see this disease transformed from one that can be treated into one that can be cured.

References

1. Fraire AE. Pathology of lung cancer. In: Aisner J, Arriagada R, Green MR, Perry MC, eds. Comprehensive Textbook of Thoracic Oncology. Baltimore: Williams and Wilkins, 1996:245–275.
2. Ries LAG, Kosary CL, Hankey BF, Miller BA, Harras A, Edwards BK. SEER Cancer Statistics Review, 1973–1994, NIH Pub. No. 97-2789. Bethesda, MD: National Cancer Institute, 1997.
3. Landis SH, Murray T, Bolden S, Wingo PA. Cancer statistics, 1998. CA Cancer J Clin 1998; 48:6–29.
4. Morabia A, Wynder EL. Cigarette smoking and lung cancer cell types. Cancer 1991; 68:2074–2078.
5. Ihde DC. Chemotherapy of lung cancer. N Engl J Med 1992; 327:1434–1441.
6. Abrams J, Doyle LA, Aisner J. Staging, prognostic factors, and special considerations in small cell lung cancer. Semin Oncol 1988; 15:261–277.
7. Martini N, Wittes RE, Hilaris BS, Hajdu SI, Beattie EJ Jr, Golbey RB. Oat cell carcinoma of the lung. Clin Bull 1975; 5:144–148.
8. Patel AM, Davila DG, Peters SG. Paraneoplastic syndromes associated with lung cancer. Mayo Clin Proc 1993; 68:278–287.
9. Schiller JH, Jones JC. Paraneoplastic syndromes associated with lung cancer. Curr Opin Oncol 1993; 5:335–342.
10. Campbell JH, Ralston S, Boyle IT, Banham SW. Symptomatic hypercalcaemia in lung cancer. Respir Med 1991; 85:223–227.
11. Dalmau JO, Posner JB. Paraneoplastic syndromes affecting the nervous system. Semin Oncol 1997; 24:318–328.
12. O'Neill JH, Murray NM, Newsom-Davis J. The Lambert-Eaton myasthenic syndrome. A review of 50 cases. Brain 1988; 111:577–596.
13. Lennon VA, Lambert EH. Autoantibodies bind solubilized calcium channel-omega-conotoxin complexes from small cell lung carcinoma: a diagnostic aid for Lambert-Eaton myasthenic syndrome. Mayo Clin Proc 1989; 64:1498–1504.

14. Zelen M. Keynote address on biostatistics and data retrieval. Cancer Chemother Rep 1973; 4:31–42.
15. Patel AM, Jett JR. Clinical presentation and staging of lung cancer. In: Aisner J, Arriagada R, Green MR, Perry MC, eds. Comprehensive Textbook of Thoracic Oncology. Baltimore: Williams and Wilkins, 1996:293–318.
16. Elias AD. Small cell lung cancer: state-of-the-art therapy in 1996. Chest 1997; 112: 251S–258S.
17. Higgins GA, Shields TW, Keehn RJ. The solitary pulmonary nodule. Ten-year follow-up of Veterans Administration–armed forces cooperative study. Arch Surg 1975; 110:570–575.
18. Shields TW, Higgins GA Jr, Matthews MJ, Keehn RJ. Surgical resection in the management of small cell carcinoma of the lung. J Thorac Cardiovasc Surg 1982; 84: 481–488.
19. Ihde DC, Harvey IP, Glatstein E. Small cell lung cancer. In: DeVita J, Hellman S, Rosenberg SA, eds. Cancer: Principles and Practice of Oncology. Philadelphia: Lippincott-Raven, 1997:911–949.
20. Chute JP, Venzon DJ, Hankins L, et al. Outcome of patients with small-cell lung cancer during 20 years of clinical research at the US National Cancer Institute. Mayo Clin Proc 1997; 72:901–912.
21. Green RA, Humphrey E, Close H, Patno ME. Alkylating agents in bronchogenic carcinoma. Am J Med 1969; 46:516–525.
22. Grant SC, Gralla RJ, Kris MG, Orazem J, Kitsis EA. Single-agent chemotherapy trials in small-cell lung cancer, 1970 to 1990: the case for studies in previously treated patients. J Clin Oncol 1992; 10:484–498.
23. Carney DN, Grogan L, Smit EF, Harford P, Berendsen HH, Postmus PE. Single-agent oral etoposide for elderly small cell lung cancer patients. Semin Oncol 1990; 17:49–53.
24. Bork E, Hansen M, Dombernowsky P, Hansen SW, Pedersen AG, Hansen HH. Teniposide (VM 26), an overlooked highly active agent in small-cell lung cancer. Results of a phase II trial in untreated patients. J Clin Oncol 1986; 4:524–527.
25. Ardizzoni A, Hansen H, Dombernowsky P, et al. Topotecan, a new active drug in the second-line treatment of small-cell lung cancer: a phase II study in patients with refractory and sensitive disease. The European Organization for Research and Treatment of Cancer Early Clinical Studies Group and New Drug Development Office, and the Lung Cancer Cooperative Group. J Clin Oncol 1997; 15:2090–2096.
26. Perez-Soler R, Glisson BS, Lee JS, et al. Treatment of patients with small-cell lung cancer refractory to etoposide and cisplatin with the topoisomerase I poison topotecan. J Clin Oncol 1996; 14:2785–2790.
27. Lynch T. Topotecan today. J Clin Oncol 1996; 14:3053–3055.
28. Masuda N, Fukuoka M, Kusunoki Y, et al. CPT-11: a new derivative of camptothecin for the treatment of refractory or relapsed small-cell lung cancer. J Clin Oncol 1992; 10:1225–1229.
29. Le Chevalier T, Ibrahim N, Chomy P, et al. A phase II study of irinotecan (CPT-11) in patients (pts) with small cell lung cancer (SCLC) progressing after initial response to first-line chemotherapy (CT). Proc Am Soc Clin Oncol, Denver, Colo., May 17, 1997.
30. Smyth JF, Smith IE, Sessa C, et al. Activity of docetaxel (Taxotere) in small cell lung

cancer. The Early Clinical Trials Group of the EORTC. Eur J Cancer 1994; 30A: 1058–1060.

31. Smit EF, Fokkema E, Biesma B, Groen HJ, Snoek W, Postmus PE. A phase II study of paclitaxel in heavily pretreated patients with small-cell lung cancer. Br J Cancer 1998; 77:347–351.

32. Furuse K, Kubota K, Kawahara M, et al. Phase II study of vinorelbine in heavily previously treated small cell lung cancer. Japan Lung Cancer Vinorelbine Study Group. Oncology 1996; 53:169–172.

33. Jassem J, Karnicka-Mlodkowska H, Van Pottelsberghe C, et al. Phase II study of vinorelbine (Navelbine) in previously treated small cell lung cancer patients. EORTC Lung Cancer Cooperative Group. Eur J Cancer 1993; 29A:1720–1722.

34. Schiller J, Von Pawel J, Shepherd F, et al. Topotecan (T) versus (vs) cyclophosphamide (C), doxorubicin (A) and vincristine (V) for the treatment (tx) of patients (pts) with recurrent small cell lung cancer (SCLC): a phase III study. Thirty-fourth Annual Meeting, American Society of Clinical Oncology, Los Angeles, CA, May 16–19, 1998.

35. Goldie JH, Coldman AJ. A mathematic model for relating the drug sensitivity of tumors to their spontaneous mutation rate. Cancer Treat Rep 1979; 63:1727–1733.

36. Goldie JH, Coldman AJ, Gudauskas GA. Rationale for the use of alternating non-cross-resistant chemotherapy. Cancer Treat Rep 1982; 66:439–449.

37. Kaufman D, Chabner BA. Clinical strategies for cancer treatment: the role of drugs. In: Chabner BA, Longo DL, eds. Cancer Chemotherapy and Biotherapy: Principles and Practice. Philadelphia: Lippincott-Raven, 1996:1–16.

38. Lowenbraun S, Bartolucci A, Smalley RV, Lynn M, Krauss S, Durant JR. The superiority of combination chemotherapy over single agent chemotherapy in small cell lung carcinoma. Cancer 1979; 44:406–413.

39. Edmonson JH, Lagakos SW, Selawry OS, et al. Cyclophosphamide and CCNU in the treatment of inoperable small cell carcinoma and adenocarcinoma of the lung. Cancer Treat Rep 1976; 60:925–932.

40. Girling DJ. Comparison of oral etoposide and standard intravenous multidrug chemotherapy for small-cell lung cancer: a stopped multicentre randomised trial. Medical Research Council Lung Cancer Working Party [see comments]. Lancet 1996; 348:563–566.

41. Souhami RL, Spiro SG, Rudd RM, et al. Five-day oral etoposide treatment for advanced small-cell lung cancer: randomized comparison with intravenous chemotherapy. J Natl Cancer Inst 1997; 89:577–580.

42. Pfeiffer P, Rytter C, Madsen EL, et al. Re: five-day oral etoposide treatment for advanced small-cell lung cancer: randomized comparison with intravenous chemotherapy [letter]. J Natl Cancer Inst 1997; 89:1892–1893.

43. Bunn PA Jr, Carney DN. Overview of chemotherapy for small cell lung cancer. Semin Oncol 1997; 24:S7(69)–S7(74).

44. Messeih AA, Schweitzer JM, Lipton A, et al. Addition of etoposide to cyclophosphamide, doxorubicin, and vincristine for remission induction and survival in patients with small cell lung cancer. Cancer Treat Rep 1987; 71:61–66.

45. Jackson DV Jr, Case LD, Zekan PJ, et al. Improvement of long-term survival in extensive small-cell lung cancer. J Clin Oncol 1988; 6:1161–1169.

46. Jett JR, Everson L, Therneau TM, et al. Treatment of limited-stage small-cell lung cancer with cyclophosphamide, doxorubicin, and vincristine with or without etoposide: a randomized trial of the North Central Cancer Treatment Group. J Clin Oncol 1990; 8:33–38.

47. Hirsch FR, Hansen HH, Hansen M, et al. The superiority of combination chemotherapy including etoposide based on in vivo cell cycle analysis in the treatment of extensive small-cell lung cancer: a randomized trial of 288 consecutive patients. J Clin Oncol 1987; 5:585–591.

48. Evans WK, Shepherd FA, Feld R, Osoba D, Dang P, Deboer G. VP-16 and cisplatin as first-line therapy for small-cell lung cancer. J Clin Oncol 1985; 3:1471–1477.

49. Bishop JF, Raghavan D, Stuart-Harris R, et al. Carboplatin (CBDCA, JM-8) and VP-16-213 in previously untreated patients with small-cell lung cancer. J Clin Oncol 1987; 5:1574–1578.

50. Evans WK, Osoba D, Feld R, Shepherd FA, Bazos MJ, DeBoer G. Etoposide (VP-16) and cisplatin: an effective treatment for relapse in small-cell lung cancer. J Clin Oncol 1985; 3:65–71.

51. Albain KS, Crowley JJ, Hutchins L, et al. Predictors of survival following relapse or progression of small cell lung cancer. Southwest Oncology Group Study 8605 report and analysis of recurrent disease data base. Cancer 1993; 72:1184–1191.

52. Fukuoka M, Furuse K, Saijo N, et al. Randomized trial of cyclophosphamide, doxorubicin, and vincristine versus cisplatin and etoposide versus alternation of these regimens in small-cell lung cancer. J Natl Cancer Inst 1991; 83:855–861.

53. Roth BJ, Johnson DH, Einhorn LH, et al. Randomized study of cyclophosphamide, doxorubicin, and vincristine versus etoposide and cisplatin versus alternation of these two regimens in extensive small-cell lung cancer: a phase III trial of the Southeastern Cancer Study Group. J Clin Oncol 1992; 10:282–291.

54. Skarlos DV, Samantas E, Kosmidis P, et al. Randomized comparison of etoposide-cisplatin vs. etoposide-carboplatin and irradiation in small-cell lung cancer. A Hellenic Cooperative Oncology Group study. Ann Oncol 1994; 5:601–607.

55. Johnson DH, Einhorn LH, Birch R, et al. A randomized comparison of high-dose versus conventional-dose cyclophosphamide, doxorubicin, and vincristine for extensive-stage small-cell lung cancer: a phase III trial of the Southeastern Cancer Study Group. J Clin Oncol 1987; 5:1731–1738.

56. Lowenbraun S, Birch R, Buchanan R, et al. Combination chemotherapy in small cell lung carcinoma. A randomized study of two intensive regimens. Cancer 1984; 54:2344–2350.

57. Ihde DC, Mulshine JL, Kramer BS, et al. Prospective randomized comparison of high-dose and standard-dose etoposide and cisplatin chemotherapy in patients with extensive-stage small-cell lung cancer. J Clin Oncol 1994; 12:2022–2034.

58. Arriagada R, Le Chevalier T, Pignon JP, et al. Initial chemotherapeutic doses and survival in patients with limited small-cell lung cancer. N Engl J Med 1993; 329:1848–1852.

59. Havemann K, Wolf M, Holle R, et al. Alternating versus sequential chemotherapy in small cell lung cancer. A randomized German multicenter trial. Cancer 1987; 59:1072–1082.

60. Wolf M, Pritsch M, Drings P, et al. Cyclic-alternating versus response-oriented

chemotherapy in small-cell lung cancer: a German multicenter randomized trial of 321 patients [see comments]. J Clin Oncol 1991; 9:614–624.

61. Joss RA, Bacchi M, Hurny C, et al. Early versus late alternating chemotherapy in small-cell lung cancer. Swiss Group for Clinical Cancer Research (SAKK). Ann Oncol 1995; 6:157–166.

62. Postmus PE, Scagliotti G, Groen HJ, et al. Standard versus alternating non-cross-resistant chemotherapy in extensive small cell lung cancer: an EORTC Phase III trial. Eur J Cancer 1996; 32A:1498–1503.

63. Murray N, Shah A, Osoba D, et al. Intensive weekly chemotherapy for the treatment of extensive-stage small-cell lung cancer. J Clin Oncol 1991; 9:1632–1638.

64. Murray N, Livingston R, Shepherd F, et al. A randomized study of CODE plus thoracic irradiation versus alternating CAV/EP for extensive stage small cell lung cancer (ESCLC). Thirty-third Annual Meeting, American Society of Clinical Oncology, Denver, Colo., May 17–20, 1997.

65. Elias AD. Dose-intensive therapy for small cell lung cancer. Chest 1995; 107:261S–266S.

66. Miller AA, Herndon JE 2nd, Hollis DR, et al. Schedule dependency of 21-day oral versus 3-day intravenous etoposide in combination with intravenous cisplatin in extensive-stage small-cell lung cancer: a randomized phase III study of the Cancer and Leukemia Group B. J Clin Oncol 1995; 13:1871–1879.

67. Loehrer PJ Sr, Ansari R, Gonin R, et al. Cisplatin plus etoposide with and without ifosfamide in extensive small-cell lung cancer: a Hoosier Oncology Group study. J Clin Oncol 1995; 13:2594–2599.

68. Ettinger DS. Ifosfamide in the treatment of small cell lung cancer. Semin Oncol 1996; 23:2–6.

69. Miyamoto H, Nakabayashi T, Isobe H, et al. A phase III comparison of etoposide/cisplatin with or without added ifosfamide in small-cell lung cancer. Oncology 1992; 49:431–435.

70. Wolf M, Havemann K, Holle R, et al. Cisplatin/etoposide versus ifosfamide/etoposide combination chemotherapy in small-cell lung cancer: a multicenter German randomized trial. J Clin Oncol 1987; 5:1880–1889.

71. Jett JR, Day R, Levitt M, Woolley G, Jacobs S. Topotecan and paclitaxel in extensive stage small cell lung cancer (ED-SCLC) patients without prior therapy. 8th World Conference on Lung Cancer, Dublin, Ireland, Aug. 10–15, 1997.

72. Miller AA, Lilenhaum RC, Lynch TJ, et al. Treatment-related fatal sepsis from topotecan/cisplatin and topotecan/paclitaxel. J Clin Oncol 1996; 14:1964–1965.

73. Hainsworth JD, Gray JR, Stroup SL, et al. Paclitaxel, carboplatin, and extended-schedule etoposide in the treatment of small-cell lung cancer: comparison of sequential phase II trials using different dose-intensities. J Clin Oncol 1997; 15:3464–3470.

74. Gatzemeier U, Jagos U, Kaukel E, Koschel G, Von Pawel J. Paclitaxel, carboplatin, and oral etoposide: a phase II trial in limited-stage small cell lung cancer. Semin Oncol 1997; 24:S12(149)–S12(152).

75. Greco FA, Hainsworth JD. Paclitaxel, carboplatin, and oral etoposide in the treatment of small cell lung cancer. Semin Oncol 1996; 23:7–10.

76. Hainsworth JD, Stroup SL, Greco FA. Paclitaxel, carboplatin, and extended schedule

etoposide in the treatment of small cell lung carcinoma. Cancer 1996; 77:2458–2463.

77. Gatzemeier U, Jagos U, Kaukel E, Koschel G, Pawel J. Phase II study of paclitaxel, carboplatin and etoposide in patients with small cell lung cancer. Proc Am Soc Clin Oncol, Denver, Colo., May 17, 1997.

78. Glisson BS, Kurie JM, Fox NJ, et al. Phase I-II study of cisplatin, etoposide, and paclitaxel (PET) in patients with extensive small cell lung cancer (ESCLC). Proc Am Soc Clin Oncol, Denver, Colo., May 17, 1997.

79. Strauss GM, Lynch TJ, Elias AD, et al. Ifosfamide/carboplatin/etoposide/paclitaxel in advanced lung cancer: update and preliminary survival analysis. Semin Oncol 1997; 24:S12(73)–S12(80).

80. Birch R, Weaver CH, Hainsworth JD, Bobo C, Greco FA. A randomized study of etoposide and carboplatin with or without paclitaxel in the treatment of small cell lung cancer. Semin Oncol 1997; 24:S12(135)–S12(137).

81. Gridelli C, Ianniello G, Brancaccio L, et al. Carboplatin plus vinorelbine: a new active regimen in extensive small cell lung cancer. Results of a multicenter phase II study. Proc Am Soc Clin Oncol, Denver, Colo., May 17, 1997.

82. Iaffaioli RV, Facchini G, Tortoriello A, et al. Phase I study of vinorelbine and paclitaxel in small-cell lung cancer. Cancer Chemother Pharmacol 1997; 41:86–90.

83. Kudoh S, Fujiwara Y, Takada Y, et al. Phase II study of irinotecan combined with cisplatin in patients with previously untreated small-cell lung cancer. West Japan Lung Cancer Group. J Clin Oncol 1998; 16:1068–1074.

84. Johnson E, Lake D, Herndon J, Green M. Phase II trial of navelbine (NVB) plus doxorubicin (DOX) in relapsed small cell lung cancer (SCLC). Proc Am Soc Clin Oncol, Denver, Colo., May 17, 1997.

85. Stewart DJ, Earle C, Cormier Y, et al. Phase I study of cisplatin, etoposide and gemcitabine in small cell lung cancer. Proc Am Soc Clin Oncol, Denver, Colo., May 17, 1997.

86. Rabmann I, Thodtmann R, Depenbrock H, et al. Gemcitabine and etoposide in small cell lung cancer: phase I and II trials. Semin Oncol 1997; 24:S7(75)–S7(78).

87. Chambers AF. Changing views of the role of matrix metalloproteinases in mtastasis. J Natl Cancer Inst 1997; 89:1260–1270.

88. Hanqing M, Avrova N, Mansson JE, Molin K, Svennerholm L. Gangliosides and neutral glycosphingolipids of normal tissue and oat cell carcinoma of human lung. Biochim Biophys Acta 1986; 878:360–370.

89. Iliopoulos D, Ernst C, Steplewski Z, et al. Inhibition of metastases of a human melanoma xenograft by monoclonal antibody to the GD2/GD3 gangliosides. J Natl Cancer Inst 1989; 81:440–444.

90. Gerardy-Schahn R, Eckhardt M, Ledermann J, Kemshead JT. Topography of NCAM antigenic epitopes recognized by SCLC-cluster-1 antibodies. A consensus view. Int J Cancer 1994; suppl 8:27–29.

91. Grant SC, Kostakoglu L, Kris MG, et al. Targeting of small-cell lung cancer using the anti-GD2 ganglioside monoclonal antibody 3F8: a pilot trial. Eur J Nucl Med 1996; 23:145–149.

92. Fuentes R, Allman R, Mason MD. Ganglioside expression in lung cancer cell lines. Lung Cancer 1997; 18:21–33.

93. Lambert JM, Goldmacher VS, Collinson AR, Nadler LM, Blattler WA. An immuno-toxin prepared with blocked ricin: a natural plant toxin adapted for therapeutic use. Cancer Res 1991; 51:6236–6242.

94. Roy DC, Ouellet S, Le Houillier C, Ariniello PD, Perreault C, Lambert JM. Elimina-tion of neuroblastoma and small-cell lung cancer cells with an anti-neural cell adhe-sion molecule immunotoxin. J Natl Cancer Inst 1996; 88:1136–1145.

95. Lynch TJ Jr, Lambert JM, Coral F, et al. Immunotoxin therapy of small-cell lung can-cer: a phase I study of N901-blocked ricin. J Clin Oncol 1997; 15:723–734.

96. Hunter T. Oncoprotein networks. Cell 1997; 88:333–346.

97. Hockenbery D, Nunez G, Milliman C, Schreiber RD, Korsmeyer SJ. Bcl-2 is an inner mitochondrial membrane protein that blocks programmed cell death. Nature 1990; 348:334–336.

98. Jiang SX, Sato Y, Kuwao S, Kameya T. Expression of bcl-2 oncogene protein is prevalent in small cell lung carcinomas. J Pathol 1995; 177:135–138.

99. Ziegler A, Luedke GH, Fabbro D, Altmann KH, Stahel RA, Zangemeister-Wittke U. Induction of apoptosis in small-cell lung cancer cells by an antisense oligodeoxynu-cleotide targeting the Bcl-2 coding sequence [see comments]. J Natl Cancer Inst 1997; 89:1027–1036.

100. Webb A, Cunningham D, Cotter F, et al. BCL-2 antisense therapy in patients with non-Hodgkin lymphoma. Lancet 1997; 349:1137–1141.

101. Stolinsky DC, Bull FE, Pajak TF, Bateman JR. Trial of 1-(2-chloroethyl)-3-cyclo-hexyl-1-nitrosourea (CCNU; NSC-79037) in advanced bronchogenic carcinoma 1,2,3. Oncology 1975; 31:288–292.

102. Eagan RT, Carr DT, Coles DT, et al. Randomized study comparing CCNU (NSC-79037) and methyl-CCNU (NSC-95441) in advanced bronchogenic carcinoma. Can-cer Chemother Rep 1974; 58:913–918.

103. Goldsweig HG, Edgerton F, Redden CS, Takita H, Garza JG, Bisel HF. Hexa-methylmelamine as a single agent in the treatment of small-cell carcinoma of the lung. Am J Clin Oncol 1982; 5:267–272.

104. Loehrer PJ Sr, Birch R, Kramer BS, Greco FA, Einhorn LH. Ifosfamide plus N-acetylcysteine in the treatment of small cell and non-small cell carcinoma of the lung: a Southeastern Cancer Study Group Trial. Cancer Treat Rep 1986; 70:919–920.

105. Jensen HS, Hansen HH, Dombernowsky P. Phase II trial of prednimustine (NSC-134087) in the treatment of small-cell anaplastic carcinoma of the lung. Cancer Chemother Pharmacol 1980; 4:259–261.

106. Dombernowsky P, Sorenson S, Aisner J, Hansen HH. *cis*-Dichlorodiammineplatinum (Ii) in small cell anaplastic bronchogenic carcinoma: a phase Ii study. Cancer Treat Rep 1979; 63:543–545.

107. De Jager R, Longeval E, Klastersky J. High-dose cisplatin with fluid and mannitol-induced diuresis in advanced lung cancer: a phase II clinical trial of the EORTC Lung Cancer Working Party (Belgium). Cancer Treat Rep 1980; 64:1341–1346.

108. Cavelli F, Goldhirsch K, Siegaltthaler P, et al. Phase II study with *cis*-dichlorodi-ammineplatinum in small cell anaplastic bronchogenic carcinoma. Eur J Cancer 1980; 16:617–621.

109. Tamura T, Saijo N, Shinkai T, et al. Phase II study of carboplatin in small cell lung cancer. Jpn J Clin Oncol 1988; 18:27–32.

110. Smith IE, Harland SJ, Robinson BA, et al. Carboplatin: a very active new cisplatin analog in the treatment of small cell lung cancer. Cancer Treat Rep 1985; 69:43–46.

111. Granfortuna JM, Newman N, Ginsberg SJ, et al. Phase II study of iproplatin (CHIP) in previously treated small-cell lung cancer. Am J Clin Oncol 1989; 12:355–357.

112. Falkson G, Van Dyk JJ, Van Eden EB, Van der Merwe AM, Van den Bergh JA, Falkson HC. A clinical trial of the oral form of 4′-demethyl-epipodophyllotoxin-beta-D ethylidene glucoside (NSC 141540) VP 16-213. Cancer 1975; 35:1141–1144.

113. Anderson G, Peel ET, Cheong CM, Broderick NJ. Etoposide—an effective single drug for treating bronchogenic carcinoma. Clin Oncol 1982; 8:215–218.

114. Issell BF, Einhorn LH, Comis RL, et al. Multicenter phase II trial of etoposide in refractory small cell lung cancer. Cancer Treat Rep 1985; 69:127–128.

115. Pedersen AG, Bork E, Osterlind K, Dombernowsky P, Hansen HH. Phase II study of teniposide in small cell carcinoma of the lung. Cancer Treat Rep 1984; 68:1289–1291.

116. Woods RL, Fox RM, Tattersall MH. Treatment of small cell bronchogenic carcinoma with VM-26. Cancer Treat Rep 1979; 63:2011–2013.

117. Knight EW, Lagakos S, Stolbach L, et al. Adriamycin in the treatment of far-advanced lung cancer. Cancer Treat Rep 1976; 60:939–941.

118. Kenis Y, Michel J, Rimoldi R, Levy P, Israel L. Results of a clinical trial with intermittent doses of adriamycin in lung cancer. Eur J Cancer 1972; 8:485–489.

119. Blackstein M, Eisenhauer EA, Wierzbicki R, Yoshida S. Epirubicin in extensive small-cell lung cancer: a phase II study in previously untreated patients. A National Cancer Institute of Canada Clinical Trials Group Study [see comments]. J Clin Oncol 1990; 8:385–389.

120. Eckhardt S, Kolaric K, Vukas D, et al. Phase II study of 4′-epi-doxorubicin in patients with untreated, extensive small cell lung cancer. South-East European Oncology Group (SEEOG). Med Oncol Tumor Pharmacother 1990; 7:19–23.

121. Cullen MH, Smith SR, Benfield GF, Woodroffe CM. Testing new drugs in untreated small cell lung cancer may prejudice the results of standard treatment: a phase II study of oral idarubicin in extensive disease. Cancer Treat Rep 1987; 71:1227–1230.

122. Von Hoff DD, Chen T, Clark GM, Callahan SK, Livingston R. Mitoxantrone for treatment of patients with refractory small cell carcinoma of the lung: a Southwest Oncology Group Study. Cancer Treat Rep 1983; 67:403–404.

123. Dombernowsky P, Hansen HH, Sorensen PG, Hainau B. Vincristine (NSC-67574) in the treatment of small-cell anaplastic carcinoma of the lung. Cancer Treat Rep 1976; 60:239–242.

124. Osterlind K, Dombernowsky P, Sorensen PG, Hansen HH. Vindesine in the treatment of small cell anaplastic bronchogenic carcinoma. Cancer Treat Rep 1981; 65:245–248.

125. Natale RB, Gralla RJ, Wittes RE. Phase II trial of vindesine in patients with small cell lung carcinoma. Cancer Treat Rep 1981; 65:129–131.

126. Higano CS, Crowley JJ, Veith RV, Livingston RB. A phase II trial of intravenous vinorelbine in previously untreated patients with extensive small cell lung cancer. A Southwest Oncology Group study. Invest New Drugs 1997; 15:153–156.

127. Lake D, Johnson E, Herndon J, Green M. Phase II trial of navelbine in relapsed small

cell lung cancer. Thirty-third Annual Meeting, American Society of Clinical Oncology, Denver, Colo., May 17–20, 1997.

128. Depierre A, Le Chevalier T, Quoix E, et al. Phase II trial of navelbine (NVB), in small cell lung cancer (SCLC). 8th World Conference on Lung Cancer, Dublin, Ireland, Aug. 10–15, 1997.

129. Havsteen H, Sorenson S, Rorth M, Dombernowsky P, Hansen HH. 5-FU in the treatment of small cell anaplastic carcinoma of the lung: a phase II trial. Cancer Treat Rep 1981; 65:123–125.

130. Simon MS, Eckenrode J, Natale RB. Phase II trial of methylglyoxal bis-guanylhydrazone (MGBG) in refractory small cell lung cancer. Invest New Drugs 1990; 8:S79–81.

131. Osborne RJ, Clark PI, Slevin ML, Wrigley PF. High-dose cytarabine in small cell lung cancer. Cancer Treat Rep 1987; 71:417–418.

132. Cormier Y, Eisenhauer E, Muldal A, et al. Gemcitabine is an active new agent in previously untreated extensive small cell lung cancer (SCLC). A study of the National Cancer Institute of Canada Clinical Trials Group. Ann Oncol 1994; 5:283–285.

133. Latreille J, Cormier Y, Martins H, Goss G, Fisher B, Eisenhauer EA. Phase II study of docetaxel (taxotere) in patients with previously untreated extensive small cell lung cancer. Invest New Drugs 1996; 13:343–345.

134. Ettinger DS, Finkelstein DM, Sarma RP, Johnson DH. Phase II study of paclitaxel in patients with extensive-disease small-cell lung cancer: an Eastern Cooperative Oncology Group study. J Clin Oncol 1995; 13:1430–1435.

135. Bunn PA Jr. Defining the role of paclitaxel in lung cancer: summary of recent studies and implications for future directions. Semin Oncol 1997; 24:S12(153)–S12(162).

136. Schiller JH, Kim K, Hutson P, et al. Phase II study of topotecan in patients with extensive-stage small-cell carcinoma of the lung: an Eastern Cooperative Oncology Group Trial. J Clin Oncol 1996; 14:2345–2352.

137. Eckardt J, Depierre A, Ardizzoni A, Von Pawel J, Fields S. Pooled analysis of topotecan (T) in the second-line treatment of patients (pts) with sensitive small cell lung cancer (SCLC). Thirty-third Annual Meeting, American Society of Clinical Oncology, Denver, Colo., May 17–20, 1997.

138. Watanabe K, Fukuoka M, Niitani H. Phase II trial of topotecan for small cell lung cancer (SCLC). 8th World Conference on Lung Cancer, Dublin, Ireland, Aug. 10–15, 1997.

139. Depierre A, Von Pawel J, Hans K, et al. Evaluation of topotecan (Hycamtin) in relapsed small cell lung cancer (SCLC). A multicentre phase II study. 8th World Conference on Lung Cancer, Dublin, Ireland, Aug. 10–15, 1997.

140. Fukuoka M, Masuda N. Clinical studies of irinotecan alone and in combination with cisplatin. Cancer Chemother Pharmacol 1994; 34:S105–111.

18

High-Dose Therapy for Small-Cell Lung Cancer with Stem Cell Support

ANTHONY D. ELIAS

Dana-Farber Cancer Institute
Harvard Medical School
Boston, Massachusetts

I. Introduction

Lung cancer is the leading cause of death from cancer in both men and women in the United States (1) and, due to growing tobacco consumption, continues to increase in incidence throughout the world. The small cell lung cancer (SCLC) histology constitutes approximately 15% to 25% of all bronchogenic carcinomas. Combination chemotherapy achieves excellent immediate palliation when using the many chemotherapeutic agents which have major activity against SCLC. Combination regimens constructed from the established agents (such as etoposide [and teniposide], cisplatin [and carboplatin], ifosfamide, cyclophosphamide, vincristine, and doxorubicin) produce almost identical short-term and long-term results. Consensus regarding conventional dose treatment consists of four to six cycles of etoposide and platinum with concurrent chest radiation therapy for the third of patients with limited-stage (LD) disease (2) and combination chemotherapy alone for extensive-stage (ED) disease. Unfortunately by 2 years only 20% to 40% of LD and fewer than 5% of ED patients remain alive (3,4). Five-year survival is about half that at 2 years. New agents which appear to have at least equivalent activity compared with these established drugs include paclitaxel, gemcitabine, and the topoisomerase I inhibitors (topotecan, irinotecan). The roles of the new active agents and resistance modulators in first-line therapy are being evaluated in ongoing trials. The underlying smoking-related cardiovascular and pulmonary comorbidity, median age of 60 to 65 years, and enhanced risk of secondary smoking-related malignancies contribute to an increased risk when applying dose-intensive therapy in lung cancer patients.

II. Dose Intensity
A. Without Cellular Support

Preclinical in vitro and in vivo experiments consistently show near log-linear dose-response relationships, particularly for the alkylating class of agents and radiation (5–8). One of the first to demonstrate higher response rates, both complete and partial, and a modestly longer median survival time, was Cohen et al. in 1977 when administering higher rather than lower doses of cyclophosphamide, lomustine, and methotrexate (9).

The contribution of dose or dose intensity of chemotherapy to response and survival remains controversial. Using the methodology of Hryniuk and Bush (10), which assumes that all drugs are therapeutically equivalent and that there are no significant drug-drug interactions, Klasa et al. analyzed numerous SCLC trials to determine whether dose intensity (expressed in drug dose administered per m^2 per week) of individual agents or regimens correlated with response or survival. Longer median survival was observed in ED patients receiving higher dose intensities of cyclophosphamide and doxorubicin with vincristine (CAV) and with etoposide (CAE), but not when receiving the regimen etoposide and cisplatin (EP). The relative differences in response and survival and the dose ranges analyzed were small (11).

Seven randomized trials have examined dose intensity in SCLC, almost exclusively in the extensive stage setting (9,12–17). While the planned dose intensity differences between the high-dose and lower-dose arms ranged between 1.2-fold and twofold, the actual delivered doses were less different between the arms. Three of these trials showed a modest survival advantage for the higher-dose therapy. Two of these three trials compared less than standard dose therapy with full-dose therapy. The trials without evident benefit generally compared full-dose to a small increment in dose intensity. Survival advantages have also not been described in trials using the currently established cytokines (e.g., GM-CSF and G-CSF), which do shorten chemotherapy-induced myelosuppression and consequent febrile neutropenia and thereby maintain dose intensity across multiple cycles (18). Due to cumulative thrombocytopenia, dose intensities are increased by only 1.5 to 2-fold with cytokine use. The effectiveness of various thrombopoietins or other cytokines to increase achievable dose intensity remains to be seen.

Arriagada et al. randomized patients to six cycles of conventional-dose chemotherapy wherein only the first cycle was modestly intensified for the high-dose arm (17). It was surprising to observe a complete response and survival advantage for the patients receiving the intensified chemotherapy, since the relative difference in the two groups was so small. While this result could reflect chance, it is possible that dose intensity, particularly if given early in the course of treatment, may be more likely to impact on outcomes in the limited-stage than the extensive-stage setting. Early intensification and treatment of earlier stage disease are two themes to consider when designing new trials.

Multidrug cyclic weekly therapy was designed to increase the number of drugs to which the cancer was exposed with less compromise of dose given the differing toxicities of the weekly agents. Although patient selection effects were evident, early Phase II results were quite promising (19,20). This optimism was unfortunately not borne out by the following randomized trials (21,22). In the randomized trials (23,24), the weekly schedules required greater dose reductions and delays than every-3-week conventional therapy, so the actual delivered dose intensities were not that different. Not only did dose and schedule differ, but so did the regimens, leading to interpretation obstacles. Follow-up is still too limited to observe late disease-free survival plateau differences.

B. With Cellular Support

Patients with small-cell lung cancer undergoing autologous bone marrow transplantation (ABMT) were analyzed if sufficient details were provided in the published reports as to their response status (relapsed or refractory; untreated; or responding to first-line chemotherapy [partial or complete response] and their extent of disease [limited or extensive]. Patients in these various categories were pooled for aggregated relapse-free and overall survival characteristics (Table 1).

Fourteen small studies (with a median of three patients, maximum eight) described outcomes in 52 patients who had either relapsed or refractory disease (25–38). Complete and partial responses were observed in 19% and 37%, respectively. The median response durations and survivals were approximately 2 to 3 months. Combination chemotherapy regimens, especially those containing multiple alkylating agents, were slightly more effective (response rate 58%, CR 26%), but more toxic (18% vs. 6% deaths). The observed high complete-response rate supported a dose-response relationship, but was insufficient to affect an abysmal survival rate.

In 103 patients with SCLC (71% limited disease) receiving high-dose therapy as initial treatment, overall and complete response rates of 84% and 42% were achieved (39–46). Relapse-free 2-year and overall survivals were comparable to treatment with conventional multicycle regimens. Seven percent achieved durable remissions. Transplantation in the newly diagnosed SCLC setting is problematic because of the frequency of life-threatening complications from uncontrolled dis-

Table 1 High-Dose Intensification for Small-Cell Lung Cancer

	Patients			
	No.	% CR	% disease free	% toxic death
Relapsed/refractory	52	19	0	13
Initial treatment	103	43	7	6
First PR/SD	189	42	8	11
First CR	110		33	3
ED	25		16	8
LD	85		38	1

Median follow-up 3 years with wide variability between studies.
PR, partial response; SD, stable disease; CR, complete response; ED, extensive
  disease; LD, limited disease.

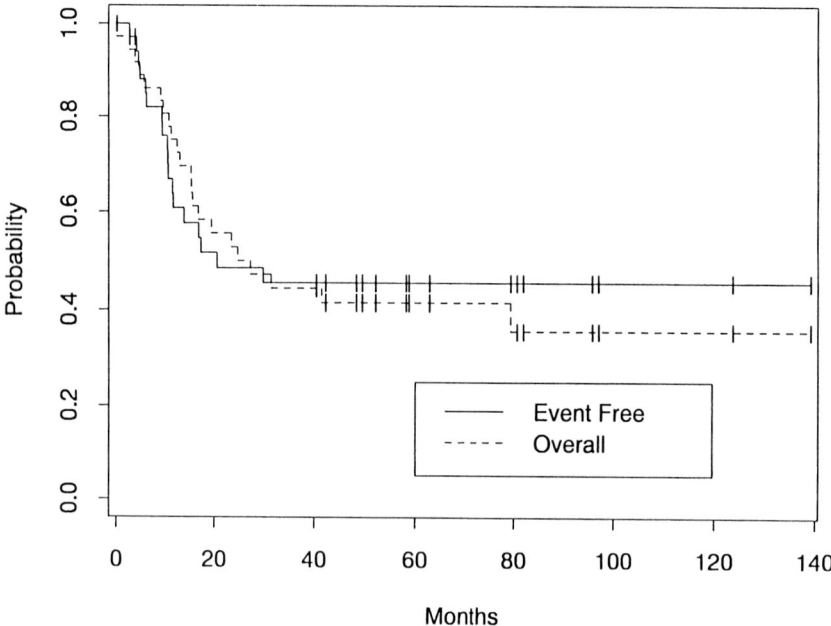

Figure 1 Event-free and overall survival. (From Ref. 62a.)

ease and the potential for tumor cell contamination in untreated autografts. On the other hand, early intensification may have greater impact on the disease.

Approximately 334 patients in response to first-line chemotherapy received high-dose chemotherapy with autologous marrow support as consolidation (47). Of patients achieving just a partial response to induction therapy, the conversion to complete response occurred in 40% to 50%, but without durable effect. The best results (35% event-free with a median follow-up >3 years at the time of publication) were reported in patients with limited disease in complete response at the time of high-dose therapy.

Much of the high-dose SCLC experience reviewed took place during the initial developmental phase of high-dose therapy for solid tumors. Suboptimal dosing compared to modern standards was frequent. Moreover, many of these high-dose trials employed either single chemotherapeutic agents (with or without low-dose agents in addition) (six series; two with chest radiotherapy) (41,42,48–53) or single alkylating agents (six series; four with chest radiotherapy) (42,44,47,54–57). Combination alkylating agents were employed in a fraction of these patients (10 series; six with chest radiotherapy) (29,32,43,58–64). Higher treatment-related morbidity and mortality were reported than is currently expected (Table 2).

Humblet et al. gave 101 patients with SCLC five cycles of conventional therapy with prophylactic cranial irradiation followed by one further cycle of either high- or conventional-dose therapy using cyclophosphamide, etoposide, and carmustine (60). No chest radiotherapy was given. Only 45 were eligible for randomization due to disease progression and morbidity of treatment. Clear dose response was demonstrated. Conversion from partial to complete response occurred in none

Table 2 Consolidation of Responding SCLC with High-Dose Chemotherapy with ABMT

	Number of trials	Subset with chest RT	Number of patients	% disease free	% mortality
Single agents	5	2	93	10	4
Single alkylator and etoposide	7	4	102	9	3
Combination alkylators	10	6	92	32	16
Without chest RT	4	—	41	17	24
With chest RT	6	6	76	39	7

RT, radiotherapy.

after conventional dose treatment compared with 77% of evaluable patients after high dose therapy. Disease-free survival was significantly enhanced, and a trend toward improved survival was observed with high-dose therapy. However, an 18% toxic death rate on the ABMT arm led the investigators to conclude that dose-intensive therapy should not be considered a standard therapy in SCLC. Moreover, since chest radiotherapy was not given in this trial, almost all patients recurred in the chest.

High rates of relapse in sites of prior tumor involvement may be explained by greater tumor burden in the chest, the possible presence of drug-resistant clones or non-small-cell lung cancer (NSCLC) elements, by poorer drug delivery, or intratumoral resistance factors such as hypoxia, or in the case of autograft contamination, the possibility of homing with microenvironmental support for the tumor in local-regional sites (41,56). After conventional dose therapy, chest relapse is reduced from 90% of individuals following chemotherapy alone to 60% of those receiving chemoradiotherapy. Thus, radiotherapy to sites of bulk disease is likely to represent an essential component in high-dose curative treatment approaches.

C. Newer Reports Using Cellular Support

A number of experiences have been reported since high-dose therapy for SCLC was last reviewed (46). Of 10 extensive-stage patients with partial responses to ifosfamide, cisplatin, and etoposide (IPE) chemotherapy, six were transplanted with high-dose methotrexate and etoposide following high-dose cyclophosphamide for mobilization. Near-complete response was obtained in all; however, all relapsed a median of 4 months later. Of note, half had tumor contamination of their peripheral blood progenitor cells (PBPC) documented (53).

In the Polish experience reported on several occasions, six LD and 20 ED patients were treated with two cycles of high-dose cyclophosphamide and etoposide as induction followed by the same drugs in six or with BCNU in 20 (63). Seven of 18 converted from partial to complete response. Seven patients were already in complete response. Five patients remain progression free 3 to 89 months later. Of the overall complete responses, 29% remained disease free >2 years (63).

Of 18 LD patients who received two cycles of vincristine, ifosfamide, cisplatin, and etoposide (VIPE) with mobilization of PBPCs, 13 (72%) received high-dose ifosfamide, carboplatin, and etoposide (ICE) with epirubicin; three non-responders and two with poor performance status were not considered candidates. With a median of 14 months follow-up, event-free survival was 69%. Nine remained progression-free. Brugger et al. updated this experience to the first 16 patients transplanted (64a). Some early-stage SCLC patients were included [stages I [1], II [3], IIIA [6], IIIB [6]), and surgical resection was performed in seven patients. None of the PBPCs collected after the second cycle of VIPE contained microscopic tumor cells as measured by immunocytochemistry using keratin and EMA-125 antibodies. At a median follow-up of 44 months, the event-free and overall survival was 56%.

At the Dana-Farber Cancer Institute and Beth Israel Hospital, over 50 patients with LD and over 25 with ED SCLC have been treated with high-dose combination alkylating agents following response to conventional-dose induction therapy. Of the original cohort of 36 limited-stage SCLC (all had stages IIIA or B disease), 29 were in or near complete response prior to treatment with high-dose cyclophosphamide, carmustine, and cisplatin (CBP) with marrow (plus peripheral blood stem cells in some) support followed by chest and prophylactic cranial radiotherapy (PCI) (62,62a). With minimum followup of 36 months after completion of high-dose chemotherapy (range 36 months to 10 years), the 5-year event-free survival is 52% (Fig. 1). Of the extensive-stage patients, 15% to 20% remain progression-free >2 years after high-dose therapy. Local regional relapse represents about 50% of all relapses.

III. Future Directions

A. Intensify Involved Field Radiotherapy

As summarized by meta-analyses of randomized trials, thoracic radiotherapy provides a 25% to 30% improvement in local-regional control and a 5% increase in long-term progression-free survival for limited stage SCLC (65,66). With the commonly used 45 to 50 Gy thoracic radiotherapy, local-regional relapse remains unacceptably high (about a 60% actuarial risk of local relapse by 3 years) (67–69) and may be underestimated due to the competing risk of systemic relapse (70). Since chest-first relapse is observed in about 40% of patients, further enhancement of local-regional control may increase the proportion of long-term survivors.

The dose intensity of chest radiotherapy has not been well studied. The Eastern Cooperative Oncology Group (ECOG) and the Radiation Therapy Oncology Group (RTOG) recently reported a comparison of 45 Gy chest radiotherapy given either daily over 5 weeks or twice daily over 3 weeks concurrent with cisplatin and etoposide chemotherapy (71). Intensified chest radiotherapy reduced chest failure from 61% to 48% actuarial at 2 to 3 years (P < .05). Further follow-up indicates a survival advantage for the more intensive radiotherapy associated with a 42% overall local failure rate compared to a 75% local failure for daily radiotherapy. Choi et al. at Massachusetts General Hospital escalated the dose of radiotherapy in cohorts of five or six patients with limited stage SCLC (72). Thoracic radiotherapy was given concurrently with cisplatin and etoposide either as daily 180 cGy fractions or as twice-daily 150 cGy fractions. Using a shrinking field technique, the maximal tolerated doses with respect to acute esophagitis appear to be 45 Gy for twice-daily administration and 70 Gy when given once daily. Thus intensification of radiotherapy dose is feasible and should be evaluated in a randomized setting.

The Cancer and Leukemia Group B and Southwest Oncology Group activated a Phase II feasibility trial stemming from the DFCI/BIH experience. Patients under age 60 with limited stage were treated with four cycles of cisplatin and etoposide with concurrent twice-daily chest radiotherapy to 45 Gy (150 cGy fractions). Patients achieving complete or near-complete response received high-dose cyclophosphamide, cisplatin, and carmustine (CBP) with autologous stem cell support. Upon recovery, prophylactic cranial irradiation was given. It is hoped that this will lead to a Phase III trial testing the concept of dose during intensification in patients with excellent initial response.

B. Intensify Induction

Induction therapy reduces tumor burden and stabilizes patients with rapidly progressive systemic and local symptoms from SCLC. It also allows selection of patients possessing chemosensitive tumors for subsequent intensification, and can reduce the level of micrometastases in the marrow and/or circulating buffy coat as discussed below. On the other hand, during this treatment time, chemoresistant tumor cells might proliferate or even be induced. As suggested by the Arriagada trial (17), initial intensification of induction may improve overall disease-free survival and overall survival. A logical extension of this concept would be to administer multicycle dose-intensive combination therapies supported by cytokines and peripheral blood progenitor cells using either repeated cycles of the same regimen (74–77) or a sequence of different agents (78–81). A growing experience with sequential cycles of stem cell–supported therapy is being reported for the treatment of good-performance status SCLC patients. Doses delivered in individual cycles range from the conventional but given more frequently to moderately intensified (about two-thirds the doses of conventional transplant doses). Thatcher and colleagues explored different methods to collect hematopoietic stem cells to achieve greater dose intensity with the ICE regimen. Conventional-dose ICE was supported by autologous hematopoietic cells given on day 3 of chemotherapy for six cycles (76). Cycle length was 3 weeks using cryopreserved pheresis products, or 2 weeks using either pheresis products or 750 cc whole blood stored at 4°C. Cycles were repeated when platelets had recovered above 30,000/µL. In this Phase I trial of 25 patients, the full planned dose intensity for each of the arms was achieved over the first three cycles, although only 56% completed all six. Mortality was 12%, complete response rate was 64%, and the median follow-up was 10 months, so the longer-term outcomes are unknown. The authors note that the collection of whole blood without cryopreservation reduced the cost and complexity of treatment substantially (76). In a subsequent randomized Phase II study, Woll et al. treated 50 "good-prognosis" patients with ICE given either every 2 or 4 weeks (75). The median dose intensity delivered over the first three cycles was 0.99 (0.33 to 1.02) vs. 1.8 (0.99 to 1.97) on the 4-week and 2-week cycles, respectively. More hematopoietic and infectious toxicity was encountered on the standard-dose 4-week arm.

Perey et al. reported a European Bone Marrow Transplant (EBMT) experience with 47 patients of whom 35 were evaluable at time of report (77). Mobilization was achieved with epirubicin and G-CSF followed by three cycles of moderately intensive ICE. Radiation to chest and head was urged but not required. Overall, complete or near-complete response was observed in 69%. Mortality was 14%.

Humblet et al. treated 37 limited-stage patients with four intensive alternating cycles of ifosfamide with etoposide, and carboplatin with etoposide (81). Concurrently with each chemotherapy administration, 10 Gy thoracic radiotherapy in five fractions was given. The median follow-up was 16 months, median event-free survival was 18 months, and 80% remained alive at 30 months. Mortality was 3%. Perhaps due to the fact that no PCI was given, eight of 13 relapses occurred in the brain.

C. Minimal Residual Tumor/Autograft Involvement

Tumor contamination of stem cells may cause relapse, particularly since stem cells must be protected from the high-dose therapy. As demonstrated by gene marking studies, residual tumor cells do contribute to relapse in certain hematologic malignancies and neuroblastoma (82–84). It is less clear whether these cells are the sole cause for relapse or rather serve as a marker to indicate the patient has increased systemic chemotherapy-resistant tumor burden. Gene marking experiments in solid tumors have not yet demonstrated gene-marked tumor cells in relapse sites (85).

In SCLC, the marrow is one of the most common metastatic sites. Of patients with untreated SCLC with histologically negative marrows at diagnosis, small trials have demonstrated that subclinical micrometastatic disease is detected in marrow in 13% to 54% of newly diagnosed LD and 44% to 77% of newly diagnosed ED SCLC by immunohistochemical techniques which have a sensitivity of detection of 1 in 10^4 cells (86–90). Two tiny series suggest two-thirds of patients in excellent chemotherapy response had residual contamination (91,92). In Leonard's series, (92) residual tumor appeared to predict relapse. In patients with metastatic SCLC or breast cancer, peripheral blood cells mobilized with G-CSF during the first cycle of IPE chemotherapy had demonstrable circulating tumor cells, although their viability was not established (93). Mobilization of tumor cells after the second cycle of chemotherapy was not observed, supporting the contention that in vivo chemotherapy induction can "purge" the patient and the autologous stem cell source (64a). In our unpublished data, up to 85% of LD patients in complete or near-complete response prior to high-dose therapy have detectable tumor cells in their marrow by keratin staining.

Numerous chemotherapeutic agents have major clinical activity against overt SCLC, though the uniform and dismal clinical outcomes suggest that differing systemic drugs fail to eradicate a central core of tumor stem cells, presumably enriched for in vivo resistance mechanisms. Characterization of these residual cancer cells may guide strategies to target these cells specifically. Thus, the detection of heterogeneity and analysis of patterns of coexpression of various markers in these cells are a critical focus. We are utilizing a confocal fluorescence microscope with automated computerized scanning with one set of fluorescent probes for detection and a second set with different fluorophores for biologic characterization (94). Prospective trials are being started to evaluate the clinical significance of marrow or peripheral blood tumor contamination and the impact of novel stem cell sources to support high-dose therapy.

IV. Conclusion

The two major strategies to administer high-dose therapy for SCLC are the initial multicycle approach and the "later" intensification. Advantages for each approach are evident. The multicycle approach can achieve early dose intensity and maintain it for about three or four cycles. Its disadvantages include lower than transplant doses, high mortality rates, general inability to deliver chest radiotherapy early (except for the Humblet trial, which provides relatively low dose radiotherapy), and the collection of stem cells early in treatment, when they are highly likely to be contaminated with tumor cells. The later intensification can take advantage of initial therapy to control the tumor-related symptoms with consequent improved performance status for the patients, the partial purge of stem cell sources, and early dose-intensive thoracic radiotherapy during an intense induction therapy. The drawback of later administration of the dose-intense cycle can be surmounted in part by intensification and shortening of induction chemoradiotherapy.

High-dose therapy kills more tumor cells and results in prolonged progression-free survival in clinical situations in which toxicity has been acceptable. An additional group of patients may achieve minimal residual tumor burden (near-cure). If additional targets of residual tumor cells can be identified for novel treatment strategies and modalities, high-dose therapy may have increased value. Most biologic strategies such as gene function replacement (retinoblastoma gene and/or p53), interference with autocrine or paracrine growth loops, or immunologic therapy (IL-2, IL-12, immunotoxins, tumor vaccines) work best against minimal tumor burden.

Acknowledgments

Supported in part by a grant from the Public Health Service, grant CA13849 from the National Cancer Institute, National Institutes of Health, Department of Health and Human Services.

References

1. Boring CC, Squires TS, Tong TT. Cancer statistics, 1993. CA Cancer J Clin 1994; 44:19–51.
2. Johnson DH, Kim K, Sause W, et al. Cisplatin and etoposide plus thoracic radiotherapy administered once or twice daily in limited stage small cell lung cancer: final report of intergroup trial 0096. Proc ASCO 1996; 15:374 (1113).
3. Seifter EJ, Ihde DC. Therapy of small cell lung cancer: a perspective on two decades of clinical research. Semin Oncol 1988; 15(3):278–299.
4. Osterlind K, Hansen HH, Hansen M, Dombernowsky P, Andersen PK. Long-term disease-free survival in small-cell carcinoma of the lung: a study of clinical determinants. J Clin Oncol 1986; 4(9):1307–1313.
5. Teicher BA. Preclinical models for high-dose therapy. In: Armitage JO, Antman KH, eds. High-dose cancer therapy: pharmacology, hematopoietins, stem cells. Baltimore: Williams and Wilkins, 1992:14–42.
6. Frei E III. Combination cancer chemotherapy: presidential address. Cancer Res 1972; 32:2593–2607.
7. Frei E III, Canellos GP. Dose, a critical factor in cancer chemotherapy. Am J Med 1980; 69:585–594.
8. Frei E III, Antman KH. Combination chemotherapy, dose, and schedule. Section XV: principles of chemotherapy. In: Holland JF, Frei E III, Bast RC Jr, Kufe DW, Morton DL, Weichselbaum RR, eds. Cancer Medicine. Philadelphia: Lea and Febiger, 1993;631–639.
9. Cohen MH, Creaven PJ, Fossieck BE, et al. Intensive chemotherapy of small cell bronchogenic carcinoma. Cancer Treat Rep 1977; 61:349–354.
10. Hryniuk W, Bush H. The importance of dose intensity in chemotherapy of metastatic breast cancer. J Clin Oncol 1984; 2:1281–1288.
11. Klasa RJ, Murray N, Coldman AJ. Dose-intensity meta-analysis of chemotherapy regimens in small-cell carcinoma of the lung. J Clin Oncol 1991; 9:499–508.
12. Brower M, Ihde DC, Johnston-Early A, et al. Treatment of extensive stage small cell bronchogenic carcinoma: effects of variation in intensity of induction chemotherapy. Am J Med 1983; 75:993–1000.
13. Johnson DH, Einhorn LH, Birch R, et al. A randomized comparison of high dose versus conventional dose cyclophosphamide, doxorubicin, and vincristine for extensive stage small cell lung cancer: a phase III trial of the Southeastern Cancer Study Group. J Clin Oncol 1987; 5:1731–1738.
14. Mehta C, Vogl SE. High-dose cyclophosphamide in the induction therapy of small cell lung cancer: minor improvements in rate of remission and survival. Proc AACR 1982; 23:155.
15. Figueredo AT, Hryniuk WM, Strautmanis I, et al. Co-trimoxazole prophylaxis during high-dose chemotherapy of small-cell lung cancer. J Clin Oncol 1985; 3:54–64.
16. Ihde DC, Mulshine JL, Kramer BS, et al. Prospective randomized comparison of high-dose and standard-dose etoposide and cisplatin chemotherapy in patients with extensive-stage small-cell lung cancer. J Clin Oncol 1994; 12:2022–2034.
17. Arriagada R, Le Chevalier T, Pignon J-P, et al. Initial chemotherapeutic doses and survival in patients with limited small-cell lung cancer. N Engl J Med 1993; 329:1848–1852.

18. Crawford J, Ozer H, Stoller R, et al. Reduction by granulocyte colony-stimulating factor of fever and neutropenia induced by chemotherapy in patients with small-cell lung cancer. N Engl J Med 1991; 325:164–170.

19. Miles DW, Earl HM, Souhami RL, et al. Intensive weekly chemotherapy for good-prognosis patients with small-cell lung cancer. J Clin Oncol 1991; 9:280–285.

20. Murray N, Gelmon K, Shah A, et al. Potential for long-term survival in extensive stage small-cell lung cancer (ESCLC) with CODE chemotherapy and radiotherapy. Lung Cancer 1994; 11(suppl 1):99 (377).

21. Furuse K, Kubota K, Nishiwaki Y, et al. Phase III study of dose intensive weekly chemotherapy with recombinant human granulocyte-colony stimulating factor (G-CSF) versus standard chemotherapy in extensive stage small cell lung cancer (SCLC). Proc ASCO 1996; 15:375 (1117).

22. Murray N, Livingston R, Shepherd F, et al. A randomized study of CODE plus thoracic irradiation versus alternating CAV/EP for extensive stage small cell lung cancer (ESCLC). Proc ASCO 1997; 16:456a (1638).

23. Sculier JP, Paesmans M, Bureau G, et al. Multiple drug weekly chemotherapy versus standard combination regimen in small cell lung cancer: a phase III randomized study conducted by the European Lung Cancer Working Party. J Clin Oncol 1993; 11:1858–1865.

24. Souhami RL, Rudd R, Ruiz de Elvira MC, et al. Randomized trial comparing weekly versus 3-week chemotherapy in small cell lung cancer: a Cancer Research Campaign trial. J Clin Oncol 1994; 12:1806–1813.

25. Douer D, Champlin RE, Ho WG, et al. High-dose combined-modality therapy and autologous bone marrow transplantation in resistant cancer. Am J Med 1981; 71:973–976.

26. Harada M, et al. Combined-modality therapy and autologous bone marrow transplantation in the treatment of advanced non-Hodgkin's lymphoma and solid tumors: the Kanawaza experience. Transplant Proc 1982; 4:733–737.

27. Lazarus HM, Spitzer TR, Creger RT. Phase I trial of high-dose etoposide, high-dose cisplatin, and reinfusion of autologous bone marrow for lung cancer. Am J Clin Oncol 1990; 13:107–112.

28. Phillips GL, Fay JW, Herzig GP, et al. Nitrosourea (BCNU), NSC #4366650 and cryopreserved autologous marrow transplantation for refractory cancer: A phase I-II study. Cancer 1983; 52:1792–1802.

29. Stahel RA, Takvorian RW, Skarin AT, Canellos GP. Autologous bone marrow transplantation following high-dose chemotherapy with cyclophosphamide, BCNU, and VP-16 in small cell carcinoma of the lung and a review of current literature. Eur J Cancer Clin Oncol 1984; 20:1233–1238.

30. Wolff SW, Fer MF, McKay CM, et al. High-dose VP-16-213 and autologous bone marrow transplantation for refractory malignancies: a phase I study. J Clin Oncol 1983; 1:701–705.

31. Pico JL, Beaujean F, Debre M, et al. High dose chemotherapy (HDC) with autologous bone marrow transplantation (ABMT) in small cell carcinoma of the lung (SCCL) in relapse. Proc ASCO 1983; 2:206.

32. Pico JL, Baume D, Ostronoff M, et al. Chimiotherapie a hautes doses suivie d'auto-

greffe de moelle osseuse dans le traitement du cancer bronchique a petites cellules. Bull Cancer 1987; 74:587–595.

33. Postmus PE, Mulder NH, Elema JD. Graft versus host disease after transfusions of non-irradiated blood cells in patients having received autologous bone marrow. Eur J Cancer 1988; 24:889–894.

34. Rushing DA, Baldauf MC, Gehlsen JA, et al. High-dose BCNU and autologous bone marrow reinfusion in the treatment of refractory or relapsed small cell carcinoma of the lung (SCCL). Proc ASCO 1984; 3:217.

35. Spitzer G, Dicke KA, Verma DS, Zander A, McCredie KB. High-dose BCNU therapy with autologous bone marrow infusion: preliminary observations. Cancer Treat Rep 1979; 63:1257–1264.

36. Spitzer G, Dicke KA, Latam J, et al. High-dose combination chemotherapy with autologous bone marrow transplantation in adult solid tumors. Cancer 1980; 45:3075–3085.

37. Eder JP, Antman K, Shea TC, et al. Cyclophosphamide and thiotepa with autologous bone marrow transplantation in patients with solid tumors. J Natl Cancer Inst 1988; 80:1221–1226.

38. Elias AD, Ayash LJ, Wheeler C, et al. A phase I study of high-dose ifosfamide, carboplatin, and etoposide with autologous hematopoietic stem cell support. Bone Marrow Transplant 1995; 15:373–379.

39. Littlewood TJ, Spragg BP, Bentley DP. When is autologous bone marrow transplantation safe after high-dose treatment with etoposide. Clin Lab Haematol 1985; 7:213–218.

40. Littlewood TJ, Bentley DP, Smith AP. High-dose etoposide with autologous bone marrow transplantation as initial treatment of small cell lung cancer—a negative report. Eur J Respir Dis 1986; 68:370–374.

41. Souhami RL, Hajichristou HT, Miles DW, et al. Intensive chemotherapy with autologous bone marrow transplantation for small cell lung cancer. Cancer Chemother Pharmacol 1989; 24:321–325.

42. Lange A, Kolodziej J, Tomeczko J, et al. Aggressive chemotherapy with autologous bone marrow transplantation in small cell lung carcinoma. Arch Immunol Ther Exp 1991; 39:431–439.

43. Nomura F, Shimokata K, Saito H, et al. High dose chemotherapy with autologous bone marrow transplantation for limited small cell lung cancer. Jpn J Clin Oncol 1990; 20:94–98.

44. Spitzer G, Farha P, Valdivieso M, et al. High-dose intensification therapy with autologous bone marrow support for limited small-cell bronchogenic carcinoma. J Clin Oncol 1986; 4:4–13.

45. Johnson DH, Hande KR, Hainsworth JD, Greco FA. High-dose etoposide as single-agent chemotherapy for small cell carcinoma of the lung. Cancer Treat Rep 1983; 67:957–958.

46. Elias A, Cohen BF. Dose intensive therapy in lung cancer. In: Armitage JO, Antman KH, eds. High-Dose Cancer Therapy: Pharmacology, Hematopoietins, Stem Cells. 2nd ed. Baltimore: Williams and Wilkins, 1995;824–846.

47. Farha P, Spitzer G, Valdivieso M, et al. High-dose chemotherapy and autologous bone

marrow transplantation for the treatment of small cell lung carcinoma. Cancer 1983; 52:1351–1355.

48. Marangolo M, Rosti G, Ravaioli A, et al. Small cell carcinoma of the lung (SCCL): high-dose (HD) VP-16 and autologous bone marrow transplantation (ABMT) as intensification therapy: preliminary results. Int J Cell Cloning 1985; 3:277.

49. Smith IE, Evans BD, Harland SJ, et al. High-dose cyclophosphamide with autologous bone marrow rescue after conventional chemotherapy in the treatment of small cell lung carcinoma. Cancer Chemother Pharmacol 1985; 14:120–124.

50. Banham S, Burnett A, Stevenson R, et al. Pilot study of combination chemotherapy with late dose intensification and autologous bone marrow rescue in small cell bronchogenic carcinoma. Br J Cancer 1982; 42:486.

51. Banham S, Loukop M, Burnett A, et al. Treatment of small cell carcinoma of the lung with late dosage intensification programmes containing cyclophosphamide and mesna. Cancer Treat Rev 1983; 10(suppl A):73–77.

52. Burnett AK, Tansey P, Hills C, et al. Haematologic reconstitution following high dose and supralethal chemoradiotherapy using stored non-cryopreserved autologous bone marrow. Br J Haematol 1983; 54:309–316.

53. Jennis A, Levitan N, Pecora AL, Isaacs R, Lazarus H. Sequential high dose chemotherapy (HDC) with filgrastim/peripheral stem cell support (PSCS) in extensive stage small cell lung cancer (SCLC). Proc ASCO 1996; 15:349 (1021).

54. Ihde DC, Diesseroth AB, Lichter AS, et al. Late intensive combined modality therapy followed by autologous bone marrow infusion in extensive stage small-cell lung cancer. J Clin Oncol 1986; 4:1443–1454.

55. Cunningham D, Banham SW, Hutcheon AH, et al. High-dose cyclophosphamide and VP-16 as late dosage intensification therapy for small cell carcinoma of lung. Cancer Chemother Pharmacol 1985; 15:303–306.

56. Sculier JP, Klastersky J, Stryckmans P, et al. Late intensification in small-cell lung cancer: a phase I study of high doses of cyclophosphamide and etoposide with autologous bone marrow transplantation. J Clin Oncol 1985; 3:184–191.

57. Klastersky J, Nicaise C, Longeval E, et al. Cisplatin, adriamycin and etoposide (CAV) for remission induction of small-cell bronchogenic carcinoma: evaluation of efficacy and toxicity and pilot study of a "late intensification" with autologous bone marrow rescue. Cancer 1982; 50:652–658.

58. Cornbleet M, Gregor A, Allen S, Leonard R, Smyth J. High dose melphalan as consolidation therapy for good prognosis patients with small cell carcinoma of the bronchus (SCCB). Proc ASCO 1984; 3:210.

59. Wilson C, Pickering D, Stewart S, et al. High dose chemotherapy with autologous bone marrow rescue in small cell lung cancer. In Vivo 1988; 2:331–334.

60. Humblet Y, Symann M, Bosly A, et al. Late intensification chemotherapy with autologous bone marrow transplantation in selected small-cell carcinoma of the lung: a randomized study. J Clin Oncol 1987; 5:1864–1873.

61. Stewart P, Buckner CD, Thomas ED, et al. Intensive chemoradiotherapy with autologous marrow transplantation for small cell carcinoma of the lung. Cancer Treat Rep 1983; 67:1055–1059.

62. Elias AD, Ayash L, Frei E III, et al. Intensive combined modality therapy for limited stage small cell lung cancer. J Natl Cancer Inst 1993; 85:559–566.

62a. Elias A, Ibrahim J, Skarin AT, et al. Dose intensive therapy for limited stage small cell lung cancer: long-term outcome. J Clin Oncol 1999; 17: 1175–1184.

63. Tomeczko J, Pacuszko T, Napora P, Lange A. Treatment intensification which includes high dose induction improves survival of lung carcinoma patients treated by high-dose chemotherapy with hematopoietic progenitor cell rescue but does not prevent high rate of relapses. Bone Marrow Transplant 1996; 18(suppl 1):S44–S47.

64. Brugger W, Frommhold H, Pressler K, Mertelsmann, R, Kanz L. Use of high-dose etoposide/ifosfamide/carboplatin/epirubicin and peripheral blood progenitor cell transplantation in limited-disease small cell lung cancer. Semin Oncol 1995; 22(suppl 2):3–8.

64a. Brugger W, Fetscher S, Hasse J, et al. Multimodality treatment including early high-dose chemotherapy with peripheral blood stem cell transplantation in limited-disease small cell lung cancer. Semin Oncol 1998; 25(suppl 2):42–48.

65. Pignon JP, Arriagada R, Ihde DC, et al. A meta-analysis of thoracic radiotherapy for small-cell lung cancer. N Engl J Med 1992; 327:1618–1624.

66. Warde P, Payne D. Does thoracic irradiation improve survival and local control in limited-stage small-cell carcinoma of the lung? A meta-analysis. J Clin Oncol 1992; 10:890–895.

67. Perry MC, Eaton WL, Propert KJ, et al. Chemotherapy with or without radiation therapy in limited small-cell carcinoma of the lung. New Engl J Med 1987; 316:912–918.

68. Bunn PA, Lichter AS, Makuch RW, et al. Chemotherapy alone or chemotherapy with chest radiation therapy in limited stage small cell lung cancer. Ann Intern Med 1987; 106:655–662.

69. Kies MS, Mira JG, Crowley JJ, et al. Multimodal therapy for limited small-cell lung cancer: a randomized study of induction combination chemotherapy with or without thoracic radiation in complete responders; and with wide-field versus reduced-field radiation in partial responders. A Southwest Oncology Group study. J Clin Oncol 1987; 5:592–600.

70. Arriagada R, Kramar A, Le Chevalier T, De Cremoux H. Competing events determining relapse-free survival in limited small-cell lung carcinoma. J Clin Oncol 1992; 10:447–451.

71. Turrisi AT, Kim K, Johnson DH, et al. Daily (qd) v twice-daily (bid) thoracic irradiation (TI) with concurrent cisplatin-etoposide (PE) for limited small cell lung cancer (LSCLC): preliminary results on 352 randomized eligible patients. Lung Cancer 1994; 11(suppl 1):172 (667).

72. Choi NC. Verbal communication. CALGB Fall Meeting, Atlanta, GA, 11/94.

73. Girling DJ, Thatcher N, Clark PI, Stephens RJ. Letter: Increasing the dose intensity of chemotherapy by means of granulocyte-colony stimulating factor (G-CSF) support in the treatment of small cell lung cancer (SCLC). Eur J Cancer 1996; 32:1263.

74. Tepler I, Cannistra SA, Frei E III, et al. Use of peripheral blood progenitor cells abrogates the myelotoxicity of repetitive outpatient high-dose carboplatin and cyclophosphamide chemotherapy. J Clin Oncol 1993; 11:1583–1591.

75. Woll PJ, Lee SM, Lomax L, et al. Randomised phase II study of standard versus dose-intensive ICE chemotherapy with reinfusion of haemopoietic progenitors in whole blood in small cell lung cancer (SCLC). Proc ASCO 1996; 15:333 (957).

76. Pettengell R, Woll PJ, Thatcher N, Dexter TM, Testa NG. Multicyclic, dose-intensive

chemotherapy supported by sequential reinfusion of hematopoietic progenitors in whole blood. J Clin Oncol 1995; 13:148–156.

77. Perey L, Rosti G, Lange A, et al. Sequential high-dose ICE chemotherapy with circulating progenitor cells (CPC) in small cell lung cancer: an EBMT study. Bone Marrow Transplant 1996; 18(suppl 1):S40–S43.

78. Crown J, Wasserheit C, Hakes T, et al. Rapid delivery of multiple high-dose chemotherapy courses with granulocyte colony-stimulating factor and peripheral blood–derived hematopoietic progenitor cells. J Natl Cancer Inst 1992; 84:1935–1936.

79. Gianni AM, Siena S, Bregni M, et al. Prolonged disease-free survival after high-dose sequential chemo-radiotherapy and hemopoietic autologous transplantation in poor prognosis Hodgkin's disease. Ann Oncol 1991; 2:645–653.

80. Ayash L, Elias A, Wheeler C, et al. Double dose-intensive chemotherapy with autologous marrow and peripheral blood progenitor cell support for metastatic breast cancer: a feasibility study. J Clin Oncol 1994; 12:37–44.

81. Humblet Y, Bosquee L, Weynants P, Symann M. High-dose chemo-radiotherapy cycles for LD small cell lung cancer patients using G-CSF and blood stem cells. Bone Marrow Transplant 1996; 18(suppl 1):S36–S39.

82. Gribben JG, Freedman AS, Neuberg D, et al. Immunologic purging of marrow assessed by PCR before autologous bone marrow transplantation for B-cell lymphoma. N Engl J Med 1991; 325:1525–1533.

83. Brenner MK, Rill DR, Moen RC, et al. Gene-marking to trace origin of relapse after autologous bone-marrow transplantation. Lancet 1993; 341:85–86.

84. Brenner MK, Rill DR. Gene marking to improve the outcome of autologous bone marrow transplantation. J Hematother 1994; 3:33–36.

85. O'Shaughnessy JA, Cowan KH, Cottler-Fox M, et al. Autologous transplantation of retrovirally-marked CD34-positive bone marrow and peripheral blood cells in patients with multiple myeloma or breast cancer. Proc ASCO 1994; 13:296 (963).

86. Stahel RA, Mabry M, Skarin AT, Speak J, Bernal SD. Detection of bone marrow metastasis in small-cell lung cancer by monoclonal antibody. J Clin Oncol 1985; 3:455–461.

87. Canon JL, Humblet Y, Lebacq-Verheyden AM, et al. Immunodetection of small cell lung cancer metases in bone marrow using three monoclonal antibodies. Eur J Cancer Oncol 1988; 24:147–150.

88. Trillet V, Revel D, Combaret V, et al. Bone marrow metastases in small cell lung cancer: detection with magnetic resonance imaging and monoclonal antibodies. Br J Cancer 1989; 60:83–88.

89. Berendsen HH, De Leij L, Postmus PE, Ter Haar JG, Popperna S, The TH. Detection of small cell lung cancer metastases in bone marrow aspirates using monoclonal antibody directed against neuroendocrine differentiation antigen. J Clin Pathol 1988; 41:273–276.

90. Beiske K, Myklebust AT, Aamdal S, Langhom R, Jakobsen E, Fodstad O. Detection of bone marrow metases in small cell lung cancer patients. Am J Pathol 1992; 141:531–538.

91. Hay FG, Ford A, Leonard RCF. Clinical applications of immunocytochemistry in the monitoring of the bone marrow in small cell lung cancer (SCLC). Int J Cancer 1988; suppl 2:8–10.

92. Leonard RCF, Duncan LW, Hay FG. Immunocytological detection of residual marrow disease at clinical remission predicts metastatic relapse in small cell lung cancer. Cancer Res 1990; 50:6545–6548.
93. Brugger W, Bross KJ, Glatt M, Weber F, Mertelsmann R, Kanz L. Mobilization of tumor cells and hematopoietic progenitor cells into peripheral blood of patients with solid tumors. Blood 1994; 83:636–640.
94. Elias A, Li Y, Wheeler C, et al. CD34-selected peripheral blood progenitor cell (PBPC) support in high dose therapy of small cell lung cancer (SCLC): use of a novel detection method for minimal residual tumor (MRT). Proc ASCO 1996; 15:341 (991).

AUTHOR INDEX

C

L

SUBJECT INDEX

A

Accelerated hyperfractionation
  stage III NSCLC, 210
Accelerated radiotherapy (AR), 363
Access port, 104
Actuarial graphs
  survival, 296f–297f
Adenocarcinoma
  CT, 53
  distant metastases, 58
Adenovirus vectors, 14
Adjuvant chemotherapy
  resected NSCLC, 140t–142t
  and surgery SCLC, 346
Adjuvant immunotherapy
  NSCLC randomized trials, 146–151
    combined modality, 146–150
    prognostic factors, 150–151,
      151t
    resected NSCLC, 148t–149t
Adjuvant krestin, 150
Adjuvant radiation therapy (XRT)
  NSCLC, 139t
Adoptive immunotherapy, 15–16
Adrenal masses

CT, 65–66, 65f
  MRI, 66, 67f–68f
Advanced non-small-cell lung cancer
    (NSCLC)
  chemotherapy *vs.* supportive care,
    248–251
  combination regimens, 242–248
    randomized trials, 246–248
  meta-analyses, 252–253
  new agents, 253–260, 254t
  paclitaxel and carboplatin, 309
  second-line therapy, 265–266
  single agents, 232–238
AFP (doxorubicin, 5-FU, cisplatin)
  Phase II trials, 246
Algorithym
  superior pulmonary sulcus tumors,
    183t
Anatomic resections
  NSCLC VATS, 108–110
Anesthesia
  VATS, 104
Angiogenesis
  measurement, 13
  and metastasis, 13–14
Anterior mediastinoscopy, 93–94